PREFACE

"Of making many books there is no end." Perhaps if writers would show cause why their book should be published, there would be a more interrupted and limited output. That stricture should apply to the present volume.

The primary motivation toward assembling the works included here was a sensitivity on the part of the authors to writings that they believe presage a revolution in the field of psychology comparable to the Einsteinian one in physics. In the wind, there are new orientations, new thoughts, new experimental approaches and findings that give promise of better things to come and that may be the forerunners of the *age of psychology*. Many of the items are isolated intellectual islands; however, when viewed from the more recently developed approaches, they make a coherent, orderly panorama.

Obviously, pioneers work at different time periods. Therefore, while there is a heavy concentration of materials from recent literature, there has been no worship of freshly dated writings as such, and the reader may occasionally meet with an article dated twenty or more years ago. For this disrespect of the calendar we make no apology. The pertinence of the findings or freshness of viewpoints is alone responsible for the inclusion of such material. Where materials were lacking, the authors did not hesitate to write suitable articles to fill the gaps. Well over half the book consists of original writings.

In such cases, a definite stand was taken which is believed to be dictated or justified by experimental or field observations stripped from traditional assumptions. However, neither these items nor the selections from the writings of others are presented dogmatically. They are meant to serve only as whetstones against which the student may sharpen his own intellectual tools. Their chief aim is to provoke the student to think about fundamental problems in psychology which have often been treated complacently or as closed matters. The authors have not lost sight of the fact that contemporary psychology is a stage in a process, and that it continues to grow. They realize, too, that in future years radical changes may be introduced into behavioral concepts and investigative techniques which are considered basic and correct today.

In some cases, the authors have included significant articles that have been generally overlooked by psychologists, e.g., Griffin and Hock's experiments on bird navigation, Marie Mason's case of Isabelle, Riesen's revolutionary studies of perception in chimps, and Spelt's conditioning of the human fetus *in utero.* One does not yet commonly encounter such articles in our general textbooks, which seem to prefer more classic illustrations. On the other hand, such excellent classical accounts of the so-called "instincts," as furnished by Kellogg's writings, are unknown to modern students. In the sense of bringing together important articles from a very scattered literature does this book hope to fill a need.

All in all, the aim was to bring together scattered nuggets from psychological literature, which, by employing the reader as a catalyst, would yield a refined and clear picture of certain developments in contemporary psychology and help in charting its future course. No attempt has been made to develop a systematic text. Therefore, the present work is, first of all, suited as a supplementary set of readings to parallel a general book. However, it may also be used as a textbook in courses where the instructor chooses to develop a theoretical orientation for his students. Its stress on origins and evolution of behavior may recommend its use in courses in child psychology.

A word of explanation is in order regarding the use of the term "empirical" in the title. With this term, we hope to call attention to the fact that the contents do not derive from armchair speculation. Indeed, whether explanations are general or specific, field or experimental, they are supported by facts "in the world of reality." The term, empirical, is also used synonymously with the contemporary usage of "operational" or as an equivalent for the phrase, "derived from actual observation." Desire for the factual, however, has not restricted us to the selection of laboratory experiments with rats. "Nature's experiments" in the everyday life settings of people, which cannot be handled with the same rigor as that permitted by rat experiments, have

EMPIRICAL FOUNDATIONS OF PSYCHOLOGY

Founded by C. K. Ogden

The International Library of Psychology

GENERAL PSYCHOLOGY
In 38 Volumes

EMPIRICAL FOUNDATIONS
OF PSYCHOLOGY

N H PRONKO AND J W BOWLES

With the collaboration of D T Herman, Harris Hill
and John Bucklew Jr

First published in 1952 by
Routledge

Reprinted in 1999 by
Routledge
2 Park Square, Milton Park, Abingdon, Oxfordshire OX14 4RN
711 Third Avenue, New York, NY 10017
First issued in paperback 2014
Routledge is an imprint of the Taylor and Francis Group, an informa company

Transferred to Digital Printing 2005

© 1952 N H Pronko and J W Bowles

British Library Cataloguing in Publication Data
A CIP catalogue record for this book
is available from the British Library

Empirical Foundations of Psychology
ISBN 978-0-415-21039-3 (hbk)
ISBN 978-0-415-75804-8 (pbk)

General Psychology: 38 Volumes
ISBN 978-0-415-21129-1
The International Library of Psychology: 204 Volumes
ISBN 978-0-415-19132-6

To
J. R. K.

nevertheless been included. All in all, the attempt has been to select items of broad scope that are substantial rather than hypothetical. Where assumption comes in, as it necessarily must, we believe that it is operationally justified and not arbitrarily imposed upon the facts, as in older psychologies. If this is a bias, then the present authors are self-admittedly biased with a vengeance.

As may be inferred from the contents of the book, the authors lean heavily upon the writings of Professor J. R. Kantor. We are also indebted to Dr. Steuart Henderson Britt for his careful reading of the manuscript and for his many helpful suggestions, and to Miss Geraldine Allbritten, Mr. Glen Allen, Mr. Fred Snyder, and Mr. and Mrs. Fred Wackerhagen for their intelligent and wholehearted help in handling the numerous details requisite to publication.

Authors and publishers from whom we have borrowed are acknowledged in the body of the text.

N. H. PRONKO

J. W. BOWLES, JR.

Wichita, Kan.
October, 1950

CONTENTS

4. BIOLOGICAL CHARACTERISTICS
OF THE ORGANISM AND EARLY ACQUISITION OF BEHAVIOR

5. BASIC PATTERNS OF BEHAVIOR

6. SOCIAL BEHAVIOR

7. PERSONALITY

8. INTELLIGENCE

9. ATTENTION

14. REMEMBERING

15. LEARNING

16. INTERRELATIONSHIPS BETWEEN PHYSIOLOGY AND PSYCHOLOGY

INTRODUCTION

I. THE SUBJECT MATTER OF PSYCHOLOGY
N. H. Pronko

There is great misunderstanding on the part of laymen as to the subject matter of psychology. Ordinarily, the man in the street is of the opinion that psychologists restrict their study to such bizarre phenomena as hypnotism, mental telepathy, and clairvoyance. On the contrary, psychologists study things that are found commonly in everyday life and that extend all over the earth.

But first, let us notice how the sciences have evolved. On this planet, there are a wide variety of occurrences taking place. "Things are happening," as we say. The different sciences have arisen as the result of man's interest in certain areas of this manifold of happenings. Thus, physicists "carved out" for their special study such "things" as water changing to ice and to steam, falling bodies, and transformation of energy (e.g., heat into power, electricity into heat, and so forth). Chemical types of changes were taken over by the chemist as his special area of investigation. But on this earth, there are also plants and animals being born, reproducing, taking materials into themselves, and growing, excreting, and moving. These events are singled out by the biologist as his special study.

Not everything that happens on the face of the earth has yet been included in the listings above.

In order to achieve a fresh viewpoint, the student might imagine himself a man from Mars come to earth for the first time. If it were morning, he would observe human beings rising and scurrying to their breakfasts and their work. Some would operate machines in factories; others would run steamships, airplanes, buses, streetcars, and bulldozers; still others would be engaged in buying, selling, preaching, writing, warring, repairing, building, painting, and composing. Should the man from Mars decide to delve further into these things, he would become a psychologist. It is these activities and, perhaps, the less complex ones of the other animals that set the stage for the psychologist's study. The student will note certain features characteristic of all the sciences: each starts with certain facts in the world of reality. This is the beginning point—to have something to study. This something may be taken into the laboratory for more painstaking analysis later on. The important point is that men observed things happening around them. These things became the subject matter for the scientist, and the divisions of the sciences are divisions of interest and subject matter only. It would be too difficult and not so profitable for one man to study storms, economic institutions, gravitation, energy, plants, and humans. This accounts for such specialties as chemistry, physics, zoology, biology, and psychology.

FACTS VERSUS THEORIES

Because the beginning student approaches the study of psychology with certain preconceptions absorbed from those about him, he is quite likely to confuse behavioral *facts* with *theories* about those facts. For example, because for him thinking is explained in such mystical terms as mental states, he comes to doubt that people do think. We suggest that by keeping facts and the explanations of facts separate, the beginning student can enter his scientific study of psychology fully confident that he does have a very definite subject matter. His legitimate field of inquiry becomes behaving organisms, and he need have not a shadow of doubt that those organisms create symphonies, atomic theories, poems, works of art, and so on. Despite the fact that he may have difficulty in understanding or explaining such events, he may be as certain of their occurrence as he is of the occurrence of storms, volcanoes, eclipses, and magnetism, or the birth, growth, and death of living things. To prove it to himself, he need only look around and see his friends, neighbors, and himself engaging in day-to-day activities of the sort mentioned above.

But let us illustrate. Suppose that the reader has solved an algebra problem. That is a fact, or datum, with which we can begin work just as definitely as can the chemist starting with a chemical interaction or a physicist with a falling object. But how shall we explain these facts? We are now in the realm of theory where description, interpretation, or explanation plays an important part, and where discrepant "stories" may be told. For example, one explanation for the solution of the algebra problem may resort to "mental states," another to brain conditions, and the like. Our job now is not to settle between them but only to call attention to the difference between a fact and a theory about that fact. The two must be kept separate.

Of course, not all descriptions of facts are equally valid. Science has a preference for theories that are derived from a study of the facts themselves rather than those that come from tradition or superstition. Furthermore, theories must be stated in such a way that one can predict or control the facts. The present book is an attempt to describe behavioral facts in operational terms. This means that our descriptions will be in terms that can actually be designated in the world of happenings and not in terms of "mind," "mental states," and "consciousness," which cannot be operationally demonstrated.

No one can show that an "insane person" has a "twisted mind." This is not an operational description. However, it is an operationally justified account to relate this person's action to a condition in his surroundings, namely a fiendish father. This is something we can work or operate with, as when we remove the boy from his father and look for changes in the boy's conduct.

Why does a child in the Soviet Union grow up to be a Communist? A possible answer would be that he "inherits Communism" from his parents. We could operationally test this explanation by importing an offspring of Communist parents into the United States and rearing him with a Republican family. At twenty-one, he is a staunch Republican. An operational account of such an incident would stick to the facts, namely that the boy's action was related to the specific life conditions surrounding him (i.e., institutions, attitudes of his adopted parents, friends, teachers, and the like) rather than upon some "inborn tendency." This latter would again be a nonoperational account.

It is the hope of the authors that the student will come to see his own, and his neighbor's, fears, angers, rememberings, forgettings, likes, dislikes, dreams, ambitions, skills, abilities, and creative acts operationally as he progresses through the present textbook.

II. THE HISTORICAL PERSPECTIVE IN PSYCHOLOGY

D. T. Herman

Just as the behaviors of a child today cannot be understood fully apart from an understanding of the particular child's unique behavioral history, so psychology today cannot be fully understood apart from its history. While concepts of human behavior have been diverse, fairly clear trends in the change and evolution of such concepts can be traced historically. It is important that the beginning student gain some perspective in which to place both the "popular" psychology with which, wittingly or unwittingly, he begins his studies as well as the more technical concepts to which he will be introduced.

Aristotle (384–322 B.C.), the ancient Greek, has a unique status. His biological training and his studies of marine biology gave him an objective observational orientation to the behaviors of organisms.[1] He noted that organisms varied in complexity of biological organization as well as in behavior. Aristotle described behavior as a functioning of the total organism. Different organisms differed in their functioning. Plant organisms functioned only by respiring, absorbing materials and excreting them, and reproducing. Animal organisms functioned by being irritable to stimuli and by locomoting. Other animals such as humans could function in still more complex ways that were called "reasoning." Further, animals were said to vary in their functioning as a result of two classes of conditions—their unique biological conditions and their unique histories. For Aristotle, it was not possible to discuss behavior of *any* organism apart from these two sets of variables. Aristotle is sometimes mistakenly assumed to have made a rigid division between organisms. Such was not the case. He described all organisms as being on a direct continuum and as differing only in complexity.

---

[1] SHUTE, CLARENCE. *The psychology of Aristotle.* New York: Columbia Univ. Press, 1941. Pp. 148.

Between Aristotle's day and the beginnings of the period of modern science, great changes took place. Migrations, wars, and political and social upheavals exercised extensive influence, directly and indirectly, upon all branches of scholarly activity. For purposes of a short historical sketch, it is possible to touch only briefly on some of the changes and developments in orientation to psychology.[2] (The interested student will find richly rewarding readings if he chooses to sample this literature.)

René Descartes (1596–1650) is generally considered to mark the beginning of the "modern" period in psychology; to have divided off the ancient and medieval periods from the modern period. Descartes was less naturalistic than Aristotle. Man was to be regarded as uniquely different from other animals. While other animals functioned on a purely mechanical level of sense organs, nerves, and muscles, man, according to Descartes, had the additional attribute of soul which regulated his behavior. No attempt was made by Descartes to describe the properties of this added factor. It was conceived, in fact, to be unobservable but to activate, control, and guide the psychological activities of man. This unobservable and unknowable entity, derived from prescientific inference, was used as the basic explanatory factor of all human psychological behavior.

Boring[3] has pointed out that Descartes in large part set the pattern of subsequent interpretations of behavior. Terminology changed, and descriptions varied in detail, but the basic orientation to psychology as being concerned with soul, mind, consciousness, and so on, each as inferred entities, persisted. Darwin's (1809–1882) publication of his monumental *Origin of Species* in 1859 constituted the first fundamental blow to this pattern. It is no exaggeration to say that Darwin's work, while primarily concerned with biology, shook the very foundation of previous psychological theory. Darwin tirelessly amassed evidence to show that no absolute differences could be drawn between man and other organisms.

2 MURPHY, GARDNER. *Historical introduction to modern psychology.* New York: Harcourt, 1949. Pp. 466.
BORING, E. G. *A history of experimental psychology.* New York: Appleton-Century-Crofts, 1950. Pp. 777.
ZILBOORG, G. & HENRY, G. W. *A history of medical psychology.* New York: Norton, 1941. Pp. 606.
3 BORING, E. G. *A history of experimental psychology.* New York: Appleton-Century-Crofts, 1950. Pp. 777.

The view of Aristotle regarding continuity of the species was supported with clear observational evidence. Darwin further showed that it was essential to an understanding of any species to include a historical dimension as well as a picture of the life conditions of the organisms. Its adaptive behavior, as well as its structure, could be understood only on the basis of its full past and present life conditions.

The full implication of Darwin's work was not immediately understood or accepted by all students of psychology. Many persisted in clinging to various forms of traditional doctrine. Others, however, soon caught the implications that man is an organism that can be studied and observed as a perfectly natural organism. A tremendous boost was given by Darwin to the study of all organisms, human as well as infrahuman.

In a series of papers and books beginning in 1913, J. B. Watson (1878–) [4] crystallized the demand for an *objective* psychology and gave it the name "behaviorism." It was Watson's proposal that psychologists very deliberately break away from the traditional dualistic orientation. The dualistic theory held that man is made up of a physical body and a psychic mind as separate entities. Each was held to function according to different laws. Watson held that such a separation of the unified organism had no basis in *scientific* observation. Psychology was to base itself on the observational method *exclusively*. Psychology would thus bring itself into line with other natural sciences. That which was not observed could not be included in descriptions of behavior.

Watson's position brings this brief historical chronicle close to our own day. Watson's work pointed to the need for a further advance in orientation to psychological facts and markedly influenced psychologists in the direction of objectivity.

A full comprehension of the trends of psychology in the contemporary phase of its historical development would take us too far afield for our present purposes. However, two principles— *relativity theory and operationism*—will help to characterize psychology's more recent developments. Both of these principles were first applied by workers in the physical sciences, but both found congenial atmosphere among those psychologists who were attempting to further psychology as a natural science.

---

[4] WATSON, J. B. *Psychology from the standpoint of a behaviorist.* Philadelphia: Lippincott, 1919. Pp. 429.

Relativity theory, as applied to psychology, stresses that behavior must be understood as events which occur in particular frames of reference. It is not possible to understand behavior fully or to describe it accurately unless it is understood and described as an intimate part of its particular frames of reference. The operational principle has served as a healthy caution upon description of behavior. It insists that any descriptive concept used must be understood in terms of concrete performances which explicitly indicate the place of the concept in the event described. Unless the concept can be understood in terms of concrete operations, it cannot be said to hold *scientific* validity. It thus becomes difficult, and under the operational principle, impossible, to cover up our lack of understanding of behavior by resorting to the facile use of mind, mental states, consciousness, ego, psyche, and other vague and mystical terminologies which do not permit of operational definition. The behavior of organisms, according to the relativity and operational principles, may be studied as real and concrete happenings and not as mere outer manifestations of some unspecifiable inner entity.

III. THE METHODS OF PSYCHOLOGY
D. T. Herman

Besides differences in the subject matter of the various sciences, there is a difference in the methods employed in their study. For example, an astronomer cannot bring Jupiter into a laboratory where he can experimentally perform operations upon it. He must view it from his *observatory*. This makes his science a field study; i.e., he studies astronomical events as they occur in nature or in the field.

FIELD METHOD. A large proportion of the data that the psychologist studies is also found in the field; i.e., people commit murder, learn to speak English, Polish, or French, pick up drinking, smoking, or chewing habits, come to pray and vote a certain way, and develop skills and techniques *in the field*. Therefore, field observation will have to be used in the study of many behaviors found in everyday life. They will be studied *as they occur* under natural conditions.

LABORATORY OR EXPERIMENTAL TECHNIQUES. While it is relatively impossible to arrange a situation in the laboratory which would allow us to study how a person develops "insanity," nevertheless this would be the best method for studying learning, remembering, and a variety of other responses. While such a technique would limit the range of behaviors studied, it would permit greater control of all the variables or factors involved. Thus, if we are interested in the time that it takes an individual to lift his foot from a brake pedal, we may set up apparatus to measure the time interval between stimulus and response. Various types of stimuli may be applied to determine whether these affect speed of reaction. Various conditions of the organism, such as fatigue, drowsiness, drugs, intoxication, and other factors, may be tested. In the same general manner, a wide variety of behaviors—learning, perceiving, feeling, reasoning—may be studied to answer specific questions regarding each. The laboratory technique, then, permits greater precision in the study of human organisms and even more so of the infrahuman animals. American universities have developed elaborate laboratories for the study of humans, apes, dogs, cats, rats, and even worms.

INTROSPECTION.   According to the older systems of psychology, it was thought that when a person reported on the intimate details of his thinkings and feelings he was looking within his mind; therefore, the term "introspection." More recently, psychologists think of this term as referring to the subject's verbal report about his own behavior which may be more easily studied in this way than by observation by someone else. It is true that a parent may know a child's "thinking" by observing his particular behavioral configuration at the moment he is lying or embarrassed, and lovers may know much about each other's thoughts by simply looking. Nevertheless, there are other subtle reactions that may be most easily studied by asking a person to report about them. This is essentially what the physician does when he asks the patient before him to report on the location of his aches and pains.

CLINICAL METHODS.   Formerly, problems arising in the school and the community spurred the study of individual organisms in an attempt to understand why they failed to make normal progress through school or why they developed delinquent behavior. More recently, the war has had a similar effect on the study of pathological behavior, with the result that, today, clinical psychology is a rapidly expanding field. The stress in this method is on the historical development of the behavior under consideration. Thus, when a 10-year-old child shows an *abnormal* fear of running water, it may be necessary to attempt to find under what conditions the fear started and how it developed in order that the fear may be alleviated. In the same manner, the numerous maladaptive behaviors of children, as well as adults, may be approached. When and how did the person acquire his troublesome reaction? In order to answer such problems, clinicians have developed testing, interviewing, and projective techniques (cf. Chapter VII).

IV. PHYSIOLOGY AND PSYCHOLOGY: A PRELIMINARY CONSIDERATION OF THEIR RELATIONSHIP

N. H. Pronko

At the very outset, the student is urged to attempt an operational exercise which we believe will throw into bold relief the fundamental characteristics of psychological facts.

Let us take two different kinds of things to work with—a muscle-nerve preparation and a child. The first, a frog's leg muscle and attached nerve, is a typical laboratory assignment for the student of physiology. This portion of the frog (the rest of the frog may be discarded) can be rigged up and experimented with in such ways as to yield precise, useful knowledge about the functioning of muscles. A weight can be hung on the leg and an electric current sent into the muscle over the nerve. In this way, the relationship between stimulus and response may be worked out.

What are some of these findings? First, we note that in physiology we can legitimately and profitably study parts of organisms —systems or even organs, such as a beating heart. The term "tissue excitation" appropriately applies to such an occurrence. Further, the responses we observe in physiology are automatic, constant, organized, and permanent. Given the same conditions, the leg muscle will always respond in the same way. It cannot do otherwise. Because the leg muscle is constructed in a certain way and because it is contractile tissue, it must contract in the way it does when it is properly stimulated.

Now, let us take a child. Say, "Good morning," to a newborn child and there is no response, nor will there be one for many months. One fine day, however, after many, many months of "stimulation," the child will respond with, "Good morning," when he is greeted.

Here we see the first big difference between the kinds of facts studied in physiology and those belonging to psychology. First of all, we must have a whole organism in psychology. Certainly, no lung, vocal cords, and head severed from an organism have ever been taught to say, "Good morning." And now we have come to the crucial difference. Teaching comes in in psychology—not in physiology. As soon as a leg muscle has been developed, it will give a reflex response *from the first contact*. It does not have to be taught, but children will have to be taught to say, "Good morning."

How important the specific details of the child's history are can be strikingly shown if we transplant our child at birth into a family in France. Lo and behold, the child now responds with *"Bon jour"* and not "Good morning." It is apparent that whether the child responds at all, or the way it responds, is conditioned by many circumstances of a social sort. Not so with a muscle-nerve preparation. The latter operates in the same fixed fashion whether the frog is raised in America, France, or the Soviet Union. Thus, a history of organisms with their stimulus objects is of prime importance in psychological study—not in physiology. Let the reader examine his own actions and test the validity of the distinction we have made here.

But the list of differences is not yet exhausted. Notice that a child may be angry and remain silent when his parent greets him upon waking. Again, leg muscles can't inhibit their response the way organisms do. When we find *inhibitions* prominently displayed in the activities of animals, let us agree to place them in a different class of activities from noninhibitable coughs, sneezes, and burps. The latter may be handed over to physiology.

Were we to study the child cited in the above examples over a period of time, we might observe that his response varies. Once, he says "Good morning"; then perhaps only "Morning," or "Howdy." Leg muscles can be counted upon not to change the patterning of their action. They will not run around in circles or zigzags. In other words, our study of a person's "good mornings" must encompass more territory if we are to understand the extra-tissue conditions to which they are sensitive.

A further difference shows up when we note that a child can

delay his response until, let us say, *after* the other person has spoken. Not so with leg muscles. As soon as the muscle is stimulated, it responds. People commonly delay their actions. When children frequently reply "Just a minute" to parental requests, they illustrate the delayability not found in other phenomena. Comparison of our two data brings out still another difference between them. Assume that the child in our example has had a teacher whom he did greet with "Good morning." The teacher moved away, and the child did not see her until 4 years later. On the occasion of their meeting after this interval, the child did not say "Good morning." His action had been modified; he had "forgotten" his teacher. Leg muscles do not "forget" stimuli with which they have been in contact 4, 10, or even more years previously. People like people and things which they previously disliked, and vice versa. In other words, their action shows modifiability. This is another way in which they differ from tissues, organs, and systems studied in physiology.

The ubiquitous child of our illustrations can also do something else that leg muscles in the laboratory cannot do. Although at first he can only concentrate on practicing the words "Good morning," in time he can *incorporate* other actions with the verbal response. For example, while he runs along, he can simultaneously take a lollipop out of his mouth and say his greeting to a person he meets while in motion and while holding the lollipop momentarily before his face. Humans perform highly integrated activity while driving, looking, and conversing, during machine operation, or while eating or dancing. Leg muscles do not act in this way.

A final important difference: If leg muscles are struck with a cardboard, hammer, reflex hammer, vulgar poster, ax, or any sharp-edged object, they react indiscriminately to these various objects. But organisms, during their historical contacts with the same objects, build up very specific actions toward them. They come to chop with an ax, to pound nails with a hammer, to be shocked at vulgar posters, to use cardboard to make a sign, and to employ a reflex hammer for testing reflexes. In other words, humans are more discriminating than leg muscles, or, for that matter, sneezing or coughing reflexes. To put it still another way, humans come to perform very specific reactions to each of these things, whereas leg muscles react in the same way to any of them.

In summary, then, psychological events will show these characteristics. They will always require an organism rather than a discrete organ or system of organs. The latter, however, can be studied in physiology. Furthermore, psychological data can be counted upon to involve a history or series of contacts between the organism and the things or people to which it responds. Thus, if a person speaks Finnish, we may be certain that during his life span he was in contact with Finnish-speaking people. Conversely, if we know that a child has grown up with Finns, we may be sure that he has built up the specific verbal reactions to things that other Finns show, and that he can be counted upon to perform them.

Finally, psychological action can be distinguished from physiological in that the former will show modifiability, delayability, variability, inhibition, integration, and high degrees of discrimination. Not every behavioral act will show all six of these features. Then, there will be borderline cases, as there always are, but the authors venture to assert that the greater bulk of human activities of a behavioral sort can be distinguished on this basis from the nonbehavioral or physiological sort.

The student should be told that a distinction between physiological and psychological data has not been attempted until recent times, and that some investigators ignore such differences. We are of the opinion that if such distinctions can be made and if they are valid, they can be tremendously helpful in delimiting a specific set of data. And, if our data are homogeneous, our principles ought necessarily to be more clean-cut and useful.

The whole purpose of this section has been suggestive. The student is urged to take such instances as coughing, belching, stomach gurgles, and swallowing, and compare them with his learning, remembering, reading, writing, running, voting, or creative activity. Operationally apply the test of the characteristics suggested above, and let the chips fall where they may. We are convinced that these criteria are practical in acquainting us with the essential features of behavioral facts.

HEREDITY AND PSYCHOLOGY

N. H. Pronko

This chapter attempts to "tease out" the relationships between the phenomena of heredity that are studied as a branch of biology and behavioral facts. Through the years, there has been a cherished *belief* to the effect that certain behaviors were inherited, or that, at least, some basis ("capacity" or "tendency") for their performance was inherited.

Such belief has not attached itself to all behaviors. For example, the least-informed psychologist would agree that talking, reading, writing, worshiping, and believing are developed during the life history of organisms. But it is a common belief of popular as well as of the older scientific psychology that the reason why organisms perform certain other behaviors (musical, artistic, and the like) must be explained otherwise. Something other than the life experiences of the organism is introduced, although these factors are also of necessity brought in.

The question may be put thus: Is it true that most behaviors are built up during the organism's life history but that a few constitute an exception to this rule? It is important how we resolve this question, for if we find that certain behaviors are somehow affected through heredity, then principles of reactional biography will not apply to them, and we must find what principles do apply. On the other hand, if we decide that the facts do not warrant two distinct sets of principles and that all behaviors may be subsumed under a principle in terms of a person's life history, we may control and predict all behavior indiscriminately. Therefore, whether for scientific understanding or for purposes of practical application, this appears to us to be a fundamental psychological problem.

Our plan is to consider first what kind of fact is designated by the term "heredity" as well as by the term "environment," both of which are brought into opposition with one another as in the proverbial "heredity or environment?" Next we examine whether even such commonly accepted beliefs as "inheritance of size" of certain human groups need be so explained. And how about behavior itself? This brings us to an attempt at resolving the question: What has heredity to do with psychology? Then, because sexual reactions are believed to be "inherited" either as "instincts" or otherwise, we examine how they operate over the range of animal species.

The remaining articles concern themselves with a question that may be put thus: Some activities of the infrahuman animals look marvelously like behavior and yet these animals could not have built up these actions because they performed them without having had opportunity to do so. On the other hand, the flying of birds appears to be genuinely psychological, since it involves complex discrimination, coordination, inhibition, and so forth. Was it, then, built up, or was it "instinctive," i.e., "inherited"? We believe that a reading of these selections will reveal that when we have under consideration such activities as the "sea-approach reaction" of the loggerhead turtle, the nest making and provisioning of the solitary wasp, and the egg-laying and mating reactions of the Chinese silkworm moth, we have a *tropistic* or physiological functioning of the animal concerned. Gone are the differential, integrative, variable, modifiable, delayable, and inhibitable characteristics so prominent in psychological facts, features which are most richly observed in human ethical, moral, affectionate, and other social conduct. The fact that sex, anger, and aggressive behavior can be inhibited, modified, and varied is well recognized, and yet these reactions are frequently erroneously identified with the elementary, reflexlike action of the lower animals.

In other words, unlearned activities, so characteristic of the "lower animals," which at first blush look so complex, are utterly simple and reflexlike in nature. In fact, they differ little from man's knee-jerk elicited by a reflex hammer. However, when we come to investigate such activities as bird migration, or merely flying itself, we find that these activities show characteristics that force us to place them in a different category from the class of reflex action.

While a newborn human infant readily responds with a knee-jerk when its patellar tendon is appropriately struck, no newborn sparrow flies around, over, and under obstacles by a blow on a tendon. Such flying requires many trials and errors; it is absent at birth. Over a period of time, it will become more finely co-ordinated. Useless movements will drop out, and the remaining ones will become specific. The essential feature will be a history in flying that is not required for knee-jerks. From the first contact, the knee-jerk operates appropriately; not so with flying. The latter will evolve only after a long series of contacts between a sparrow and the trees, buildings, air, and ground in his surroundings. When the actions of organisms, human or infrahuman, have only the characteristics of knee-jerks, we suggest that they be called physiological. When they show the more complex features of an evolution or history and variability, modifiability, inhibition, and a high degree of discrimination, we suggest that such acts be placed on a continuum toward the other end which we would characterize as behavior. These statements should not be considered as dogmatic but rather provocative and a spur to the student's thinking about some very fundamental problems of psychology that have not yet been settled.

I. THE NATURE OF HEREDITY [1]

If pressed for a concrete definition of heredity, many psychologists will suddenly leave the area of behavior resemblances and differences which they have been studying, and with a quick change of scene introduce the biological mechanism of the genes. The genes are thus regarded as the mechanism for the inheritance of psychological traits, by a sort of analogy with their demonstrated role in the transmission of structural characteristics. Regardless of how heredity is defined, however, all psychologists would undoubtedly agree that the genes play an important role in their concept of heredity. But the exact role will vary in different concepts. Some will maintain that heredity is "carried" by the genes or that it is

[1] ANASTASI, ANNE & FOLEY, J. P., JR. A proposed reorientation in the heredity-environment controversy. *Psychol. Rev.*, 1948, 55, 239–249. (Reprinted by permission of the authors and the American Psychological Association.)

"determined" by the genes. Others will insist that heredity *is* the genes, thus defining heredity as the specific material with which the individual begins life at conception.

From a realistic, objective point of view, the genes obviously consist of specific chemical substances. They are not filled with "potentialities," "tendencies," "influences," "determiners," or other mystical entities. As Jennings puts it, "That which is directly inherited . . . is the set of genes, with the accompanying cytoplasm . . . certain substances in certain combinations, which under certain conditions give rise to the individual, having certain later characteristics." Similarly, Holt writes: "No potential character ever is 'already contained' in anything; and the notion of potentiality, wherever used, is a mark of finalistic thinking. The contents of the germ-cell are not potential characters at all, whether bodily or mental; they are actual proteins and other substances, and to call these substances 'potential' this or that is to flout the truth."

The fact that adult individuals differ from species to species, as well as within species, is undoubtedly related to the specific chemical constitution of the germ cells out of which each individual developed. In the same sense, an iron knocker differs from a brass knocker because of the difference in the original material out of which it was fashioned. But it would be pointless to insist that the original piece of iron contained the potentialities of the knocker, or that as the result of proper handling by a skilled worker (i.e., "favorable" environment), its normal knocker potentialities were realized. It would have been equally "normal" for the iron to become a horseshoe.

THE NATURE OF ENVIRONMENT

Psychologists have not only been frequently remiss in failing to sharpen and clarify their concept of "heredity" as applied to behavioral phenomena, but have often been equally vague in their use of the term "environment." Recognition of the implications of this term is of basic importance for an understanding of the heredity-environment problem.

"STIMULATIONAL" VERSUS "LOCATIONAL" ROLE. Environment has been all too frequently envisaged as a *passive place* or *"locus"* in which the organism's behavior is said to occur. In other words, the environment is regarded as a setting for behavior, rather than as an *active stimulating agent.* The former, passive sense of the term seems to be that characteristically implied by sociologists as well as by many psychologists. Actually, however, from a psychological point of view the environment consists of a myriad of specific stimuli which act upon the behaving organism.

SPECIFICITY. The layman's notion of environment is usually a rather general or superficial geographical one, as illustrated by such descriptions as a city slum, a suburb, or a French village. A somewhat more discriminating, *familial* definition is implied in the frequent popular assertions that any differences in ability, interest, emotional adjustment, and the like between siblings in the same home must be the result of heredity, "since the environments were the same."

An *individual* definition of environment recognizes the marked differences in personal relationships, participation in various activities, and the like, among individuals in the same home. It is apparent that from a psychological point of view, environment must be regarded as a complex of stimuli which is unique for each individual. Finally, the consideration of *inter-cellular* and *intra-cellular* environment and their role in the processes of growth has further modified the concept of environment and has dispelled the notion of environment as an "external" force in contrast to heredity operating "from within" [pp. 243–245].

II. THE FALLACY OF THE "SAME ENVIRONMENT"

N. H. Pronko

The student who is heavily steeped in popular psychology, with its superficial attitude toward behavioral events, is puzzled by the differing personalities that result often even where individuals have been reared under the same roof. Since neither the customary hereditary type of explanation nor the theory which alleges that individuals have had the "same environment" helps him much, he seeks aid in answering this conundrum.

In trying to throw light on the problem, we must first emphasize that there is no such entity as "environment" affecting or pushing around humans as though they were puppets. Behavioral study requires following the succession of events that involve the organism and all the factors that constitute its surroundings. What contact the student has had with behavioral study should have taught him the need for detailed analysis. The unit of the "behavioral segment" must drive home the necessity for a painstaking dissection which accounts for behavior in terms of reactions consuming fractions of a second. Surely a difference in any of these is sufficient to account for the resulting behavioral differences. Consider, for example, how a few of the more important behavioral segments conditioned the reactional biographies of Mary and Molly, identical twins reared together.

From birth on, the twins have been identically dressed and have had identical cribs, high chairs, and toys, and have lived in the same house with their true parents. At the age of five, Mary contracted pneumonia. During her illness, she was attended faithfully by her mother. As a result, she demands more attention and affection from her parents. The situation was aggravated by grandma, grandpa, and Uncle Jim who showered Mary with gifts, at the same time ignoring Molly.

During Mary's illness, Molly spent long hours with her father in his basement workshop. She would try to use the tools and has developed a genuine mechanical interest. Recently, she took apart the family alarm clock and is often found unscrewing the bolts inside the family car. Also, as the result of their long hours of contact, Mary and her mother have a preference for each other's company. There is a definite family alignment. Incidentally, Mary does not show interest in mechanical things. One summer day while Mary was in the house getting a drink of water, Molly was badly frightened by a neighborhood dog. Ever since that occasion, Molly has run to her mother at the sight of a dog. Mary shows no fear of dogs.

When the twins started school, a girl engaged Molly in sexual play, for which the teacher punished her. Since then, she has been shy and withdrawn and never volunteers to recite in class. By contrast, Mary is more spontaneous and is making a satisfactory social adjustment.

It will be interesting to follow the personality development of the twins. Even the scanty account presented here has pointed out differences that have given each twin a certain slant in the direction of a highly individualistic reactional biography or psychological history, which may cause greater divergence as time goes on. In the example cited, one of the twins happened to experience an illness which was a factor in her personality development, but note that without any such complications, Molly has also developed difficulties.

Mary and Molly live with the same father and mother under the same roof and get the same toys for birthdays and Christmas, but this is obviously not psychological talk. We are not interested in a list of things surrounding developing humans but in the specific *occurrences* or *reactions* that take place between people and those things. Note that although Mary and Molly were both surrounded by the same parents, mechanical objects, neighborhood dogs, and school circumstances, they nevertheless came to react differently to them because of the reactions that they built up to them.

Behavioral differences between two sisters born two years apart would be even greater. Make it a brother and sister, and the situation has even greater possibilites for behavioral divergence. If the boy is born first, the geographic, social, and financial conditions of the family may be very different than when the little girl is born. Note, too, how different the two parents may be by the time the second child comes along. The family may have moved in between times, and the social, financial, and health circumstances of the family may be much improved or worsened. And, finally, note that when brother was born he had no older brother in the family, but when the girl is born, her parents are older and she also has a 2-year-old brother to cope with. It should be apparent, then, that to talk in terms of "environment" is quite meaningless in behavioral discussion, although the term may be useful in a biological framework.

III. ARE SHAPE AND SIZE INHERITED?

A variation of the well-disseminated view that individuals' structures are inherited is illustrated by the following quotation regarding the sharp anatomic differences that exist between the True Negroes of West Africa and the Pygmies in the interior. The investigators offer a simpler theory for morphologic divergences than the traditional hereditary theory.

Stockard and Bean [2] are inclined to believe that the anatomy of the True Negroes is due to their nearness to the seacoast and the resulting large intake of iodine, which acts as a stimulant to the thyroid. On the other hand, the Pygmies are in the deep forests of central Africa, where there is a dearth of iodine, a fact which may be related to the striking similarity of the features of these people to those of the cretin. Pygmies are

---

[2] LEWIS, J. H. *The biology of the Negro.* Chicago: Univ. of Chicago Press, 1942. Pp. 433. (Reproduced by permission of the publisher.)

likely to be underfed, in general. They are victims of conquests of other African tribes and have been driven into parts of the continent where food is least accessible. The result of repeated generations of underfed people is probably represented by physiques not of normal proportions [pp. 25-26].

IV. "BEHAVIOR" IS NOT INHERITED

There is a growing realization of the fact that while one may speak loosely of "inheriting" structures, the same does not hold for behaviors, even when the latter *involve* such structures, for obviously behavior is always *action* that must be acquired; it is not "stuff." Stoddard [3] appears to have made the distinction in the excerpt here presented.

Whenever one speaks of hereditary factors in intelligence, he must speak of hereditary *structures*. There can be no such thing as hereditary behavior in the biological sense. If similar structures lead to similar behavior, it is still not precise to speak of the inheritance of the behavior. A mechanism conducive to walking on two legs is inherited by man, but walking as a complex motor activity is not. A child could take this inherited mechanism and devote it entirely to walking on four "legs," if that was what social models and pressures demanded. The Ubangi lip is more striking than the Hapsburg. The fastest way to get an extraordinarily long neck is not through breeding, but through the collar customs of certain African tribes. The inheritance of these persons, like our own, leads to a standard type of neck under certain environmental controls; under other external controls, the outcome is long necks. To say that refraining from hanging rings about the neck is hereditary is to argue in a circle. The human race, if deprived of its present choices in clothing, food, shelter, and social custom, would choose and stamp in different genetic potentialities. The truth is that man has overemphasized his individuality. If, like the corn plant, he were imbedded in the earth as one of many corn plants, drawing sustenance from the same soil and sunlight, he might get a better idea of himself, not only as a genetic series going back to the beginning of life, but as an item with cross-sectional reference [p. 68].

---

[3] STODDARD, G. D. *The meaning of intelligence.* New York: Macmillan, 1947. Pp. 504. (Reproduced by permission of the publisher.)

V. WHAT HAS HEREDITY TO DO WITH PSYCHOLOGY?

N. H. Pronko

The article by Anastasi and Foley shows in what confused fashion the term "heredity" has been used. SEMANTICS. The term "heredity" did not, as a matter of fact, originate in scientific investigation. For example, chemists worked in laboratories and stumbled across facts which they called "heavy water" and "radium." In such cases, they discovered "something" *and then* named it. Two points are important here: (1) they discovered a clean-cut datum, and (2) they gave it a distinctive name so that other things would not be confused with the newly discovered one. As a result, disagreement was eliminated, for everybody knew what such terms meant; or, conversely, when they dealt with such "things," experimentally or otherwise, there was only one way of referring to them.

This has not been the case in either biology or psychology in regard to the term "heredity." In fact, the situation is reversed. Long before the sciences of biology and psychology developed, the term "heredity" was in widespread use in everyday language. It has been used loosely to refer to a wide variety of things and conditions. Examination of old dictionaries reveals usage of the term to refer to the "inheritance" of the crown, property, money, and office. Sinfulness, gout, idiocy, various diseases, and temperament were said to be "hereditary." The theological notion of "infant damnation" is to the point. All of the preceding suggests that superstition and old wives' tales are responsible for the dissemination of a belief that has been culturally transmitted from the Dark Ages down to the present time. We may take it as a general formula that whenever facts are not readily understood they are referred to the mysterious operation of "heredity."

The situation then is opposite to that of the chemists of our example, for in the present case the word came first. The everyday term with its manifold but vague usages got incorporated into biology and psychology. Then these workers got busy and tried to find "something" to which the term *might* refer. It is as if these investigators heard the term "heredity" used and were scrambling about in an effort to find something in the world of reality to go with it. The question "What is heredity?" illustrates the point. Let the reader substitute "mermaid" or "centaur" for "heredity" and he will get the full force of the argument. Small wonder that as long ago as 1924 Jennings,[4] a pioneer in the study of genetics, said:

Possibly we should be better off with no such concept as heredity; then analysis would be correctly directed toward understanding, in organisms as in other things, in what ways there is dependence on the stuff they are made of; in what ways on the conditions in which that stuff is found. [pp. 225–226].

In our opinion, Jennings is saying that it is too bad that students of genetics did not start with facts. Then, we would not have the contemporary unholy mixture of scientific facts and the superstitious connotations of the term.

What could the term "heredity" possibly "mean"? But let us accept the challenge to find in the "world of reality" some facts for which we could possibly use the label "heredity." First, we would call attention to the illustration that attempts to portray the broad sweep of succeeding generations of any species. Just incidentally, we should indicate the complexity and interrelatedness of various portions of this "stream of life," all of which could never be represented even for the small segment included here.

The striking feature of the series of individuals is their origin from a single cell contributed by two individuals of that series. This *material* we may call hereditary. It is the link between one generation and another. Since it is actually a portion of the contributing animals (egg and sperm cells), it is not surprising that offspring look like their parents. True, they are not "spit'n' images" of the parents, and even unrelated individuals may look very much alike, as everyday observation and the popular press prove. Perhaps this variability simply reflects the principle of individual differences that operates in both biology and psychology, while the occasional similarity of unrelated people points to the limited possibilities that the hereditary material has in the way of end products. Thus, members of one species will bear a closer resemblance to one another than to members of another species. That each species looks different from another species is

---

[4] JENNINGS, H. S. Heredity and environment. *Sci. Mon.*, N.Y., 1924, **19**, 225–238. (Reproduced by permission of the publisher.)

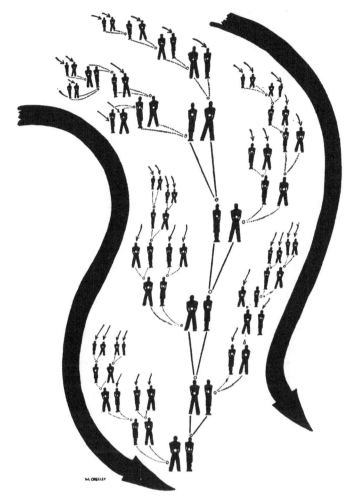

FIG. 1 How "heredity" operates. This picture attempts to convey the per-
petuation of the organisms of a species through "heredity." The reader may
catch the suggestion of a mighty stream which is nevertheless bounded. Its
complexity can be realized by attempting to trace back the complex known as
ancestry for any individual. The continuity, which is an essential feature of
"heredity," is indicated by the small circle before each individual which
eventually becomes that individual, the cell (which he carries around) becoming another individual upon mating, etc., etc. The stability of cellular material and of developmental and post-natal conditions gives a certain over-all
stability to the succession of generations.

obviously related to the material from which their respective members originate. In a certain sense, then, "heredity" (i.e., the original material) plays an important role in the eventual appearance of animals (or plants) in a given succession.

This is all that we can say. For, following conception, each individual undergoes an embryologic evolution which after 9 months yields a finished product. Insofar as conditions here are stable, the offspring will resemble the parents within the limits mentioned above. But change these conditions experimentally, or let various accidents supervene, and the end product may be a monstrosity only remotely resembling the parents. In other words, there is not the rigid operation of "heredity" (however defined) as is popularly believed. It is only similar material under similar developmental conditions that yields the similar individuals of a given species. Just because embryologic conditions are more or less stable, we should not discount their importance. The orientation suggested here would tend to give all the factors their proper place in the total picture. Heredity (the original material) is only one of many factors that account for the appearance of any individual.

DEVELOPED STRUCTURES AND BEHAVIOR—THEIR RELATIONSHIP. Now our purpose is to show how various organisms, having started with different materials and subsequent embryologic histories, fit into behavioral study. At a certain stage of their respective reactional biographies, let us take a duck and a chicken. It is obvious that the duck's webbed foot *makes it possible* for it to learn to swim, while the chicken's structures act to discourage the acquisition of swimming behavior. Another case would be the wings of the bird as compared with the arm and hand appendages of human animals. Note how the anatomy of the former *facilitates* the building up of flying behavior, while that of the latter *prevents* it. This is a far cry from the oversimplified statement of the man in the street to the effect that birds "inherit" flying and man does not. In fact, as we have seen, it is not even scientifically correct to say that the animals in question inherit their structures. The more correct statement would be to the effect that, having started with different initial materials *and* having undergone certain embryologic histories during which they elaborated various anatomic structures, their *subsequent* behavioral development is conditioned by all of these factors. In distorting the importance of the factors started with, the term "heredity" prevents us from comprehending the continuity of the various classes of events and their relation to one another. Regardless of where one puts the stress, nevertheless, one cannot relate "heredity" directly with behavior. The two have only a thin and indirect relation; namely, an animal's structure *permits* his acquisition of reactions involving such structures, or absence of organs *prevents* his learning things that he could learn if he were an organism possessing them. Viewed in this way, the problem becomes a simple one in which the investigator notes behavioral advantages and disadvantages that come to individuals as members of certain species. The opposable thumb, binocular vision, and bipedal construction are among the distinctive anatomic advantages that belong to humans (barring embryologic failures). These give humans advantages in learning acts involving these structures. Infrahumans are at a definite disadvantage in this regard. The theoretical advantage in handling the problem as presented here is that it leads to clarification instead of mystification.

Next, we examine how popular psychology handles those behaviors that are alleged to be "inherited." The most common ones are related to musical composition or performance and mathematical activities. It is interesting to note that no one claims that language behavior or racial prejudices are inherited. On the contrary, there is general agreement that individuals build up practically all the behavior that they perform. The exceptions lie in the fields mentioned above.

It is our contention that this state of affairs is the result of a lack of understanding. Because psychology up until very recent times could not interpret these reactions, they were simply attributed to heredity. In the same way, before medicine had learned the details of such diseases as tuberculosis or syphilis, they were alleged to be inherited. Where ignorance has reigned, heredity has always been invoked to "explain."

FALLACIES OF THE HEREDITARY DOCTRINE. Note that to assert that a certain activity is inherited illustrates purely circular reasoning.

"Why did Haydn compose and play so well?"
"Because he inherited a capacity."
"How do you know?"

"Because he composed and played so well," and so on.

The beginning student of elementary classical logic learns to detect such logical monstrosities in the study of fallacies in reasoning.

If we should then point out that both on his mother's and his father's side for two generations back there was not a single musician in Haydn's ancestry, but only blacksmiths, wheelwrights, and farmers, the defender of the hereditary dogma would resort to statement making that would involve further hypothetical assumptions leading to deeper obscurity.

But let us take the Bach family which did produce a succession of generations of able musicians. We do not need any additional principle to explain musical as opposed to other behaviors. These are not "out of this world" but of a piece with all other reactions.

The argument that the musical activity of the Bachs was hereditary because it "ran in the family" should hold just as consistently for their German-speaking activity. By what criterion can one possibly discriminate what is hereditary and what not when all "run in the family," including (in some families) Methodism, Catholicism, Buddhism, medical practice, weaving, skiing, voting Republican, Whig, Tory, and so on? The argument is an obvious *reductio ad absurdum*.

It is obvious that whether the Haydns or Bachs composed or performed, they were interacting with stimulus objects—pianos, organs, notes, and teachers. Furthermore, they were not geniuses from the very beginning. Their genius behavior was the culmination of a series of events of their reactional biographies involving long hours of practice and other labor. The following quotations [5] clearly demonstrate this point.

What is true of today's composers was probably equally true of most of the great musicians of the past. We know that many of them toiled and struggled, often sweated blood over their music. We have only to look at Beethoven's sketchbooks to see how he chiseled and hammered away, wrote and rewrote most of his greatest compositions, before he got them right. Bach, asked what was the secret of his art, responded, "I have worked hard." There is no question that he and all the great masters labored con-

---

[5] SIEGMEISTER, ELIE. *The music lover's handbook.* New York: Morrow, 1943. Pp. 817. (Reproduced by permission of the publisher.)

stantly and with intense application—they had to in order to get all that work done [p. 56].

Even Wagner, whose autobiography tends to give the impression that his life was one endless series of adventures, intrigues, love affairs, and his music the product of the famous raptus, must have spent years and years sitting stock-still at his desk or piano. The sheer labor of setting down the hundreds of thousands—if not millions—of notes contained in the orchestral scores of the "Ring" alone is appalling, and could never have been achieved without the months and years of patient, systematic work old Richard put in . . . [p. 56].

For three years Haydn's efforts to stave off hunger were no more interesting or distinguished than those of any young man in his position; he sang in church choirs, took part in street serenades, and helped out the music at weddings, funerals, and other festal occasions. All this time he studied hard; he learned theory backward and forward, and practiced the clavier. He got hold of six of Karl Phillipp Emanuel Bach's clavier sonatas, and studied them so thoroughly that they became the backbone of his own style [p. 378]. For the long journeys in his traveling coach, he [Haydn] carried with him a little silent clavier to keep in daily technical training [p. 485].

A contemporary artist has estimated that he has practiced 75,000 hours over a 40-year period. This averages about 5 hours per day, day in, day out.

These are reactions, then, that we are dealing with in music as elsewhere, and even from the superficial account presented above, it is obvious that the music masters built up these responses and as concert performers kept them well practiced. While it may be possible to stretch the scientific facts to say that organisms "inherit" structures, how could one possibly claim that action is inherited?

Stated in this fashion, the hereditary dogmatists usually assert that, of course, definite interaction with stimulus objects is necessary and that these factors must be included in their interpretation, but they would add X, an unknown quantity, verbally labeled as a "talent," "capacity," or "tendency." We must point out that, if we can do with conditions of the reactional biography alone what they do with conditions of the reactional biography plus other unspecifiable variables, then theirs is a radical theory. In terms of scientific method, the *simpler* of two explanations for a given event is to be preferred. We believe that our factually derived account is thus in accord with the principle of parsimony.

Another criticism of popular psychology's resort to hereditary forces or powers in explaining reactional superiority is its utter uselessness. Since it is derived from folklore rather than the facts, it can never be used to predict or control facts. Note that the theory of allegedly inherited talents or tendencies is brought forth only *after* the individual in question has attained reactional superiority. No one has stood over Paderewski's or anybody else's cradle and predicted that he would be a genius. Since by very definition talents and tendencies are unknown and unknowable sorts of things, one can do nothing with them.

In contradistinction, the hypothesis of the reactional biography works with behavioral variables (parents, teachers, musical instruments, notes, and so forth) all of which are demonstrable and which, in regard to prediction and control, limit us only to the extent to which we can devote effort to them.

This is a practical matter, not one of theoretical embarrassment, as is true of the competing hereditary theory. When one considers how many family lines do not show a succession of geniuses but only a sporadic individual showing behavioral superiority, one wonders how the traditional hereditary dogma can persist in the face of such facts. Note that most often there is only one Beethoven, one Tchaikovsky, one Edison, Bell, Marconi, Toscanini, da Vinci, Gutenberg, and so on, in an otherwise consistently mediocre lineage. Indeed, it is a commonplace observation that the world's outstanding men have come from humble ancestry. Who can formulate the hereditary "principle" that operates in such a strange, erratic manner?

Here another point of valid criticism obtrudes itself. Biology has long ago given up the theory of the inheritance of acquired characteristics. Nevertheless, "psychohereditary" doctrine persists in full force. The belief that parents "pass on" their "traits" to their offspring is an unwitting assumption of popular psychology's stand on this problem. Several interesting questions suggest themselves. Have the "genes" representing these "capacities" always been present in the human species or (assuming a theory of evolution) in its precursors? If so, have there always been "genes" for musical and mathematical ability even before these disciplines came into being? And do humans today possess "genes" for performances on yet-to-be-discovered instruments? How did these "genes" get in? When? Are they not just so many words—terms without referents?

SUMMARY. This brief treatment of the relationship of heredity and psychology has pointed out how an error was perpetrated when the term "heredity" was taken into science with all its non-scientific connotations. We then tried to find some fact in nature to which this term might refer, and we showed that animals that begin life as a cell contributed by members of a certain species will look (more or less) like other members of that species. This material might be called hereditary. Since it differs in different species, it gives rise to animals with different structures which enter into behavioral events as factors of advantage or disadvantage in the acquisition of various behaviors.

Popular psychology has claimed that musical and certain other behaviors must be treated differently from most other reactions in that the former have a hereditary basis. Examination of this theory reveals circular reasoning—*reductio ad absurdum;* it shows dependence upon factors of reactional biography in addition to hereditary ones, which violates the principle of parsimony; the theory is a derivative of the long-discarded doctrine of inheritance of acquired characters; and, finally, it is both scientifically and practically useless. In general, this traditional theory succeeds only in obscuring that which it sets out to explain.

Again, the foregoing is not asserted dogmatically but is offered as a rebuttal to the hereditary dogma with which every student approaches the study of psychology. At least, it will be apparent that the relationship between heredity and psychology is not, by any means, a closed case.

VI. THE PLACE OF SEX IN THE STUDY OF PSYCHOLOGY
N. H. Pronko

Because the following article deals with sex behavior, it deserves an extra comment for the following reasons. The data of psychology are more closely connected with moral and ethical considerations than are the materials of such sciences as chemistry and physics. It is obvious that the chemist does not blush or stammer when referring to CO_2 or HCl. Even in biology, the student attains a certain degree of objectivity in handling all the anatomic features of living things. In psychology, we are under obligation to deal with every variety of behavior, excluding none nor stressing one above another. We must be neutral to all in our scientific analysis of them.

The primary reason for including the present paper, however, is to illustrate the vast difference between physiological reactions as demonstrated in the "lower" animals and genuine psychological interbehaviors which are most complexly developed in the human animal. In the former, the reactions discussed here are pretty much the simple functioning of certain structures. In the latter, these reactions are clearly conditioned by the reactional biography of the individual, and they show all the characteristics of psychological interactions including their inhibition or total absence as a result of failure to build up such behavior. Certainly, in between the end points of this continuum are reactions which begin to take on some of the characteristics of behavior. Insofar as they do, to that extent are they psychological.

VII. PHYSIOLOGICAL SEXUAL REACTIONS VERSUS SEXUAL BEHAVIOR

N. H. Pronko

The ante-pituitary personality is educable for intelligence and even intellect, provided the proper educational stimulus is supplied. Men of brains, practical and theoretical philosophers, thinkers, creators of new thoughts and new goods, belong to this group. The distinction between men of theoretical genius, whose minds could embrace a universe, and yet fail to manage successfully their own personal everyday lives, and the men of practical genius, who can achieve and execute, the great engineers, the industrial men, lies in the balance between the ante-pituitary and the adrenal cortex primarily. Men like Abraham Lincoln and George Bernard Shaw belong to this ante-pituitary group [3, p. 213].[6]

Such unrestrained psychologizing regarding behavior was ushered in when a new explanatory mechanism was afforded by

---

[6] The numbers in brackets refer to the numbered items in the bibliography on pp. 40–41.

the recent expansion of the science of endocrinology. But behavioral explanations in terms of the magic secretions of the glands have not been restricted to the normal personality. Writers [19, pp. 174–193], [7, pp. 216–218], and [12] have allowed their imaginations free reign in explaining even psychopathic actions of individuals, with little or no evidence to support their interpretations. More recently still [6, pp. 209–224], endocrinological treatment has been proposed as a possible avenue for improving the intelligence of the race.

With many such extravagant claims of endocrinic powers, it would behoove the psychologist to examine the experimental literature in an effort to orient himself with respect to the role of the endocrines in the explanation of behavior. This paper is an initial effort in that direction, the purpose here being to examine the part played by hormonal products in mating behavior by a comparative approach to the problem.

Behavioral studies of the lower animals are generally scarce, particularly in regard to the participation of hormonal secretions in the reproductive activity of invertebrates. The role of endocrines in color changes of the Arthropoda and in the development of insects is pretty well established, but the question of an active role of sex hormones in invertebrates is still controversial [16, p. 383]. Stone's [17, pp. 828–879] chapter in Allen's excellent treatise deals only with classes above the Aves; nor is sexual behavior in the subavian groups adequately treated in the various textbooks on comparative psychology.

AMPHIBIA. It may be well, therefore, to begin this discussion with a common laboratory observation on Amphibia. It is a well-known fact that under certain appropriate conditions of age of subject, of surrounding temperature, and the like, injection of anteropituitary hormone will elicit mating behavior in the male frog, even in the late winter months. An analysis of such action shows the typical mounting and clasping reflex. It is hardly necessary to point out that the endocrinal secretion in this case is not a source of power or "sex drive." Rather, it is to be considered an indispensable condition in the operation of a sheer reflex type of action. But it must be emphasized that such behavior is at the same time a definite response to a stimulus object—in this case, the female frog.

It appears to be a rare occurrence for a male to clasp another male. Noble [13] has made an analysis of the factors that are operative in the situation. One factor is the female's responsiveness to the male's croaking. Then, too, the rapid hopping about of the male makes him difficult for another male to hold. It is suggested, also, that the croaking of males causes them to be released; females remain silent once they are clasped. In addition, there are differences in the shape of male and female bodies which may serve as important cues in sexual selection. That such is the case has been shown by Noble and Farris [14] who found that wood-frog males, injected with water until they resembled the egg-swollen females in size and firmness, were clasped and held as readily as were the females.

Along the same lines, the work of Hinsche [9] has shown that male toads would grasp and continue "to hold pieces of rubber sponge and other objects that gathered fairly well into the arms," indicating that the stimulus function for the mating behavior of the male frog may be present in many objects only distantly resembling the female. In summary, while the data are admittedly brief, it would seem that they at least permit the generalization regarding the frog member of the Amphibia that endocrinal secretions are important factors in facilitating a type of reflexive mating behavior easily elicited by a variety of stimulus objects in addition to the female.

BIRDS. Since studies of endocrinological factors in the sexual behavior of reptiles is not available, our next consideration will be directed toward the birds. In an attempt to determine the relative importance of glandular and environmental factors, Carpenter [4] observed the sexual behavior of male pigeons that had been castrated at the age of 1 month. While frequency of copulation was greatly reduced, the important point is that such behavior still continued. Charging behavior was next reduced, but billing and preening could be elicited in castrated birds, providing that social stimulation was sufficiently intense.

In a somewhat earlier study, Craig [5] studied the appearance of the separate responses—bowing, cooing, preening, and mouthing—in four male doves reared in absolute isolation. As in the frog, reflexlike acts appeared in response to a wide variety of stimulus objects, particularly in response to the experimenter's hand at feeding time, the human foot, and other objects. Only gradually were these responses transferred to a female presented on later occasions, which shows that "normally it is previous companionship with other birds of the species that mainly accounts for the greater potency of the more submissive female as a stimulating object to the sexually excited male" [5, p. 257].

In a recent study by Noble and Zitrin [15] in which the investigators injected male chicks with testosterone propionate, a synthetic male hormone, it was shown that this hormone caused the chicks to exhibit all the sexual behavioral patterns of the adult cock.

Crowing appeared as early as the 4th day of age and treading was seen on the 15th day. The copulatory pattern was identical to that of the sexually mature male bird. Injected males raised in isolation crowed and treaded as early as other treated birds [15, p. 327].

It is important to observe that there is no one-to-one correspondence between the injection of the hormone and the response. Note that crowing appears only as early as the fourth day of age; treading only after the fourteenth. In other words, injection does not eliminate the necessity for development of such behavior; rather, it is to be considered as a means of greatly stimulating physiological mechanisms which make such responses possible. That such is the case is shown by the authors' statement: "Chicks in which hormone treatment was initiated on the second day did not exhibit this behavior" [15, p. 334]. While the hormonal conditions described above must be recognized as necessary factors in the type of responses observed, we must not carelessly overlook the presence of a stimulus object in each case.

Again the stimulus function for eliciting the copulatory act is found to reside in a number of different things. For example, on the twenty-fourth day of the experiment, it was noted that one of the isolated males extended the sex invitation to the hand of the observer inserted through the cage, then mounted it, and went through all the movements of the copulatory act. A dead chicken had exactly the same stimulus function for another cock who went through all the movements exhibited by the adult rooster during copulation. We must repeat that for the chick as for the frog, hormonal factors are powerful ones in permitting a sexual type of behavioral occurrence which, however, appears to be somewhat more complicated with its context of such "secondary sexual acts" as billing, preening, and charging, as compared with the solitary, simple clasping reflex of the frog. Furthermore, historical conditions become more important in this "higher" animal group.

MAMMALS—RODENTS. Most of the mammalian work in endocrinology has utilized the very convenient laboratory rat. As a result, there is an embarrassing wealth of data, extensive consideration of which would lead to an overemphasis of this order. Hence, only the most pertinent of the representative studies need be considered here.

Stone [17, pp. 828–879] has pointed out the difficulty of getting some reliable index of the "strength of sexual behavior," although surgical and therapeutic measures such as castration, injection of sexual hormones, transplantation of glands, and other extreme measures have been resorted to in an attempt to discover the importance of gonadal and nongonadal factors of sexual activity. An indirect approach has been to use the activity cage; peaks of spontaneous activity every 4 or 5 days, that is, correlated with sexual receptivity in the female as well as with ovulation as determined by the vaginal smear technique, have been observed. Other experimenters report marked decrease in activity following castration and are reluctant to accept the validity of this measure. That possible uncontrolled factors have been overlooked is suggested by Hoskins [10] who found that when his castrated rats were subjected to 4 or 5 days of starvation, spontaneous activity increased almost 200 per cent, indicating perhaps that the usual decrease in the activity of castrates is conditioned by the accumulation of fat. Other similar studies have been generally vague and superficial and have yielded little significant evidence.

Among the more behavioral investigations are those of Josephine Ball [1]. This investigator castrated six male rats at weaning and gave them injections of the female sex hormones, estrogen, during the following 1½ to 3 months. Their sex behavior was compared with that of three litter-mate sisters, similarly injected with estrogen, and with normal brothers and sisters. All the castrates showed a female type (?) of mating behavior—lordosis—when mounted by a male; the rest of the female behavior was never elicited in the males, only in the females; nor did the females show any masculine behavior. Such results only show how the same substance permits the development of one type of behavior in one animal, another type in a sexually different animal —again supporting the view that such injections provide necessary conditions for sexual responses but that they do not "cause" them. In a follow-up study [2], ten normal, young, adult female rats were injected with testosterone and testosterone propionate over a period of 2 months. Sex behavior was tested, and vaginal smears were made throughout this time and for several weeks before and after it. Vaginal cycles and high degrees of heat behavior were suppressed, but eight of the ten rats continued to accept aggressive males throughout the injection period in spite of diestrous smears. A striking change was observed in the clitorides of injected females; these were hypertrophied to such an extent as to resemble male penes. In other words, the sex hormone stimulated the growth of the female sexual apparatus. Ball [2, p. 164] concludes:

. . . the male copulatory pattern in more or less rudimentary form is part of the equipment of the normal female rat. The threshold of this behavior pattern is very high normally but it can be lowered by testosterone administration which, however, although suppressing vaginal cycles, does not completely eliminate female sex behavior.

Instead of adopting Ball's explanation of an (ostensibly) inherited generalized male-female sex-behavior equipment, we should argue that the facts may be explained in a less hypothetical manner. In concrete terms, if one injects a substance which develops a malelike copulatory organ in an organism, he will thereby permit that organism to behave similarly to a male.[7] Another outstanding result of Ball's investigation is that suppression of the vaginal cycle does not necessarily eliminate sexual behavior. Here is a hint of the increase in relative detachment of sexual behavior from hormonal secretions—an independence which will be seen to culminate in man.

The fallacy of directly connecting behavior as effect with hormonal secretion as cause is excellently pointed out in a timely discussion by Wiesner and Sheard [20] who were able to set up maternal responses in virgin rats by injection of gonadotropic substances from the anterior lobe of the pituitary.

But these investigators show the need for cautious inference since Noble, Kumpf and Billings induced maternal behavior in the pearl fish by corpus

---

[7] It is only adherence to an outmoded "cause-effect" viewpoint which forces Miss Ball to connect injection of testosterone with behavior, with utter disregard of other perhaps more directly concerned concomitants of the observed event (in this case, the hypertrophied clitorides).

luteum hormone and to a lesser degree by thyroxine and a .5% solution of phenol. Moreover, recent experiments by Leblond and Nelson show that hypophysectomized young rats and mice may be induced to display maternal behavior, as do normal animals, by putting suckling young with them for short periods of time daily [20, p. 376].

In an earlier period of armchair speculation and easy generalization from crude observation, it was maintained that castration inevitably resulted in a cessation of reproductive activity. However, Stone [18] has recently restored sexual activity in ten inactivated castrated male rats by subcutaneous injection of testosterone propionate. Copulatory frequency in the most active castrates closely approached that of their precastration records and also the records of the controls. Such facts insistently affirm the need for a relativistic approach to the complex endocrinological and other conditions associated with mating behavior and definitely show that, for the rat, there is a greater departure from the one-to-one correlation of pituitary injection and clasp reflex shown in the frog.

THE UNGULATA AND CARNIVORA. Strictly experimental data on these orders are lacking, but observations on behavior at time of estrus are presented in a recent review by Young [23]. The nonpregnant cow is reported as coming into heat every 19 or 20 days. Sexual behavior at this time is more marked "when a bull or other cows are present." [8] There is a marked restlessness, twitching of the tail, and wandering off in isolation or with another cow, with occasional attempts to ride her.

A cow in heat frequently lowers the hips and small of the back and raises the tail end. She will frequently play with the bull by horning him. Cows in heat commonly jump other cows and bulls. This behavior reaches its extreme expression in nymphomania when the cow not only jumps other cows and bulls repeatedly but may even attempt to mount other species including man [23, p. 146].

"Of the Carnivores for which data exist, all except the dog show a heat behavior which in one way or another is more elaborate from the standpoint of display than that encountered in the other (lower) orders" [23, p. 149], but this behavior is still depend-

_____
[8] Is this not just another way of indicating that such behavior consists of very specific acts toward stimulus objects, and that the objects which elicit sexual responses to a most marked degree are bulls or cows?

ent upon a certain physiological condition because no trace of the response can be elicited by vaginal stimulation in cats which are not in heat. Nor is there a specificity of stimulus object since in some cats presence of a male cat is not essential, the response being operative with slight stimulation of the external genitalia or of the skin surrounding the vulva.

The infrahuman primates. Regarding Macacus rhesus, workers [23] are in agreement that members of this species copulate *at all times,* but that mating is more frequent when the sexual skin is active. Indeed, it is here that we find a great gap between the lower orders—a gap which foreshadows the increasing importance of the psychological factors that reach a climax in man. An earlier study of Yerkes and Elder [22] forced the conclusion that copulation does not necessarily imply female receptivity (i.e., as conditioned by heightened endocrinal secretions during estrus). These investigators describe the situation as follows:

> The female chimpanzee is cautious, discreet, accommodating at all times and as a rule she seeks to avoid arousing the male to violence by antagonizing him. Whether or not in estral phase, she may offer herself to the male at his command, or when pursued by him, for sexual intercourse. Conversely, the male may refuse to accept a receptive female, either because he is *not attracted to her* or because her cycle phase does not suit him. Males differ markedly in sexual selectiveness, preference, dominance, and aggressiveness. . . . Our S's offered instances of what in human life would unhesitatingly be designated frigidity and nymphomania, shyness and self-assertion, indifference and coquetry, weak and strong sex appeal, marked sexual preference and lack of it, affective attachment and coldness [22, pp. 37–39].

In a more recent study, Yerkes [21] observed that in a food-competition situation in which pairs of chimpanzees of both sexes were reared in the same cage, the priority of food acquisition varied between the male and female in apparent relation to the menstrual cycle of the female cage companion. For example, it was conclusively demonstrated that the ordinarily submissive female obtained much more food when in the maximal phase of genital swelling. At such times, she belligerently stationed herself at the food chute without a murmur from the *ordinarily* aggressive male. Occasionally, this spot was surrendered to the female in exchange for sexual surrender by the latter. ("Prostitution" behavior?) We find here a clear instance of the importance of situational factors determining a positive response when it would not otherwise occur, or inhibiting it despite strong sexual desire in both consorts. Similarly, such factors as strangeness, hostility, devotion, and desire for food may compare with physiological factors and in some instances may even dominate them.

THE HUMAN PRIMATE. Experimental studies of endocrinological participation in the sexual behavior of the human are necessarily limited. Clinical cases have been reported, but these are of little significance in a scientific determination of the role of hormones in sexual activity, since they are for the most part empirical investigations aimed at achieving some particular practical end. In a general way, Grollman [8] discusses the effects of castration in the following manner:

> Complete castration of the adult does not always lead to impotence, and the sexual instinct may persist. The earlier the age of castration, the less marked is the subsequent sexual desire. Eunuchs may copulate up to 25 or 30 years after castration [*sic.!*]. Among soldiers castrated by war injuries, sexual vigor remains undiminished in some cases, but in most cases, it is decreased from normal, and in many there is almost complete suppression of the libido and potentia [8, p. 356].

As a last bit of evidence in support of the thesis developed here, we refer to the study of Kinsey [11] who points out the fallacy of a recent attempt to connect a particular type of sexual behavior (homosexuality) in the human with a specific endocrine product of the urine. Kinsey has emphasized that any endocrinological explanation of such behavior must consider the fact that homosexuality and heterosexuality may both occur coincidentally in a single life period of a particular individual; that the two may exist simultaneously or successively in every sort of combination or pattern; and, finally, that it is a prevalent form of sexual behavior. In conclusion, this investigator suggests that "in the adolescent individual there is only a *gradual development* [9] of the exclusively homosexual or exclusively heterosexual patterns which predominate among older adults" [11, p. 428].

There is a proper recognition here of the weight of cultural factors in determining in which direction an individual will develop sexually. As Kinsey and other investigators point out, in-

---

[9] Italics mine.

dividuals reared on isolated farms are in contact with situations which lead to the acquisition of sexual acts that are labeled as "zoophilia." On the other hand, such behavior is almost nonexistent among urban dwellers. It has also been noted that homosexuality was more prevalent among the boys of European aristocracy—thrown into intimate and (in many cases) exclusive contact with male servants and tutors—than it was among the children of peasant families in which heterosexual contacts were assured. Note, too, the wide prevalence of homosexuality in certain periods of Greek history. And, finally, one must insist on the dominating influence of social, economic, and structural factors in determining whether or not a particular individual shall perform any sort of sexual behavior during his or her lifetime, the frequency and the manner in which such acts are performed (if they are performed at all), and the subtle conditioning of attitudes toward such behavior.

SUMMARY

An exhaustive treatment of the thesis developed here would require a complete volume by itself. It does appear to be a valid generalization, though, that sexual behavior becomes progressively more independent of endocrinal secretions as one goes up the animal scale. There appears to be a corresponding dependence upon behavioral conditions.

The attempt was made to show that in the lower orders such as the frog, the sexual responses closely approximate a reflex type of behavior—a simple kind of interaction with a variety of objects only remotely similar, but also one strongly dominated by hormonal products. In the birds, more complex acts (billing, preening, charging) were associated with mating behavior in relative independence of endocrinological factors, although, here, too, stimulus functions were seen to inhere in a number of objects besides the female. The sexual behavior of rats, while still showing dependence, at least in the female, upon a certain physiological condition, could also be elicited toward the end of estrus ("when the response is difficult to elicit") by a dominating male. But it is in the lower primates that sexual behavior is seen to be completely free of the estrus cycle. While in man, social, cultural, economic, geographical, and structural factors were shown to condition his sexual activity over a latitude which permitted an extreme degree of plasticity, ranging from nonperformance of sexual behavior through all possible patterns of reflexlike, and homosexual, homosexual-heterosexual, and heterosexual activities; these human acts are most independent of endocrinal secretions.[10] But even such gross and crude ways of regarding human sexual performances only hint at the infinite variety of acts subsumed under this class of behaviors and suggest that their complete understanding can only be achieved by investigating particular organisms in their specific life situations.

BIBLIOGRAPHY

1. BALL, J. Male and female mating behavior in prepubertally castrated male rats receiving estrogens. *J. comp. Psychol.*, 1939, **28**, 273–284.

2. BALL, J. The effect of testosterone on the sex behavior of female rats. *J. comp. Psychol.*, 1940, **29**, 151–165.

3. BERMAN, LOUIS. *The glands regulating personality.* New York: Macmillan, 1921. Pp. 300.

4. CARPENTER, C. R. Psychobiological studies of social behavior in Aves, *J. comp. Psychol.*, 1933, **16**, 25–97.

5. CRAIG, W. Male doves reared in isolation. *J. Anim. Behav.*, 1914, **4**, 121–133.

6. DISPENSA, J. & HORNBECK, R. T. Can intelligence be improved by prenatal endocrine therapy? *J. Psychol.*, 1941, **12**, 209–224.

7. DORCUS, R. M. & SCHAFFER, G. W. *Textbook of abnormal psychology.* Baltimore: Williams & Wilkins, 1945. Pp. 549.

8. GROLLMAN, A. *Essentials of endocrinology.* Philadelphia: Lippincott, 1941. Pp. 480.

9. HINSCHE, G. Uber brunst-und-kopulations reaktion von bufo vulgaris. *Psych. Vergl. Physiol.*, 1926, 4, 564–606.

10. HOSKINS, H. G. Studies on vigor, II. The effect of castration on voluntary activity. *Amer. J. Phys.*, 1925, **72**, 324.

11. KINSEY, A. C. Homosexuality. *J. Clin. Endocrin.*, 1941, I, 424–428.

12. McCARTNEY, J. L. Dementia praecox as an endocrinopathy with clinical and autopsy reports. *Endocrinology*, 1929, **13**, 73.

13. NOBLE, G. K. *The biology of the Amphibia.* New York: McGraw-Hill, 1931. Pp. 577.

14. NOBLE, G. K. & FARRIS, E. J. The method of sex recognition in the

---

[10] Unless we stretch to the breaking point the concept of abnormality of endocrinal secretion in the general population.

wood frog, *Rana sylvatica* Le Conte. *Amer. Mus. Novit.,* 1929, No. 363, 1–17.

15. NOBLE, G. K. & ZITRIN, ARTHUR. Induction of mating behavior in male and female chicks following injection of sex hormones. *Endocrinology,* 1942, 30, 327.

16. SCHARRER, BERTA. Endocrines in invertebrates. *Physiol. Rev.,* 1941, 21, 383–409.

17. STONE, C. P. Sexual drive, in ALLEN, EDGAR. *Sex and internal secretions.* Baltimore: Williams & Wilkins, 1934. Pp. 951.

18. STONE, C. P. Copulatory activity in adult male rats following castration and injections of testosterone propionate. *Endocrinology,* 1939, 24, 165–174.

19. WATSON, J. B. *Psychology from the standpoint of a behaviorist.* Philadelphia: Lippincott, 1919. Pp. 429.

20. WIESNER, B. P. & SHEARD, N. M. *Maternal behavior in the rat.* Edinburgh: Oliver & Boyd, 1933. Pp. 425.

21. YERKES, R. M. Social behavior of chimpanzees; dominance between mates in relation to sexual status. *J. comp. Psychol.,* 1940, 30, 147–186.

22. YERKES, R. M. & ELDER, J. H. Oestrous receptivity and mating in chimpanzee. *Comp. Psychol. Monogr.,* 1938, 13, 39.

23. YOUNG, W. C. Observations and experiments on mating behavior in female mammals. *Quart. Rev. Biol.,* 1941, 16, 135–156.

VIII. HOW THE NEWLY HATCHED LOGGERHEAD TURTLE FINDS ITS WAY TO THE SEA [11]
N. H. Pronko

How is it that the newly born turtle just emerged from its shell goes promptly and directly to the ocean without any benefit of previous experience from its parents? Does this indicate that it has an "ancestral memory of the sea"? Is this an exception to the hypothesis of a reactional biography which states that all behavior originates during the life history of the organism?

The answer to this question comes from a study carried out by Daniel and Smith on the east coast of Florida. These investigators observed that, after an incubation period of about 50 days,

[11] DANIEL, R. S. & SMITH, K. U. The sea-approach behavior of the neonate loggerhead turtle (Caretta caretta), *J. comp. Phys. Psychol.,* 1947, 40, 413–420.

the young turtles hatch in a nest which is essentially a 2-foot hole in the sand about 1 foot in diameter, containing from 50 to 200 eggs. The young turtles spend from 3 to 5 days in the nest, then emerge from it, make a straight path toward the water, and swim immediately for the ocean, as shown in the accompanying figure. The experimenters observed that the young turtles usually emerged at night. Suspecting that the water-locating reaction was a visual one, they placed turtles individually and by groups in a pit about 15 feet from the water's edge. The animals could see nothing but the uniformly lighted sky, and although they were active in the pit, they did not show signs of orientation toward the ocean. However, when they were removed from the pit and placed on the beach, they went directly toward the water. Apparently, not the sound or smell of the water but the sight of the water was the crucial factor.

That the experimenters' hypothesis seemed to be correct was indicated by several tests that they carried out on the beach. Once a turtle had started for the surf, a black hood slipped over its head would effectively prevent it from completing the trip to the water. Furthermore, when four animals were released from the pit on a moonless night, their tracks showed mere random movement. None reached the water under these circumstances, but when these same turtles were later released from the same point on the beach *after* the moon had risen, they all found their way to the surf within 2 or 3 minutes after release. Finally, it was discovered that turtles would follow a beam of light from a flashlight in any direction on the beach. As a matter of fact, those that had made their trip to the water on the basis of reflected moonlight from the surf could be stimulated to go back to the land again by directing a beam of light at them. At this point in the study, it was clear that the stereotyped action of the turtle was specifically related to stimulation by light.

Accordingly, Daniel and Smith carried out laboratory investigations in order to get at the details involved. They first observed that turtles kept in the dark were quiescent, and that illumination directed upon them made them very active. They also found that their approach to lighted areas was positively accelerated. Moderately lighted areas gave moderate speeds of approach, and more intense areas of light, faster speeds. The phototropic nature of the turtles' response was indicated by the circular crawling that

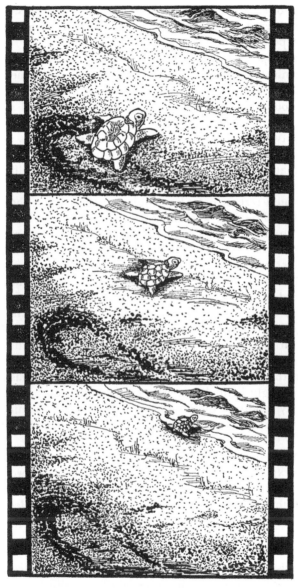

FIG. 2 Drawn from photos loaned by Dr. R. S. Daniel. The "snapshots" shown above represent a sequence in the straight path to the sea made by a newly-hatched loggerhead turtle on its first excursion from the nest. This reaction is a light or phototropic response rather than an acquired (i.e. psychological) response. (Daniel, R. S. & Smith, K. U., Sea approach of the neonate loggerhead turtle.)

turtles showed when they were illuminated from above while one eye was covered. This circus movement occurred toward the side of the exposed eye.

The response was not found to be related to effects of gravity on the animal (geotropism), nor was it related to the smell of sea water. The latter situation was tested by experiments in which turtles could select between a path to an illuminated stimulus card and another path which led first to a tank of sea water interposed between the animal and an illuminated stimulus card. By changing the position of the sea water from trial to trial, they found that five turtles given 50 trials each showed no differential response to the two paths.

Because certain preceding students believed that the expansiveness of the ocean was the crucial variable in the turtles' approach to the sea, Daniel and Smith explored this possibility. "Openness" of the visual field or the degree to which it is broken by shrubs, trees, and so forth, was represented by cards with vertical black and white stripes behind which was a uniformly illuminated wall. Five turtles released in the test situation went promptly to the cards without attempting to explore the "open country" beyond. Another interesting item that turned up showed that, with older turtles, there might be a reversal of this phototropic response, for it was found that turtles 3 weeks old would swim in the darker portions of an aquarium when it was illuminated by bright light. Apparently, circumstances of the reactional biography condition the phototropic response of this animal, for turtles not treated in this fashion swim toward light rather than dark.

THE SIGNIFICANCE OF DANIEL AND SMITH'S STUDY. In our opinion, the experiment reported above gives a clear-cut answer to the question posed at the beginning of this article. First of all, it is obvious that the response of the newly hatched turtles is not learned because there are no opportunities for acquiring that reaction.

The next question is: Is it behavior? Does it show the usual characteristics of psychological occurrences? Can one detect here a high degree of discrimination, variability, modifiability, inhibition, integration, or delayability such as the reader can easily discern in his own learned responses? Is this not more like the constant and somewhat automatic reflex activities, with the exception that the tropistic action here described is an organismic response rather than the operation of a part of an animal? In our estimation, the migratory response of the loggerhead turtle toward the ocean is best described as a stereotyped physiological operation of the total animal to a physical stimulus (light reflection) striking a sensitive portion of the animal (the eye). That it is not a psychological adjustment is shown by the fact that when the necessary light condition is lacking (as on moonless nights), the animal may fail to reach its natural habitat and perish. The same thing may happen if the turtle should come into contact with an accidental light source such as a flashlight in a direction away from the ocean. In other words, let the reader set up a string of lights along the Florida beaches to the landward side of the loggerhead-turtle nests, and he can cause a rapid extinction of these animals.

IX. THE NEST MAKING AND PROVISIONING OF THE SOLITARY WASP

Kellogg [12] long ago described the tropistic response of the digger wasp, Ammophila. During September, along the western shores of the long southern arm of San Francisco Bay, the female wasp may be seen digging a hole in the salt-encrusted ground. When finished, she caps the hole with a bit of salt crust and flies away. She then returns with a dead looper or inchworm held in her mouth, puts it alongside the recently prepared nest, removes the salt-crust cover, and drags the inchworm down into the hole, going head first and coming up backward.

This process may be repeated five or more times, after which she deposits an egg on the surface of the worm, replaces the cover, and flies away. Such activity appears to be highly psychological, yet when one analyzes it further, it shows up its strictly biological character. The following quotation from Kellogg clearly classifies the Ammophila's action as a tropistic response.

Interrupt her chain of activities in the nest-making and provisioning performance and she is lost. If, for example, we quietly remove one of the inchworms, after she has brought it and laid it on the ground near the nest,

---

[12] KELLOGG, VERNON L. *Mind and heredity*. Princeton: Princeton Univ. Press, 1923. Pp. 108. (Reproduced by permission of the publisher.)

and place it a few inches farther away while she is engaged in getting the salt-crust off of the hole, what happens? When she turns about to seize the worm to drag it down into the hole and does not find it where she placed it, she is non-plussed. She moves about distractedly. She doesn't search. She simply flutters about, perhaps happening by chance on the worm; perhaps not. She doesn't seem to use her powers of sight and smell which she has certainly used in finding the same inchworm in the pickleweed, to find the nearby worm now on the ground in plain sight or smell of her. So if she doesn't happen to find it promptly by chance, she simply gives up further work on this burrow. If she goes on with her nest-making at all, she starts a new hole. In other words, she starts the chain of performance all over again from the beginning. Fabre found in a case of another kind of solitary wasp which stores its burrow with individuals of a certain kind of wingless ground cricket, that if he merely turned around one of these crickets brought by the wasp to the side of the hole, and which she deposited with the long hind legs nearest the hole so that she always seized the cricket by these legs preparatory to dragging it down, that the wasp failed to put the cricket in the hole although the antennae projecting from the head, which was now nearest the hole, were about as good handles to seize it by as the legs [pp. 9–10].

X. THE EGG-LAYING AND MATING REACTIONS OF THE CHINESE SILKWORM MOTH

With a final example again taken from Kellogg's [18] writing, we conclude our discussion of unlearned reactions in the infrahuman animals. While superficially, these activities resemble behavioral action, closer analysis will always show them to be stereotyped, mechanical action of the total animal which can be treated satis-factorily as physiological stimulus response—in other words, as an activation of the animal by a certain kind of physical energy with-out benefit of a complicated history. The egg-laying and mating reactions of the Chinese silkworm moth are excellent illustrations of a nonpsychological type of action.

The Chinese silkworm moths issue from their cocoon-covered, pupal cases as full-fledged insects, sexually mature. They have four wings, but

---

[18] KELLOGG, VERNON L., *Mind and heredity.* Princeton: Princeton Univ. Press, 1923. Pp. 108. (Reproduced by permission of the publisher.)

can not fly, or can only in exceptional cases, and then for but a few feet or yards. They take no food; indeed they can not feed, for their mouth parts are atrophied. They have done their eating, and plenty of it, as larvae (silkworms). They take enough food then, not only to provide energy for their six or seven weeks of active larval life, but to store up food in the body, mostly as fat, to provide for their inactive pupal life of twelve to fourteen days and their active life as moths, which lasts, however, only a few days, usually not more than a week. Having no need, or even means, of feeding; having no bird or toad or lizard or insect enemies to avoid, because they are entirely protected, as their ancestors have been for the past five thousand years, by the silk-growers; and the males not having to search widely for their female mates which issue from cocoons within a few inches of them; and these females, once mated, not needing to search for a particular food plant on which to deposit their eggs, as most moths and butterflies do, so that the hatching larvae will find proper food ready to mouth; without having, thus, to do any of these various things usually necessary for moths to do, the silkworm moths have just two essential activities to achieve, namely, mating and egg-laying.

Here, then, we have a highly developed insect, of different order, but of little less structural specialization than the solitary wasps and honeybees, whose behavior, however, is extremely limited and very simple, although no less important to the persistence of its own species than the elaborate behavior of the bees and wasps is to the maintenance of theirs. Under these advantageous circumstances, perhaps, we can discover, as we did in the case of the swarming of the honey-bees, an explanation, or better put, a description, of the behavior of the silkworm moths in terms of definitive response to physio-chemical stimuli; in other words, a mechanistic explanation or description.

After the female moths issue from their cocoons, with bodies already heavy and swollen because of the mass of eggs in them, they move about but little and only slowly. The males, on the other hand, of more slender and lighter body, are active and restless in their movements, which soon culminate in bringing them to the females. Now, these movements might be described as resulting from an intention to find the females, if we cared to ascribe the power of conscious intention to these creatures; or as an instinctive search for their mates, if we preferred to explain their behavior as controlled by unconscious instinct. But if we go further in our observation, and add a little experimentation to it, we shall find basis for a third kind of description.

The females bear, in the posterior end of the abdomen, a pair of scent glands which are occasionally, and in some cases continuously, protruded from the body. The males have organs of smell—many minute pits with a free nerve-ending at the base of each—on their antennae. They smell the odor from the female scent-glands; or, put as the mechanists would put it, the scent particles proceeding through the air from these glands strike and stimulate these nerve-endings, which in turn results in a positive stimulation of the males to move in the direction of the source of the scent particles. This brings them to the females. They do not find the females by sight, for they find them in darkness as well as in day time and with their eyes totally blinded as well as with their eyes untreated. If one antenna of a male moth standing near a female is removed, the movements of this male will constitute a series of circles, or a spiral, turning always toward that side on which the intact antenna lies, this devious movement, however, also usually bringing it finally to the female. Finally, if the scent-glands be cut from a female, and a male, with eyes and antennae intact, be put equidistant between the female moth and the removed glands, or even much nearer the female than the glands, the male will inevitably move toward the glands and reaching them remain there and go through the motions of an attempt at mating. It doesn't distinguish the difference between the cut-out glands and the female moth, and it thus doesn't mate at all. The male silkworm moth is, say the mechanists, positively chemotropic; its movements are simply a positive and inevitable physical reaction to a chemical stimulus. That accounts for practically all of the behavior of a male silkworm through all of its adult life.

As for the egg-laying, very soon after mating the female begins to lay its eggs, in small batches, until all of the 300 or more in its body have been deposited. This is, of course, a very useful performance; it is a necessary one for the persistence of the species. Does the female moth know of this usefulness, this necessity? Or is egg-laying an unconscious performance due to an inherited instinct? Or can it, too, be seen as a positive and inevitable result of a mechanical reaction to a certain specific and immediate physico-chemical stimulus? If the abdomen, or even just that posterior part of it containing the eggs, is cut off from a female moth, thus leaving the head, with brain, eyes and sense-organs on the antennae, and the thorax with its large mid-body ganglion, quite separated from the egg-laying organs (ovaries, oviducts, muscles) with the small posterior abdominal ganglion and its nerves which run from the skin and to the muscles of the hinder part of the abdomen, this cut-off hinder fraction of the body, if its ventral side is brought in contact with the bottom of the tray in which the moths are kept, or if this fragment of the body be turned over and its ventral side is rubbed, will extrude the eggs. The performance of egg-laying will be carried on just as it would be by an unmutilated female. In other words, the interesting and useful egg-laying behavior of the adult female moth—which is practically all of its behavior in its whole adult life—is, the mechanists would say, simply an inevitable physical or mechanical reaction by a small mass of living substance to a group of physicochemical stimuli [pp. 16–30].

This last illustration indicates that our description of tropisms as reactions of the total organism is not always required, for the egg-laying reaction of the moth apparently operates as a "part reaction"—in other words, it is no different than a reflex.

XI. EXPERIMENTS ON BIRD NAVIGATION [14]
Donald R. Griffin and Raymond J. Hock
Department of Zoology, Cornell University

Students of bird migration have generally assumed that birds head straight toward their goal, even when flying across wide stretches of ocean or other areas devoid of landmarks. Since natural migrations do not readily lend themselves to experimental study, most of our knowledge of bird navigation has stemmed from artificial homing experiments. In such experiments birds are captured, usually at their nests, and carried to a distance before release. Many species have returned from hundreds of miles, sometimes from territory which the individual birds had almost certainly never visited before, and to the sensory physiologist these homing flights have generally appeared to pose the same problems as natural migrations. Nevertheless, one of us concluded recently, after considering all the evidence then available (1), that the basic assumption of an essentially straight flight path might be incorrect. Indeed, it was possible to account for most of the recorded data by assuming (a) that birds have a well-developed topographical memory, so that, having flown over an area in migration or natural wanderings, they could thereafter orient themselves within it by means of landmarks, and (b) that, when artificially transported to unknown surroundings, they explore wide areas until they reach familiar territory.

Clearly, the critical test of this exploration hypothesis would be to

14 GRIFFIN, D. R. & HOCK, R. J. Experiments on bird navigation, *Science*, 1948, 107, 347–349. (Reproduced by permission of the authors and publisher.)

trace the actual flight paths of homing birds; if they fly essentially straight toward home when released in unknown territory, the hypothesis can be discarded. Gannets (Morus bassanus) were selected as the best available species for this experiment, since they are large white birds, easily observed from an airplane, and since they are strictly marine and virtually never fly more than a very short distance inland. Thus, we could be sure that the 17 gannets which we released more than 100 miles from the nearest salt water were in completely unknown territory. Nine of them were followed from an airplane, the remainder being controls against the possibility that the presence of the airplane 1,500′–2,000′ above the bird would influence its homing performance. Since both groups showed roughly the same speed (average, 99 miles/day) and the same percentage of returns (63% of those released in good physical condition), it seemed clear that the airplane had no detrimental effect on their homing. Furthermore, this speed and percentage of returns was comparable to the results obtained with other wild birds [1].[15]

The performance of gannets is compared, in Table [1], with other species which have been transported in sufficient numbers to equivalent distances to permit a valid comparison.

Table 1

Species	Returns (Per Cent)	Average Speed (Miles per Day)
Herring gull (inland releases)	97	90
Swallow	67	141
Gannet	63	99
Leach's petrel	61	38
Starling	54	17
Noddy and sooty tern	52	114
Common tern (inland releases)	29	109

The gannets fall in the middle of this series with respect to speed and per cent returns, and they might well have ranked higher in per cent returns but for the fact that overland flights were quite unnatural for them. They can not take off from the land without an appreciable head wind and an open space of 100 yards or more, so that any which were forced down over land from fatigue or other causes would almost certainly be lost. This probably reduced the number of returns in comparison with the other species listed in the table.

---

[15] The numbers in brackets refer to the numbered items in the bibliography on p. 53.

With these considerations in mind, it is appropriate to turn to Fig. [3], which shows the actual routes flown by 9 gannets followed by us for portions of their return flight ranging from 1 to 9½ hours and from 25 to

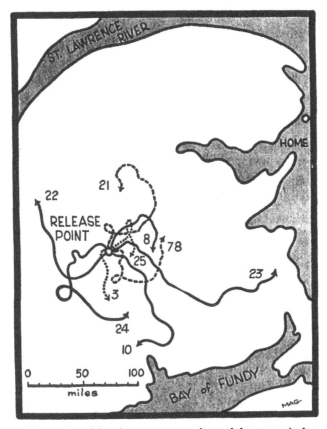

FIG. 3 Flight paths of homing gannets as observed from an airplane. Note that none of the gannets headed directly home. Five of these birds were back at their nests after the following times: No. 10, 70 hours; No. 22, 45 hours; No. 23, 45 hours; No. 25, 24 hours; and No. 78, 75 hours. The rest (Nos. 3, 8, 21, and 24) never returned home. It is quite likely that during previous fishing trips or annual migrations these gannets had flown along the entire coastline shown here. (Griffin, D. R., & Hock, R. J., Experiments on bird navigation.)

230 miles. It is obvious that they did not head at all directly home. On the contrary, their flight paths radiate in many directions from the release point, with a suggestion of spiraling.

Five of these birds were back at their nests after the following periods of time: No. 10, 70 hours; No. 22, 45 hours; No. 23, 45 hours; No. 25, 24 hours; and No. 78, 75 hours. The rest did not return; but it should be noted that No. 24 was released in poor physical condition. It is quite likely that during previous fishing trips or annual migrations, these gannets had flown along the entire coast-line shown in Fig. [3] (with the exception of the upper Bay of Fundy). If so, this coast would be familiar territory within which they might be expected to orient themselves by means of landmarks remembered from their previous experiences.

A detailed description of these experiments, together with an interpretation of the results, will be presented elsewhere, but it seems clear that for this species at least, *the actual flight paths suggest exploration rather than any absolute "sense of direction."* Since the performance of gannets is comparable to that of most other wild birds, it is quite possible that their homing ability is also based largely on exploration for visual landmarks.

What of natural migrations, particularly those which cross long stretches of ocean, or those in which young birds seem to migrate along the route characteristic of the species without adults to guide them? Clearly, one should not speculate too widely on the basis of one experiment with a single species, but it would perhaps be pertinent to re-examine the evidence concerning the directness of natural migratory flights. Could it be that trans-ocean migrants, for example, do *not* fly straight in the absence of landmarks—or such cues as wind direction—but rely, under difficult conditions at least, on some type of exploratory searching for their goal? Since observations of the usual type tell us little or nothing about the actual flight paths of individual birds, we can not safely infer from them that a migrant flies along an essentially straight course, although this has generally been assumed to be the case, just as it has been assumed for the return flights of homing birds.

To be sure, the important experiments of Rowan [4], Ruppell [5], and Schuz [6] have shown that inexperienced young birds may migrate in approximately the correct direction even without adults to guide them. These flights were over land with many landmarks available, the problem being to explain how the birds selected the appropriate cues to guide their first fall migration southward. But it seems unnecessary to conclude as many have done [2, 3, 7], that birds must possess an unknown sensory mechanism capable of informing them of their latitude and longitude, or the equivalent, so that they can travel to their nest or winter range, as the case may be, without reliance on such mundane cues as landmarks, the position of the sun, or wind direction. Neither the observed flight paths of homing gannets and herring gulls nor the indirect evidence that other homing birds rely on landmarks and exploration [1] are consistent with these theories. Merely as an example of an alternate explanation for the results obtained by Rowan, Ruppell, and Schuz, it should be noted that the birds were released north of 50° latitude, where even in summer the sun is always perceptibly south of the zenith. Rowan's releases were made in Alberta during November, when the sun never rises more than 20° above the horizon. Thus, a tendency to fly toward the sun could perhaps account for the southward movement of these inexperienced birds.

Insofar as our conclusions are relevant for other species under other conditions, they suggest that birds do not possess a special "sense of direction" or any sensitivity to the earth's magnetic field. The behavior of the gannets reinforced our impression that birds navigate by means of environmental cues which lie within the scope of the known receptors. When landmarks (rivers, coastlines, mountain ranges, etc.), prevailing winds, or the direction of the sun are not available as guiding influences, or when birds are released in unknown territory where the environmental cues have no meaning, they may well reach their goal by a process of exploration. There is need, however, for more observations from the air of the actual flight paths of other birds, both during homing flights and during migration, and one can perhaps look forward to a solution of this classic problem of biology as investigators make greater use of aircraft and other fruits of modern technical ingenuity.

REFERENCES

1. GRIFFIN, D. R. *Quart. Rev. Biol.*, 1944, **19**, 15–31.
2. ISING, G. *Arch. Math., Astron., Eys.*, 1946, 32A (4) No. 18.
3. MAYR, E. *Bird Lore*, 1937, **39**, 5–13.
4. ROWAN, W. *Trans. Roy. Soc. Can.* (3rd Ser., Sec. V), 1946, **40**, 123–135.
5. RUPPELL, W. *J. Ornithol.*, 1944, **92**, 106–132.
6. SCHUZ, E. *Vogelzug*, 1934, **5**, 21–24.
7. YEAGLEY, H. L. *J. appl. Phys.*, 1947, **18**, 1035–1063.

XII. DO BUZZARDS INHERIT AN INSTINCT TO FLY?

N. H. Pronko

Dennis [16] chanced upon two immature turkey buzzards which he removed from the nest on June 22. They were still covered with white down, could not stand erect, and were unable to run away from their captor. Furthermore, they did not flap their wings or attempt to fly.

Immediately after their capture, the birds were placed in a small cage, but they had to be moved to larger quarters with continued growth. However, there was never room enough for them to flap their wings or to fly. They ate a variety of raw meats, were in good health throughout the experiment, and became quite tame.

Six days after their capture, the birds were taken individually from the cage for a few minutes. Held under the wings, the birds flapped their wings synchronously one or more times. While Dennis does not discuss the significance of this action, we believe that it merely shows that an organism's structure will be moved if it is given the opportunity to do so. An infant's slashing action of arms and kicking of legs illustrates the point.

The birds were given no tests or further opportunity to fly until August 30, a little over 2 months following their capture. By this time, they were approximately adult size and had attained full adult plumage. The larger bird now had a wingspread of 60 inches and the small bird one of 46 inches.

FLYING TESTS. The birds were individually placed on the ground in a pasture. Both were relatively inactive and when approached would run away but could be recaptured easily. Occasionally, the larger bird flapped its wings as it ran, which succeeded in carrying it off the ground for a horizontal distance of 2 feet. This occurred in two instances. The smaller bird reacted similarly.

The next test attempted to determine whether the birds could balance themselves from a perch and fly from it, since neither subject had had an opportunity to perform either reaction. Thus, each bird was placed on a fence post 6 feet high. On two

---

[16] DENNIS, WAYNE. Spalding's experiment on the flight of birds repeated with another species. *J. comp. Psychol.*, 1941, 31, 337–348.

successive trials given each bird, both subjects fell to the ground. Thinking that if the birds were once in the air, flight might come more easily, Dennis tossed them lightly in the air. The larger bird could be given only one trial because it was feared it might injure itself. The smaller bird spread its wings but did not flap them and landed 6 feet away, the first time on its feet and the second time heavily on its breast.

A second test 2 weeks later showed no improvement in flying and only a slight advance in perching, the smaller bird still falling off the post on both trials. In flying after being tossed into the air, the smaller bird performed more poorly than on the previous test, although his wingspread was now 50 inches. The larger bird, with a wingspread of 62 inches, showed a little improvement. Three more tests yielded no impressive progress despite the fact that the tests themselves constituted opportunities for practice.

The birds were then given their liberty during the day, attempts being made to return them to the cage at night as long as possible. The smaller bird, which died October 1, never flew more than a few feet but succeeded in gliding approximately 15 feet along a sloping lawn. The larger bird was able to fly into treetops and onto housetops but was never observed to soar or fly more than 100 yards at a time. Frequently, other birds landed in the tree where Dennis' subject was perched, but when they flew away and soared, he was unable to follow. Eventually, he joined them in their flight and was never recognized again.

IMPLICATIONS. According to Dennis, observations on these two buzzards indicate that the flying of birds is not something that is native or that simply "matures." He believes that lack of practice rather than physiological immaturity was responsible for their failure to exhibit normal flight reactions and adds that he observed nothing that resembled a "sudden maturation of function." "This interpretation is further strengthened by the fact that even as late as October 1 neither bird could fly more than short distances, and neither could soar in the manner which is so characteristic of the turkey buzzard" [p. 344].

In our opinion, Dennis' study shows that birds do not inherit a flying instinct or ability, but that flying, which involves discrimination, integration, inhibition, variability, modifiability, and delayability, in such acts as soaring, gliding, swooping down on prey, and pursuing or being pursued, demands an early, long, and complicated history. Prevent such a history either totally or to some degree or other and you prevent the development of flying behavior. Thus, we have prediction and control.

In summary, we should point out that when we consider such reactions as flying and fully determine that they are behavioral facts, we can rest assured that they were developed during the life history of the organism. We can likewise be certain that if an organism performs reactions without a prior history (as in the moth and loggerhead turtle), the activity will not show the customary characteristics of behavioral events. Rather it will belong to the tropistic or physiological class of events. If behavioral, then history; if no history, then physiological.

3

THE REACTIONAL BIOGRAPHY:

THE PSYCHOLOGICAL LIFE HISTORY OF ORGANISMS

I. INTRODUCTION
N. H. Pronko

Old-fashioned psychology had a ready explanation for behaviors by conveniently calling them instincts. Thus, there were religious instincts, antisocial instincts, instinctive attitudes, and so forth. In the twentieth century, such pseudoscientific explanations have been gradually discarded because psychologists generally have recognized the importance of the life history or reactional biography of the individual. This chapter calls attention to the manner in which behavior does or does not become acquired, depending upon the circumstances surrounding the particular organism, and also the role of maturation in understanding how organisms act as they do.

According to the concept of the reactional biography, all behavioral happenings have a zero point somewhere in the life history of the animal. For every individual, there was a stage in his life span when he did not yet perform the acts which he now performs. No one talks or reads, operates automobiles or airplanes, or plays instruments at birth. As a matter of fact, this is the zero point as far as the development of all these activities is concerned. The individual will remain in this zero point for a long time. When he has managed to say his first word, then he has left behind the zero point of his language reactions and is launched on a definite program of behavioral acquisition. Conversely, if we could have a complete motion-picture recording of an individual's behavioral performances and could run it backward, we would see that person performing many complex responses at the beginning of the film. As we ran it through, simpler stages of those same acts would be observed until we would reach stages of his life history when those acts were not performed at all. In the case of many sorts of actions, such as walking, talking, or solving arithmetic problems, the zero points are easily observable. The zero point for all behaviors is, however, less readily fixed. That it may, in some instances, be located in the fetal-life period is apparent, however, from the study here included on conditioning of the fetus *in utero*. It will be evident that the organism is sufficiently complete sometime before birth to engage in simple psychological reactions if it comes into contact with appropriate stimuli. Behaviors do not, however, "automatically" evolve at any time prior to or following birth, as the following selections demonstrate.

II. REACTIONAL BIOGRAPHY AND MATURATION
J. W. Bowles, Jr.

Maturation has been a troublesome problem in psychology. Some investigators have dispensed with it entirely; others employ it as an explanatory tool. The following discussion is aimed at helping the student reach some conclusion of his own on this point.

A vigorous inspection of biological happenings reveals no set of data warranting the special label "maturation" outside of the subject matter of embryology. Embryology is the science which studies "biological histories" or "organisms" in their progressive elaboration from the unicellular stage at fertilization to developmental completeness and eventual deterioration. Notice that such development does not cease at birth; this is only a temporal phase or nodal point in the history known as an "organism." Maturation, then, is coincident with the subject matter of embryology, although typically more attention is paid to pre- than to postnatal development. This does not indicate that there are different subject matters here, but only that development is less dramatic following birth.

The next question is, "How does the developing organism relate to behavioral phenomena?" Is there evidence that any behaviors simply "mature" or come into being without a history of organism-object contacts? Can such actions as walking, trotting, running, dancing, and climbing; talking, singing, choral reading, shouting, and chanting; fearing dogs, snakes, mice, failure, evil, and the unknown be adequately described as the maturing of some structure-function mechanism? We think not. Notice that in the human even such reflex actions as sex responses cannot be treated as the maturation and operation of the reproductive apparatus. Although fertility and conception must wait upon biological development, human sex happenings cannot be understood except in terms of the details of the reactional biography. Sex responses may occur at any time following birth, and they become attached to a multitude of stimuli, but if they do, we may be certain that such reactions developed and did not simply "mature."

Biological structures and physiological functions are best regarded as necessary factors in the more complex organism-object interactions. And, certainly, undeveloped organisms are handicapped or prevented from entering into organized and complex interactions with things. This by no means ensures that complete development of structures determines that behaviors necessarily will occur. The distinction between "possibilities for behaviors" and "determiners of behaviors" is clearly seen in the case of Isabelle, who did not learn to speak until after 6½ years of age, Anna, who was deprived of complex behavioral development by virtue of living in isolation in an attic for the first several years of her life, the chimpanzees reared in darkness, and the children who walk on all fours. Yet, all these organisms had mature structures.

It is asserted that behaviors do not "come into being" through maturation. The progressive development of the animal's structures work so as to permit more complex adjustments, but, without the reactional history, without the series of contacts between the organism and objects, behavioral events do not evolve. Consider Metfessel's [1] study of singing in roller canaries. Species songs did not "mature." Birds kept in soundproof cages did not develop the species song, but they did modify their singing in the direction of whatever tones were introduced into their cages. Thus, singing was not inherited. Instead, the life history of these birds determined the specific way in which they came to sing.

---

[1] METFESSEL, M. Relationships in heredity and environment in behavior. *J. Psychol.*, 1940, 10, 177–198.

Experimental, field, and clinical observations clearly show the relationship between behavior and development. If the organism is not sufficiently complete biologically, he is prevented from behaving in certain ways. On the other hand, neither do behavioral events occur if the stimulus objects are missing. For example, most infants are not developed sufficiently before the age of 1 year to engage in walking actions. But, infants may be well beyond the stage of development necessary for walking and still go about on all fours or hands and knees until parents force them to assume upright postures. In most cases creeping behaviors are possible by a chronological age of 6 to 8 months, but some infants never creep because of lack of stimulation. They may be denied opportunities or confined to a play pen. Quite young children, i.e., under 3 years of age, are sufficiently developed biologically to permit precisely coordinated manual activities, as illustrated by handling hammers, screw drivers, pliers or wrenches, but individual differences in such performances are extremely great. In fact, some adults, lacking the necessary reactional biography, are less effective in manipulating such objects than are some preschool children.

Our own conclusion on the question of maturation may be put thus: It is obvious that organisms, even after birth, are not completely developed. Until certain stages of structural development are reached, a particular organism cannot begin a series of contacts with stimulus objects which will enable it to acquire reactions to such objects. However, the mere presence of vocal structures will not dispose an organism to speak, and, undoubtedly, there are humans with sexual structures who do not necessarily perform sexual behavior. Something more is needed—opportunities to develop such behavior. For that reason, it is doubtful if behavior ever simply unfolds or matures, although not all psychologists agree.

III. THE CONDITIONING OF THE HUMAN FETUS *IN UTERO*

N. H. Pronko

While newly born and even "premature" human infants show behavioral development soon after birth, psychologists have been interested in the possibility of demonstrating behavioral modification in the human fetus. Recently, Spelt [2] was able to show experimentally that human infants can "learn" even while they are in the uterus. The essential condition is a definite interaction with stimulus objects. This does not mean, of course, that infants come into the world with a large repertoire of behavioral acts. The extremes to which Spelt went to contrive the situation described here indicate what an impoverished behavioral circumstance the uterus must be. Obviously, there are no toys, buses, streetcars, sisters, and parents, but a rather quiet, dark, and uniform set of conditions which do not easily stimulate acquisition of behavior. This study is important in showing that, at a certain time prior to birth, the human infant is sufficiently complete (mature) as a biological organism to permit it to participate in events of a behavioral order.

APPARATUS. Essentially, Spelt's setup was a conditioning apparatus. The unconditioned stimulus was an oak clapper 5 inches wide, $22\frac{1}{2}$ inches long, and 1 inch thick, which was released through an arc of 85 degrees so as to strike the face of the box sharply, thus producing a loud noise, and simultaneously closing a circuit through a dry cell and signal marker, which was recorded on the kymogram.

The conditioned stimulus was furnished by means of a doorbell, the gong of which had been removed and the striker so adjusted as to strike perpendicularly to the surface of any part of the abdomen. The instance of application of the conditioned stimulus was also recorded on the smoked paper.

Three pairs of tambours with thin rubber diaphragms were fastened next to the mother's abdomen. A kick of the fetus would thus depress the rubber diaphragm and increase the pressure of

---

2 SPELT, D. K. The conditioning of the human fetus *in utero*. *J. exp. Psychol.*, 1948, **38**, 338–346. (Reproduced by permission of the author and the American Psychological Association.)

the air column of the rubber tube joined to it. At the other end of the tube, there was another diaphragm with a writing pen resting on its surface, so adjusted as to record upon the glazed paper the changes in the air column resulting from any fetal kick as indicated in the drawing. A push button in the mother's hand was wired so as to record the instant she could feel a kick of the fetal infant. A breathing record of the mother was also secured. A time line was recorded simultaneously with the rest. A screen hid the experimenter and apparatus from the mother.

SUBJECTS AND PROCEDURE. Except for one pregnant and three nonpregnant control subjects, the sixteen experimental subjects were all patients of an obstetric clinic of an urban hospital. All but two were past the seventh month of pregnancy. They were not informed that they were to participate in an experiment, but were simply told that certain observations would be made of fetal movements, providing that they were willing. The only incentive was guarantee of free care in the obstetric ward when patients came to term.

In the experimental sessions, the subjects were prepared in the manner indicated above. X-ray data, external manual examination, and fetal heart sounds were used to locate the position of the fetus. One pair of receiving tambours was then taped to the abdomen over the fetal head, another over the fetal arms, and the third over the fetal legs. The apparatus was then set in operation.

RESULTS. In Group I, three subjects were given from 8 to 16 successive unconditioned stimuli alone (loud noise) followed by 3 to 10 successive conditioned stimuli alone to show that the former elicited fetal response and the latter, not. The doorbell vibrator never elicited the response from the fetus, but the clapper regularly did so. It should be noted that since the mothers were warned of the noise of the clapper, very few were startled even on the first day. The conditioning series was arranged so that the vibratory stimulus (CS) operated for 5 seconds, terminated by the loud noise (US).

One fetus gave evidence of a conditioned response by the eighth session (8 to 16 trials constituting one session). Subject No. 16 showed the first fetal response to the CS (buzzer) *without* the

FIG. 4   Sketch of apparatus arrangement for fetal conditioning study. (Spelt, D. K., The conditioning of the human fetus.)

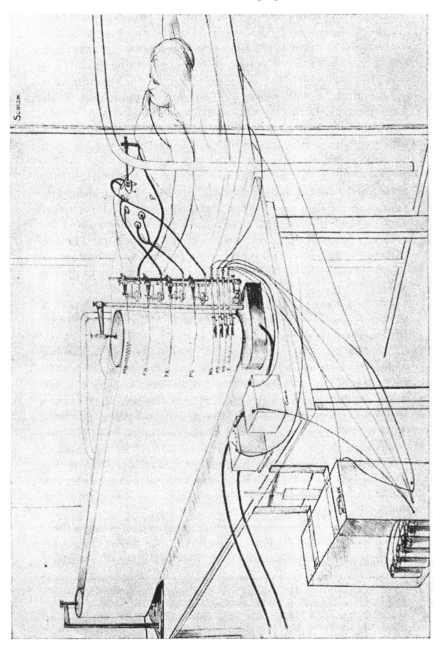

FIG. 4

accompanying loud noise (US) after only 21 paired presentations. In the sixth session, 7 CR's occurred in succession after 59 reinforced presentations of the vibratory stimulus. On the next morning, 4 more CR's were recorded without any reinforcement. Another subject showed presence of a fetal conditional response in the seventh session after 21 paired stimulations. At the beginning of the ninth session, 2 CR's appeared, but when 4 successive conditioned stimuli no longer gave any response (extinction), the session was terminated in order to test for spontaneous recovery. After a 24-hour rest, the subject was given a series of conditioned stimuli alone. Out of a total of 11 trials, there were 6 clean-cut CR's, and on 2 other trials the mother pressed the button to indicate that she felt kicks, although no direct record of a fetal kick was obtained. The subject then left the hospital and returned again so that work was resumed 3 weeks later. The conditioned stimulus was presented alone 12 times in succession and elicited 7 responses in the first 9 trials, being ineffective in the last 3 trials.

There is evidence here that despite the short training period, the conditioned response was stable enough to survive a considerably lengthy time interval.

GROUP II. The subjects of this group were all in the late eighth or ninth month of pregnancy and were given a series of 4 to 7 trials of the vibratory stimulus (CS) alone in order to determine whether this stimulus by itself was effective in eliciting a fetal response, especially as the fetus approached greater maturity. This control showed that none of the vibratory stimuli (unaccompanied by the loud noise) operated to elicit a fetal response.

GROUP III. Three nonpregnant subjects also served as controls to show that the two stimuli in various arrangements and combinations produced no records remotely resembling those that demonstrated fetal conditioning.

GROUP IV. The two pregnant subjects of this group showed that the response of the fetus to the loud noise does not occur before the eighth month, indicating that this stage of biological

FIG. 5   Sample kymograph records from fetal conditioning study. A, showing response to both stimuli, and B, showing response to CS, obtained from the same S. C is a record from a non-pregnant control S. D shows result of applying CS alone in late pregnancy without previous conditioning trials. (Spelt, D. K., The conditioning of the human fetus.)

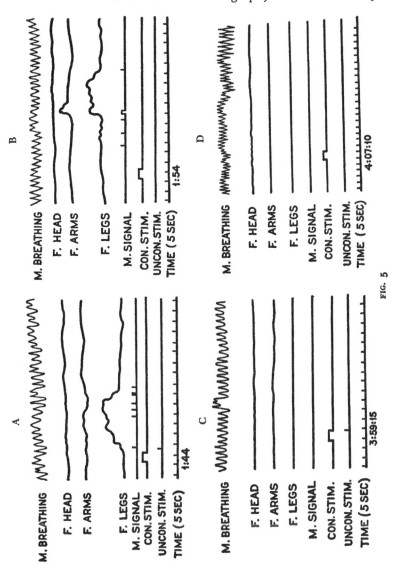

FIG. 5

maturity must be reached before the organism can interact with such stimulus objects.

CONCLUSION. By use of a vibratory-tactile stimulus as a conditioned stimulus and a loud noise as an unconditioned stimulus, Spelt was able to establish a CR (conditioned response) in the human fetus while it is in the uterus during the last 2 months prior to birth. After as few as 15 to 20 paired presentations, it was possible to establish the response to the point where one could expect a series of 3 or 4 successive responses to the (CS) vibratory stimulus alone, but additional practice would give as many as 11 successive CR's. Experimental extinction, spontaneous recovery, and retention of the conditioned response over a 3-week interval show that a more stable response either to the kind of stimuli employed here or to other appropriate stimuli is only a function of proper experimental conditions. These features and the fact that the reactions studied here showed modifiability as a result of changing historical conditions place these fetal reactions very definitely with the class of conditioned responses.

IV. EXTREME SOCIAL ISOLATION OF A CHILD

Certain kinds of behavioral acquisition can be prevented effectively by keeping the organisms from getting into contact with stimulus objects. Organism-object interbehavior cannot occur if the organism is not given opportunities for contacts with the various objects, situations, and happenings that constitute his surroundings. When this psychological and physical deprivation is extreme, behavioral evolution is severely limited, as is revealed in Davis'[3] study of extreme isolation in the case of "Anna."

Anna, from the age of less than 1 year, was confined for approximately 5 years in one room. The child was resented by her mother and received almost no attention during this time. She was fed milk, and eventually thin oatmeal, but had never learned to eat solid food. As her undernourished condition became severe, she became apathetic and was left reclining in a chair. Here she was ignored except for feeding. Her contacts with others were limited to this feeding by the mother and occasional mistreat-

---

[3] DAVIS, K. Extreme social isolation of a child. *Amer. J. Sociol.*, 1940, **45**, 554–565. (Reproduced by permission of the author and the publisher.)

ment by an older brother. Both children were illegitimate. The mother resided with her father and other relatives. The father objected to even seeing the second child, hence Anna was kept in an out-of-the-way room. The following quotations from the Davis study reveal marked improvement in behavioral equipment as Anna is provided with increased opportunities for contacts with stimuli.

By the time we arrived on the scene, February 7, Anna had been in her new abode, the county home, for only three days. But she was already beginning to change. When first brought to the county home, she had been completely apathetic—had lain in a limp, supine position, immobile, expressionless, indifferent to everything. Her flaccid feet had fallen forward, making almost a straight line with the skeleton-like legs, indicating that the child had long lain on her back to the point of exhaustion and atrophy of her foot muscles. She was believed to be deaf and possibly blind. Her urine, according to the nurse, had been extremely concentrated and her stomach exceedingly bloated. It was thought that she had suffered at one time from rickets, though later medical opinion changed the diagnosis to simple malnutrition. Her blood count had been very low in haemoglobin. No sign of disease had been discovered.

Since Anna turned her head slowly toward a loud-ticking clock held near her, we concluded that she could hear. Other attempts to make her notice sounds, such as clapping hands or speaking to her, elicited no response, yet when the door was opened suddenly, she tended to look in that direction. Her feet were sensitive to touch. She exhibited the plantar, patellar, and pupillary reflexes. When sitting up, she jounced rhythmically up and down on the bed—a recent habit of which she was very fond. Though her eyes surveyed the room, especially the ceiling, it was difficult to tell if she was looking at anything in particular. She neither smiled nor cried in our presence, and the only sound she made—a slight sucking intake of breath with the lips—occurred rarely. She did frown or scowl occasionally in response to no observable stimulus; otherwise, she remained expressionless.

Next morning the child seemed more alert. She liked food and lay on her back to take it. She could not chew or drink from a cup, but had to be fed from a bottle or spoon—this in spite of the fact that she could grasp and manipulate objects with her hands. Toward numerous toys given her by well-wishers all over the country, she showed no reaction. They were simply objects to be handled in a distracted manner; there was no element of play. She liked to have her hair combed. When physically restrained, she exhibited considerable temper. She did not smile except when coaxed and did not cry . . . [pp. 555–556].

On a subsequent examination, 10 days later, some broadening of behavioral equipment was apparent. She was more alert to objects and to changes in conditions about her. She would attend to these longer, showed more varied facial responses, and handled herself better generally. "The doctor claimed that she had a new trick every day." On the 2-year-level Stanford-Binet test items, she showed only very limited responsiveness. Six months after the first visit, she showed further improvement physically, was beginning to make vocal noises, and would make walking movements if held. Her responsiveness to other persons increased and was more definite and discriminating.

Until removed from the county home on November 11, there were few additional changes. By this time she could barely stand while holding to something. When put on a carpet she could scoot, but not crawl. She visibly liked people, as manifested by smiling, rough-housing, and hair-pulling. But she still was an unsocialized individual, for she had learned practically nothing.

If we ask why she had learned so little—not even to chew or drink from a glass—in nine months, the answer probably lies in the long previous isolation and in the conditions at the county home. At the latter institution, she was early deprived of her two little roommates and was left alone. In the entire establishment there was only one nurse, who had three hundred and twenty-four other inmates to look after. Most of Anna's care was turned over to adult inmates, many of whom were mentally deficient and scarcely able to speak themselves. Part of the time Anna's door was shut. In addition to this continued isolation, Anna was given no stimulus to learning. She was fed, clothed, and cleaned without having to turn a hand in her own behalf. She was never disciplined or rewarded, because nobody had the time for the tedious task. All benefits were for her in the nature of things and therefore not rewards. Thus she remained in much the same animal-like stage, except that she did not have the animal's inherently organized structure, and hence remained in a more passive, inadequate state.

On our visit of December 6, a surprise awaited us, for Anna had undergone what was for her a remarkable transformation—she had begun to learn. Not that she could speak, but she could do several things formerly considered impossible. She could descend the stairs (by sitting successively on each one), could hold a doughnut in her hand and eat it (munching like a normal child), could grasp a glass of tomato juice and drink it by herself, could take a step or two while holding to something, and could feed herself with a spoon. These accomplishments, small indeed for a child of seven, represented a transformation explainable, no doubt, by her transference from the county home to a private family where she was the sole object of one woman's assiduous care . . . [pp. 559–561].

Still later, on March 19, 1939, her accomplishments were the following: she was able to walk alone for a few steps without falling; she was responsive to verbal commands of her foster-mother, seeming to understand in a vague sort of way what the latter wanted her to do; she definitely recognized the social worker who took her weekly to the doctor and who therefore symbolized to her the pleasure of an automobile ride; she expressed by anxious bodily movements her desire to go out for a ride; she seemed unmistakably to seek and to like attention, though she did not sulk when left alone; she was able to push a doll carriage in front of her and to show some skill in manipulating it. She was, furthermore, much improved physically, being almost fat, with chubby arms and legs and having more energy and alertness. On the visit prior to this one, she had shown that she could quickly find and eat candy which she saw placed behind a pillow, could perform a knee-bending exercise, could use ordinary utensils in eating (e.g., could convey liquid to her mouth in a spoon), could manifest a sense of neatness (by putting bread back on a plate after taking a bite from it).

On August 30, 1939, Anna was taken from the foster-home and moved to a small school for defective children. Observations made at this time showed her to have become a fat girl twenty pounds overweight for her age. Yet she could walk better and could almost run. Her toilet habits showed that she understood the whole procedure. She manifested an obvious comprehension of many verbal instructions, though she could not speak . . . [pp. 561–562].

This study is important in demonstrating what devastating effects early and extreme behavioral deprivation may have if continued for a period of years. Nevertheless, once opportunity for development was provided, acquisition of behavior went forward. Obviously, we would not expect the same rate of development in Anna, confined in a room for 5 years, as in other children who had a 5-year lead building a rich basis for subsequent behavior.

V. THE CASE OF ISABELLE [4]

Isabelle came to the attention of the authorities at the age of 6½ years—the illegitimate child of a mother who, as the result of injury to her eye and ears, had been apparently deaf since infancy, and so had failed to learn to talk, read, or write. The mother was completely uneducated and could communicate with the family only by means of crude gestures of her own invention.

During the mother's pregnancy and for 6½ years after Isabelle's birth, the mute mother and the child were kept locked in a room with drawn shades. Lack of hygienic conditions resulted in Isabelle's developing a serious rachitic condition which eventually justified her removal to a hospital for treatment.

It was here that she came in contact with Dr. Marie Mason of the Ohio State University Speech Clinic, who won the child's confidence. At first, Isabelle lacked both speech and language comprehension, so that administration of an intelligence test was quite futile. From here on the story is told in Dr. Mason's own words.

The general impression was that she was wholly uneducable and that any attempt to teach her to speak, after so long a period of silence, would meet with failure. In spite of this, I decided to make the attempt on my own assumption that Isabelle's failure to speak was due to the six and a half years of isolation with a mute and deaf mother; that, in spite of her hearing acuity, she had either heard speech not at all or at such distance and with such indistinctness as to have established no auditory impressions of speech or language forms.

The first important problem to confront me in my endeavor to teach Isabelle to speak was the choice of some satisfactory method of procedure. Gesture was her only mode of expression. In her characteristic descriptive motions with which she tried to make clear what she wanted, I noted a similarity to the sign language used by deaf children. She seemed to have had no acquaintance with simple childhood toys. She was apparently utterly unaware of relationships of any kind. When presented with a ball for the first time, she held it in the palm of her hand, then reached out and stroked my face with it. Such behavior is comparable to that of a child of

[4] MASON, MARIE K. Learning to speak after six and one half years of silence. *J. Speech Disorders,* 1942, 7, 295–304. (Reproduced by permission of the author and the publisher.)

six months. She made no attempt to squeeze it, throw it, or to bounce it. These observations prompted me, therefore, to adopt an educational approach combining gesture, facial expression, pantomime, dramatization, and imitation.

Isabelle made her first attempt at vocalization one week after my first visit to her. I sat with her at a small table on which I had placed a ball, a toy automobile, a horn, and a bell. She seemed interested in each object as I presented it, but their spoken symbols seemed to make no impression on her. In the form of play, I held up the ball and said, "Ball," close to her ear. This seemed a pleasurable sensation, but she gave no response other than a smile. Repeating the performance and again saying, "Ball," I placed my ear close to her mouth and in pantomime indicated that I wished her to make a vocal response, whereupon she gleefully said, "Buh" (ba), . . . Her joy in successful performance was similar to that of a baby whose first "coo" elicits his parents' surprise and approval. My praise of her attempt immediately prompted her to say "Ah," in response to my word, "Car." Thus, Isabelle's first imitative utterances were made. While apparently proud of her first vocal sounds, Isabelle seemed disinclined to repeat the attempt on the following day, and it was only after many repetitions that these two words were correctly spoken and became for her the verbal symbols of the objects represented.

Thus began my laborious task of devising resources to assist her in establishing relationships between symbolization and concrete objects. Independent word concepts were introduced at first, and Isabelle was taught to make individual oral responses. The habit of silence was so ingrained that the mere fact that she could speak a word was not a sufficient stimulus to motivate its spontaneous and automatic reproduction.

Simultaneous with her attainment of independent word concepts, phrases, and short sentences were used in addressing her, but with no expectation of demanding that she reproduce them. Nouns were naturally the first concepts introduced. Verbs were represented in the form of action and dramatization. This was limited to certain activities because of her difficulty in walking as a result of the bowed leg condition and also to the post-operative cast on both legs which held her bedfast from December 13, 1938 until March 13, 1939.

Isabelle's first language concepts were developed exclusively through experience with actual objects. Whenever this was impossible, brightly colored pictures, sketches, and diagrams of various types were utilized. Action games, such as throwing a ball, holding up an object as its name was spoken, were begun as early as November 26, 1938, and similar games involving more complicated dramatic action grew out of these as Isabelle's vocabulary increased. By December, 1939, Isabelle participated in the dramatization of many of the nursery rhymes and children's songs involving both the spoken word and pantomimic or imitative action. Music was first introduced on December 5, 1938. Hoping to encourage her to use newly acquired word concepts, I used them in little home-made songs for which I improvised piano accompaniment. Victrola records were next introduced, and Isabelle was taught to clap her hands to the music. On February 4, 1939, she had her first experience in beating the rhythmic tempo of a musical selection, using percussion instruments, such as tambourines, bells, triangles, drums, etc. Soon after March 13, 1939, when the removal of the plaster casts allowed free motor leg and foot activities, skipping, hopping, marching, and dancing were performed to music, in order to develop in Isabelle a rhythmic response to motor stimuli in preparation for stress and accent in speech and for continuity of articulation and modulation in phonation. Isabelle's love of music was further fostered by teaching her to play some simple melodies.

Other educative materials such as those used in pre-school classes, kindergarten and first grade, were utilized in order to build up Isabelle's speech vocabulary and to prepare her for future reading, writing, and numerical accomplishment. Attractive pictures to be colored, cut out, and the printed name pasted under it were used as early as March 9, 1939. The use of a clock, calendars, and geographical maps gave Isabelle an idea of temporal and spatial relations.

Isabelle's acquisition of speech seemed to pass through successive developmental changes. While it is true that her earliest vocal utterances at the age of six and a half were those of a child of a year and a half or two years, it is also true that she passed through each successive stage more rapidly. . . .

Summarizing the twenty-two months of Isabelle's speech and linguistic development, we find that she has progressed from her first spoken word to full length sentences, intelligent questioning, recitation of nursery rhymes, story-telling, and songs. She has a reading readiness vocabulary of words and sentences; she counts to a hundred; identifies coins; recognizes their numerical values; and performs arithmetical computations to ten. She has a well-defined sense of form in manuscript writing and evidences taste and discrimination in crayon work and painting.

She is aggressive, often to the point of stubbornness; under certain conditions she shows extreme negativism. She has an excellent sense of humor and is an inveterate tease; she is given to temporization which she utilizes to delay an undesirable task, to divert attention from her mistakes or lack of knowledge, or to enjoy in others the exasperation which her actions provoke. She is highly imaginative and has an acute sense of the dramatic. She is very affectionate and lovable. Her first unsocial behavior which betrayed itself in antagonistic and often animalistic reaction, in the richness of her newly-acquired experiences, has changed to one capable of making adjustments in social situations.

Here is a little girl now eight years old, who, in a period of less than two years, has made striking social adjustments to a living and hearing world after six years in a world of silence, fear, and isolation; a child, who can communicate with others in speech after six and a half years of primitive gesturing to a mute and deaf mother; a child who at six and a half years, bearing the semblance of a mental defective, after two years of changed environment, enriched experience, unremitting instruction, improved physical condition and appearance, is at eight years considered a child of normal intelligence.

The factors of major importance which have been instrumental in effecting this change are: medical therapy, administered by the orthopedic surgeon, Dr. Harlan Wilson, and the staff of physicians and nurses of Children's Hospital; enriched environment which, under the capable hands of Miss Eva Jansen, Superintendent of the Hospital, and her corps of attendants, unfolded to this child a new world of joyous and fruitful living, social adjustments to changed conditions, and a new experience in community life; education, directed by the author with the assistance of a group of fifteen student teachers in training.

The long route by which this goal has been reached and the arduous task of selecting the proper educational techniques to bring about this change, together with the infinite patience and perseverance in overcoming the many obstacles which impeded the progress, have been but briefly suggested in this short article. A future and complete report could draw upon the wealth of data accumulated during this two-year educative period.

Speech has come to Isabelle. To what extent, if any, will her future adjustments in a speaking world be jeopardized by the years of isolation which delayed her acquisition of speech and language concepts? Who can say [pp. 299–304]?

We wish to stress one point in the case of Isabelle. Singing, reciting poems, and talking did not "mature" during her 6½ years of silence. Her structures were ready for use in such ways, but until a definite set of conditions was brought about for developing such reactions, they did not occur. Organs are not enough. Factors of the reactional biography are indispensable to acquisition of behavior.

VI. FACTORS INFLUENCING SEXUAL BEHAVIOR IN THE HUMAN ORGANISM

In the initial report of their extensive interview study of sexual activity in humans, Kinsey, Pomeroy, and Martin [5] present statistically treated case-history data on 5,300 white males. A variety of factors was found to influence sexual activity. Perhaps as clear as any other finding is the fact that sexual behavior cannot be understood clearly apart from the influence of a variety of nonorganic variables. Among these factors, each of which was found to have a greater or lesser influence upon actual frequency and manner of sexual activity, were the following: race and cultural grouping, marital status, educational level, occupational class, occupation of parent, rural-urban background, religious affiliation, degree of religious adherence, and geographical origin.

The sexual behavior of the human animal is the outcome of its morphologic and physiologic organization, of the conditioning which its experience has brought it, and of all the forces which exist in its living and non-living environment. In terms of academic disciplines, there are biologic, psychologic, and sociologic factors involved; but all of these operate simultaneously, and the end product is a single, unified, phenomenon which is not merely biologic, psychologic, or sociologic in nature. Nevertheless, the importance of each group of factors can never be ignored.

Without its physical body and its physiologic capacities, there would be no animal to act. The individual's sexual behavior is, to a degree, predestined by its morphologic structure, its metabolic capacities, its hormones, and all of the other characters which it has inherited or which have been built into it by the physical environment in which it has de-

---

[5] KINSEY, A. C., POMEROY, W. B., & MARTIN, C. E. *Sexual behavior in the human male.* Philadelphia: Saunders, 1948. Pp. 804. (Reproduced by permission of the authors and the publisher.)

veloped. Two of the most important of these distinctively biologic forces, age and the age at onset of adolescence, have been examined in the earlier chapters of the present volume.

But through all of the previous chapters, constant consideration has been given to the significance of the psychologic factors which affect sexual behavior, and it should be apparent by now that the experience, the conformance or non-conformance of that experience, with the individual's personality, attitudes, and rational thinking, and a great variety of other factors make the psychologic bases of behavior even more important than the biologic heritage and acquirements.

It is evident, however, that psychologic processes depend, to a considerable degree, upon the way in which external forces impinge upon the animal. For a creature with as highly organized a central nervous system as is found in the human animal, the most important external force is the social environment in which it lives. In the human species, the environment consists of one's family, his close friends, his neighbors, his business associates, and his mere acquaintances. It also includes the thousands of other persons whom he has never seen but whose attitudes, habits, expressed opinion, and overt activities constitute the culture in which he moves and lives. These are the social forces which contribute to the individual's behavior. There is, of course, no part of the individual himself which is social in nature, in quite the way that morphologic, physiologic, or psychologic capacities may be identified and localized in an organism. Occasionally social forces provide physical restraints on individuals, or facilitate their physical activities; but more often they operate only as they affect the individual psychologically . . . [pp. 327–328].

VII. AN EXPERIMENT TO COMPARE THE RE-ACTIONAL DEVELOPMENT OF AN APE AND A CHILD
N. H. Pronko

Because their subjects are human beings, psychologists are not so free to experiment as are other scientists. Otherwise, the hypothesis of the reactional biography could be very easily put to experimental test. One could then take a human infant at birth, rear it under conditions of almost absolute lack of stimulation, and demonstrate the resulting product as an idiot. Better still, one could take identical twins, rear one to be a genius, and keep the other at a near zero level of behavioral development. But such an experiment would be scandalous and inhuman, and, therefore, impossible. The answer must come from elsewhere.

Kellogg [6] decided to ask the question contrariwise. Instead of attempting to find out what the result would be if a human animal were reared under nonhuman conditions, he decided to take an infrahuman animal and rear it under the same human circumstances as those surrounding a typical human infant.

Of course, there have been observations of "cupboard children" and "feral children" reported elsewhere in this book which do throw light on this subject, but only as "nature's experiments" and not as planned investigations.

As one of his subjects, Kellogg selected a young female chimpanzee named Gua from the colony of the Anthropoid Experiment Station of Yale University at Orange Park, Florida. The animal was separated from her mother at the age of 7½ months and taken into the Kellogg home to be reared with the other subject, their own son, Donald, who was then 10 months of age. Ideally, the chimp should have been separated from her mother at birth and brought together with the human child, also at the point of birth, but such conditions are difficult to arrange. Under the circumstances, each of the subjects had a considerable reactional biography prior to the beginning of the experiment.

At any rate, the two subjects lived together under the same roof as companions and playmates for a period of 9 months. During this period their surroundings and treatment were as nearly alike as it was humanly possible to make them. This means that for no part of the day or night was the chimp caged or treated as a zoo animal. Both subjects were petted, scolded, and corrected as children in families have been down through the ages. Nor were they drilled as animal trainers "train" their subjects to perform a certain routine. On the contrary, behavioral opportunities for both were casual or "natural," such as might exist for brother and sister in a normal family even to the point where each had his own crib, high chair, walking chair, bib, and the like.

SOME RESULTS OF THE EXPERIMENT. It is obvious that the subjects were members of different species, with differences in anatomic structures, relative proportions, rate of growth, and so

---

[6] KELLOGG, W. N. & KELLOGG, L. A. *The ape and the child.* New York: McGraw-Hill, 1933. Pp. 341. (Reproduced by permission of the author and the publisher.)

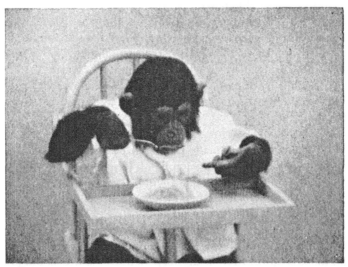

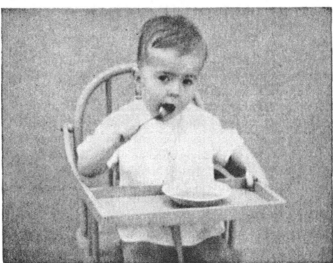

FIG. 6 If one were assigned the task of "teaching an animal to eat with a spoon," this picture shows that it would make little difference whether one selected a human child or a young ape. Both learned to perform this reaction, the ape being considerably in advance in the rate at which she learned to perform this behavior. (Kellogg, W. N., & Kellogg, L. A., *The ape and the child.*)

on. Clearly, such differences permit or prevent acquisition of different behaviors in the two animals. On the other hand, in such cases as walking, even such unfavorable anatomic conditions as existed in the case of the chimp were surmounted, for although Gua found it convenient to use her unusually long arms as "leaners" in her locomotion, she eventually achieved a bipedal form of walking as the result of holding on to the experimenter's trousers during her learning period.

MANUAL COORDINATION. Handedness tests showed that the total number of reaches made by the two subjects was equal for the right as compared with the left hand. In manual dexterity, Gua suffered anatomic disadvantages in that the joints of her fingers and hands prevented the range of movements permitted the human child so that the former often resorted to seizing small objects with her lips. However, in tests of coordinated arm movements, Gua compared favorably with the human subject. In fact, upon the first application of the "cap-on-head" test, Gua did practically everything that Donald did by the time he was 18½ months old, removing the cap in less than 2 seconds with either or both hands.

WALKING AND CLIMBING. In comparison with the child, the chimpanzee, although quite wobbly, was advanced in locomotion from the very start of the experiment. However, she showed such rapid improvement that she could outrun Donald. More important, she learned to stand and walk with more erect posture than that characteristic of chimps whose anatomy causes them to bend forward at the hips to an angle of 30 or 40 degrees and to support themselves by placing their hands on the ground.

As might be predicted from a knowledge of comparative anatomy, the chimpanzee excelled the human subject in developing climbing behavior. Powerful musculature of arms and shoulders facilitated the ape's superior performance. Indeed, with Gua's stimulating example, Donald soon built up climbing behavior superior in quality to that found in children of his own age group. It should be pointed out that, in walking upstairs, the chimp also outstripped Donald, but her most outstanding feat was in chinning herself up to her customary place in the family perambulator in preparation for a ride while Donald stood helplessly by until lifted into his place.

PLAY. Playful activity of a distinctly human sort was just as basic to the ape as to the child, and both played almost continually alone, with each other, or with elders. After a few months of human companionship, the two subjects of the experiment had such an interest in playing together that one of them could not be induced to eat a meal if the other should be playing at the time.

Here are listed other forms of play which Gua built up as the result of her human surroundings and which she could never have built up in the "normal" ape environment of the jungle and zoo.

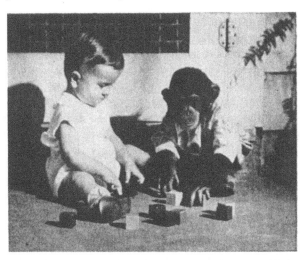

FIG. 7 Both subjects reacted similarly to play with blocks, manipulating, examining, throwing and chewing them. Other more complex forms of cooperative play behavior were also acquired by the subjects during the course of the experiment. (Kellogg, W. N., & Kellogg, L. A., *The ape and the child.*)

1. Dropping objects from the high chair to the floor in the traditional manner of human babies.
2. Playing with her feet and examining them while lying on her back or swinging or kicking them against the rungs of a chair while sitting in it.
3. Draping or wrapping herself in various articles of clothing and trailing them behind her.
4. Hanging from doors as she pushed them to and fro or rocking in a rocking chair or baby rocker.
5. Pushing the perambulator or walker back and forth.
6. Making marks in the fogged portion of windows upon which the moisture of her breath had condensed.

7. Picking up sand and letting it run through her fingers, wiping off what might adhere to her palm with the tips of the fingers of the opposite hand. Digging holes in the sand.

8. Playing a game resembling tag in which she would seize some plaything of Donald's, running ahead of him far enough to invite him to pursue her.

9. Developing a social form of peekaboo.

10. Cooperating with Donald in a game of ball by rolling it back and forth.

11. Imitating Donald as when the latter would drum on a radio bench to produce a noise, or opening and closing cabinet doors, or "brushing" her hair with a hairbrush.

SOCIAL AND AFFECTIONATE BEHAVIOR.   The early and intimate contact of the ape and the child might be expected to provide opportunities for development of affectionate reactions between them. As a matter of fact, in this respect, the situation was not different from that of most human families. Even after only 3 months' residence together, Donald would often cry when Gua screamed. Later, if Gua were required to stay in her chair as punishment, Donald came to her, reached up, and embraced her, while Gua would put her head on his shoulder and hug him with one or both hands.

Later, Donald would go to Gua as soon as he was dressed in the morning and hug her. On her part, Gua soon adopted a protective attitude toward her human companion, especially if they were out of doors. If he cried while being carried by someone, she would attack the latter. When Donald and she walked together, they constantly held each other's hand.

With other children, Gua was somewhat reserved, although she entered freely into social intercourse with a little girl of 3½ years, sitting with her, holding hands, and engaging in other play even upon first acquaintance. Toward older and bigger children who pointed at her and giggled, she became hostile and would pour out doglike barks at them, often slapping them on the shins. Adults had a difficult time being accepted, except, of course the experimenters. She developed an extreme emotional dependence toward the male experimenter, running to him in every emergency, and was quite uncomfortable out of his sight.

LEARNING.   Under the casual learning opportunities provided in the home, the chimp learned a considerable repertoire

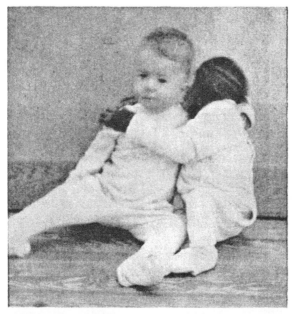

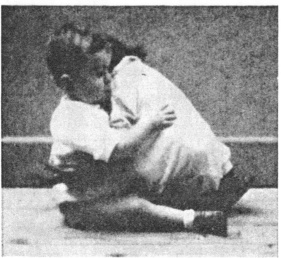

FIG. 8 Shown here are the common affectionate responses built up mutually by the two subjects of the experiment. When Gua was punished, Donald would run up and hug her and she would do likewise. Gua even adopted a protective attitude toward her human companion attacking anyone threatening him. (Kellogg, W. N., & Kellogg, L. A., *The ape and the child.*)

anlike reactions. Among other things, she learned to wear (see Fig. 10 for bladder-training curve) and shoes and oc-lly a romper suit. She soon mastered the operation of a swinging door and could unlatch other doors as well as manipulate light switches. Both subjects learned to use implements, and although many human children cannot eat with a spoon before the

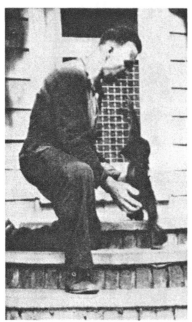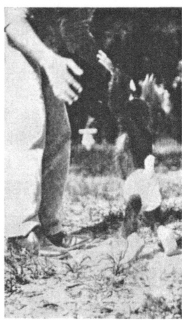

FIG. 9 Emotional dependence and a "need" for security are indicated here. The picture on the left was taken two days after Gua's separation from her mother, the other one week later. The ape showed a great "emotional dependence" upon the experimenter and ran into his arms when there was any sort of trouble. (Kellogg, W. N., & Kellogg, L. A., *The ape and the child.*)

eighteenth month (even with some spilling of food) Gua had made considerable progress before the thirteenth month, and was eating alone and quite well some weeks later. In this respect, she showed superior performance over Donald.

INTELLIGENT BEHAVIOR. As one basis for comparison of the two subjects in their more complex behavioral acquisitions, they were administered a form of intelligence test known as the Gesell Tests for Preschool Children. The graph shows the number of test items passed by both subjects during the series of monthly testings. In general, where one might excel, the other fell down, and vice versa. Where Gua lacked human structures, as for lifting movements, she was at a serious disadvantage in comparison with Donald. In general, however, the human child surpassed Gua, although the experimenters draw no general conclusion regarding the relative performance of other chimps and humans.

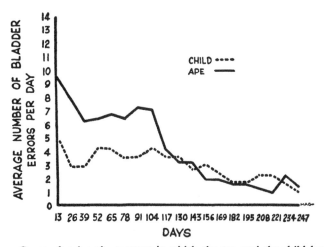

FIG. 10 Curves showing the manner in which the ape and the child learned to inhibit bladder voidings. Progress of training in units of 13 days is shown along the base line while the average number of errors per day is represented along the vertical line. Voiding while subject was not on nursery chair or toilet constituted an error. During the latter half of the period both subjects were about equal in the superiority of their performance, although in the case of the child there were more bed-wetting errors than in Gua's case. (Kellogg, W. N., & Kellogg, L. A., *The ape and the child.*)

LANGUAGE REACTIONS. Although the experiment was not continued for an extended period of time, nevertheless interesting observations were made both of the language usage and comprehension of the subjects. Donald showed superior acquisition of articulate sounds, although Gua did develop vocalizations which conveyed specific meanings.

As for comprehension language, the ape was considerably superior to the child in responding to human words in the first few months. Even in the fifth month, she surpassed Donald with a comprehension vocabulary of 21 words as compared with his score of 20. With a sudden development of locomotion, however, Donald soon took the lead so that the final comprehension score was 107 for Donald and 95 for Gua. Finally, both subjects reacted appropriately to pictures, both in picture books and as intelligence-test items on the Gesell test. One of the intelligence-test performances is to point out objects represented on a card. At 17½ months, Donald reacted appropriately to the command "Show me the bow-wow," but he did not pick out either the shoe or any

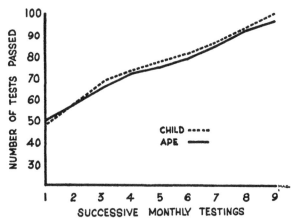

FIG. 11 The relative performance of ape and child on an intelligence test is shown in the total number of items passed on the Gesell Tests for Pre-School Children during each of the nine months of the experimental period. Although the child shows a slight advantage over the ape, nevertheless the latter does give evidence of remarkable progress in intelligence development. (Kellogg, W. N., & Kellogg, L. A., *The ape and the child.*)

other objects. However, at 15 months, Gua correctly pointed out both the dog and the shoe.

IMPLICATIONS OF THE APE AND CHILD EXPERIMENT. In our opinion, the significance of the experiment described above may be put as follows. We start with animals who are members of different species. As such, they do not possess the same structures. Since they are different, we should not expect to rear them so that they are behaviorally alike. It is not possible to make an ape into a human, and vice-versa, i.e., not in every behavioral detail.

The only legitimate question would appear to be: What happens behaviorally to these different animals when they are subjected to similar conditions of reactional biography. One of the

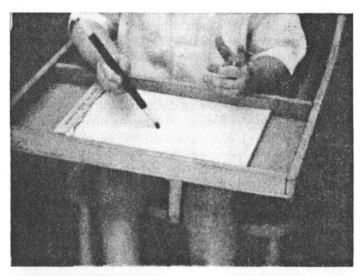

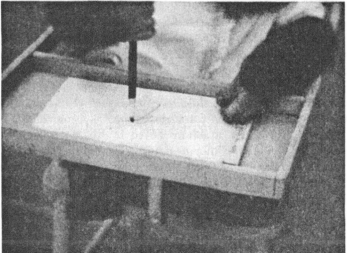

FIG. 12 Both subjects get a "pass" on the Gesell (Intelligence) Test for Pre-School Children which requires a scribble going in two different directions. Note that for scribbling the ape has a distinct disadvantage in its clumsy hand structure, yet surmounts this difficulty. (Kellogg, W. N., & Kellogg, L. A., *The ape and the child.*)

outstanding results points to the behavioral factors of advantage or disadvantage given or withheld by the anatomic make-ups of the two subjects. The ape walks earlier and climbs better than the human, while the latter can seize objects with pincerlike movements of index finger and thumb, hence his superiority on intelligence-test items demanding such movements.

Perhaps more important is the finding that, despite their membership in different species, nevertheless they learn to react similarly when given similar opportunities. Thus, although, zoo or jungle apes do not learn to walk on twos, Gua did because she had human surroundings of the sort that also stimulated Donald to build up such locomotion. Only in the human surroundings under which Gua actually developed could she have learned to play tag, peekaboo, ball, and other cooperative human games. Nor does one find sympathetic and affectionate responses of the sort here described occurring in apes developing in nonhuman circumstances, yet it is correct to say that Gua developed distinctly human "needs" of "security" and "affection." Furthermore, wearing shoes and learning to keep diapers dry are barred to chimps raised in nature, as are eating human food with human utensils. And lastly, Gua would never in the jungle have learned to scribble with a pencil, or to point out objects in pictures when she was referred to them with noises that constitute human language. But, for that matter, would the child have performed all the things he learned to do had he been reared in a jungle environment? This is the most provocative question raised by this experiment. In other words, is not the "human nature" of human animals conferred upon them exclusively by their residence among humans?

4

BIOLOGICAL CHARACTERISTICS

OF THE ORGANISM AND EARLY ACQUISITION OF BEHAVIOR

I. INTRODUCTION
N. H. Pronko

The infant at birth is essentially nothing more than a biological organism. With the exception of possible reflex conditioning in the uterus, behavioral events do not take place prior to birth. This means that behaviors evolve during the course of the postnatal life of the individual. Since that is the case, the period immediately following birth is a time of *transition*. The newborn infant begins to get into contact with the many objects around him, and happenings that have the distinctly psychological characteristics of differentiation, integration, variability, modifiability, delayability, and inhibition develop. That is to say, such action as discriminating milk bottles from rattles and the crib begins to develop soon. Reaching for a milk bottle is attempted first one way, then another, and so on until the act is accomplished. Likes and dislikes develop so that the cod-liver oil, which at first may be poured "down the hatch" with no more difficulty than milk, is later discriminated and rejected. Gradually, toilet habits are evolved that may permit delay and inhibition. By this stage, the infant is well launched on his psychological career, but not without a complex and very gradual evolution. The beginnings of that career are much simpler.

In the absence of behavioral happenings, reflex actions are prominent features of infant activity. Although essentially physiological at birth, these reflexes undergo modification and conditioning, as some of the following selections illustrate. Thus, they eventuate in performances that are distinctly psychological.

Random-movement action also characterizes the new born child and it is from these activities that many complex behaviors evolve by slow degrees. This period is highlighted by the progressive development of discriminations of objects and their qualities, such as sizes, weights, colors, temperatures, tastes, odors, and so on. The materials in this chapter illustrate the development of such fundamental forms of behavior as reflex actions, random movements, and more complex interactions in the earliest portion of the organism's life history.

II. THE ELABORATION OF THE ORGANISM

The infant does not come into being at once. In fact, it is only through a long series of events that the union of the sperm and egg cell culminates in an organism capable of independent existence. It attains this terminal status after approximately 9 months of embryologic evolution during which the egg cell, fertilized at conception, increases in size and complexity. Gradually, structures and functions are elaborated, these are integrated into systems, and the systems themselves are eventually coordinated into a functional unit, the organism. The final upshot is a level of organization permitting ingestion and digestion of food, circulation, respiration, and other activities of living on a relatively independent basis.

A premature birth occurring before this organismic stage has been attained means inability to carry on independent existence and, therefore, death. However, a degree of organization sufficient to ensure a separate existence may be attained even within 28 weeks after conception. It is from an extensive observational and cinematographic study that Dr. Gesell [1] of Yale University has uncovered interesting stages of the development of the human animal. This study involved a series of eighty observations of "incubator" and "full-term" babies. The following "snapshot" descriptions at various stages of embryologic evolution are quoted from Dr. Gesell's book. The alert student will note the unfolding of simple acts that form the foundation for later psychological

---

[1] GESELL, A. *The embryology of behavior.* New York: Harper, 1945. Pp. 289. (Reproduced by permission of the author and the publisher.)

responses and which will become definitely incorporated into genuine behavioral events.

Biologists use conception, the time of origin of the living organism, as a convenient reference point from which to calculate subsequent stages. Thus, the first 2 weeks following conception are called the "germinal period," from the second to the eighth week, the "embryonic period," and the eighth week to the fortieth week, the "fetal period." The term "neonate" designates the newborn child during its first 2 weeks following birth, after which he enters infancy which lasts until he is about 2 years of age.

THE FETAL PERIOD. The fetal period is a period of preparation. The first eight weeks of his embryology are given over to the formation of the constituent organs of the future infant. During the twenty weeks which follow, these organs acquire their specific functions and are consolidated into a total pattern. Nature adds one finishing touch to another; the nostrils reopen; the eyes are unsealed; the anal plate becomes perforate; a sucking fat pad for each cheek is laid down to cushion the buccinator muscles; the epidermis is cornified; the skin becomes a true integument providing both protection and communication. These are final improvements for the impending crisis of birth. Every organ system is essential to meet the test of that crisis, but the autonomic-somatic nervous system is supreme. It is the over-all integrator which before and after birth finally determines whether the organism will live and breathe and have its being.

THE FOURTH DAY. In the chick, as in man, the heart begins to beat very early—only 30 hours after incubation. It develops, as in man, from a single tube from which the ventricles, the auricles, and the sinus differentiate, not simultaneously but in sequence. The several regions of the heart begin to beat in the same sequence in which they are formed. The timing and rhythms of the beat change with the developmental sequences. These progressive changes are clearly reflected in electrocardiograms— Serial studies show that during the fourth day of incubation the electrocardiogram settles into a pattern which is strikingly like that of the adult. This is a remarkable fact, because at this stage of development no nerve control has yet been established over the heart [*sic.*] [pp. 37–39].

THE SECOND MONTH. 1. Muscular Development—Muscles . . . are peculiarly sensitive to environing influences. They tend to twitch at an early stage of their embryonic development when the ions in the surrounding medium are unbalanced. They may contract feebly and intermittently, without the stimulus of nervous impulses [*sic.!*]. In the heart, as we shall see, this contraction becomes a peristaltic sweep and settles into a rhythmic beat before nerve connections are established. Smooth muscles of intestine, stomach, and blood vessels are capable of similar myogenic activity [p. 30].

2. Postural Reactions—Equilibrium . . . is not a general ability which is mastered once and for all. It always functions in relation to the motor system which is operative at the time. In the post-natal period, specific equilibrium patterns must be acquired for the maintenance of head station, sitting posture, standing, and walking. The human infant does not balance himself independently on his two feet until he is about 56 weeks of age. The equilibrium of the embryo has a different economy, but in part it depends upon the same mechanisms which will be used by the infant in the assumption of the upright posture. Man begins his life-long contest with gravity even before he is born. All told, it takes about a hundred weeks before he stands and walks erect. Most of the basic organization of this distinctly human posture is laid down during the fetal period [p. 32].

THE FETUS AT 12–16 WEEKS.   Twelve lunar months hence, at the post-fetal age of 20 weeks, he will rotate his head repeatedly and avidly, through an arc of 180 degrees. This pattern comes to a peak of intensity at that age. But it is anticipated and to a modest degree actually fabricated in the fourth fetal month.

This month is in many respects the most remarkable in the embryology of behavior; because the fetus exhibits (even though he does not yet command) an extremely varied repertoire of elementary movement patterns. Almost his entire skin is sensitive to stimulation. Crude generalized responses give way to specific reactions. Arms and legs show more motility at every joint and make excursions into new sectors of space. Within the confines of the amniotic sac, these movements are probably mild, and vary from episodic twitches to variably prolonged tonic contractions which wax and then wane into nothingness. Their vigor and incidence must also vary with constitutional and with passing biochemical conditions. As in all growth patterning, the primary impulses come from within.

The daily course of these natural activities is not conspicuously ordered by rhythms of work and rest. It must depend rather on the meandering distribution of the metabolic foci of growth. Accordingly, now the head and mouth, now the feet, now the hands, emerge into action, somewhat as ripples rise here and there upon a placid surface. Reactions seemingly detached are nevertheless patterned and all have their morphogenetic determination in a unitary growth plan. So this fetus in the course of a day or fortnight (between 14 and 16 weeks) would display a changing succession of patterns with successive intervals of quiescence. He moves his upper lip. When a little more mature, he moves his lower lip. Later he moves both lips in unison. Still later he opens and closes his mouth. He swallows with closed mouth, but at times he also swallows amniotic fluid. His tongue moves, or he moves his tongue. (We have no semantics to take care of this distinction.) He may also rotate his head in association with the "oral reflex"; for complex patterns of feeding behavior are in the making. Peristaltic waves sweep over his lengthening digestive tube [pp. 68–69].

Arms and legs occasionally move in diagonal alternation in a manner which suggests locomotion, whether aquatic or terrestrial—small movements which may, however, displace the position of the fetus. But human arms and hands are ultimately meant for manipulation as well as locomotion and the fetus accordingly foreshadows long in advance the patterns of a higher order. He elevates the upper arms, he extends his drooping hands. Elbows formerly fixed are mobile. He deploys his hands in the median plane; sometimes they almost touch the mouth. His movements are less stilted than they were in the previous month, when his palms assumed a stiff pat-a-cake attitude or were retracted far apart. He now rotates his forearm medially. He opens and closes his hands. He moves his thumb independently, or curls it fistlike under the conjoint digits, a token of late opposability.

We do not suppose that these movements are executed with decision; but it has been demonstrated that they are part of the behavior equipment of the fetus at this stage, and like other growing functions they soon express themselves in natural self-activity. Such activity, with its varying emphasis and intensities, is a normal accompaniment of the growth process. Structures are being laid down which will again come to expression in a different context at a later stage of maturity. Some of the activities, however, may have a retrospective significance. The foot, for example, is especially nimble. It dorsiflexes at the angle, with exaggerated dorsiflexion of the great toe and fanning of the other toes. The deviation and excess mobility of the great toe, the orientation of the soles toward the sagittal plane, and some of the leg-foot patterns hark back to quadrumanual ancestory and arboreal brachiation. But basically, the behavior of the fetus even at this age harks forward. The developmental tide is flowing into the future [pp. 69–70].

DEVELOPMENT AT 16–20 WEEKS.   The mother experiences this quickening at first as an almost imperceptible fluttering. The onset of motion is gentle; the occurrences are few, perhaps only one or two a day in the beginning. The amount and intensity of the activity tend to increase steadily during the last half of gestation, and in some instances, they become extremely vigorous. Toward the end of pregnancy, over 200 movements may be experienced in a single day.

There are many movements, however, which are too small to be experienced as quickening. As early as the 12th week, the eyeballs have begun to move, and somewhat later the fused eyelids blinked, the corrugators of the brow contracted, and the upper lip drew up in a sneer-like manner. Such movements and concealed movements of tongue, pharynx, and larynx doubtless occur in increasing abundance during the fourth fetal month [p. 70].

BREATHING RESPONSES. To what extent the human fetus executes respiratory movements while in utero is not precisely known. Atmospheric respiration being an impossibility, does he none the less prepare for breathing by a kind of fore-exercise? Use is not a necessary stimulus to growth; it may, however, play a role in the early establishment of function. As early as 1888, Ahlfeld described a slight, rhythmic rising, and falling of the maternal abdominal wall toward the end of pregnancy. The movements occurred in short runs, interrupted by quiescence, at a rate of from 60 to 80 per minute. Objective records show that these prenatal movements bear a close resemblance in rate and depth to the respiratory movements of a five-day-old infant. Some of them even show a Cheyne-Stokes type of respiration.

Strictly speaking, the prenatal movements should be called prerespiratory rather than respiratory, because they have no direct relation to oxygen consumption. In fact, they aspirate fluid rather than air into the air sacs. If the amniotic fluid is contaminated, this may produce an intrauterine pneumonia. On the other hand, a sterile fluid may serve a beneficial function by bringing about dilatation of the alveoli and facilitating the growth of their pavement epithelium [p. 80].

THE FETAL-INFANT. The fetal age of 28 weeks approximately demarcates the zone between viability and non-viability. The fetal-infant at this stage weighs only about two pounds. He is so diminutive that he can be held in the palm of the adult hand. When so held, he feels very much like a loosely articulated manikin. The head is so flaccidly attached to neck and shoulders that it scarcely seems part of a single anatomy. Arms and legs, too, are flaccid, but they seem a little more definitely joined to the torso [p. 108].

The eyeballs move conjointly both laterally and vertically. But positive visual responses are scanty or quite absent. The fetal-infant will, however, make mild avoidance responses to a bright light, frowning, and flinching slightly. Even this response, however, soon peters out and diminishes to a tired blink, or the eyes simply remain closed [p. 112].

The reaction to sound, when a small hand bell is tinkled near the ear is similar. There may be a slight frown, a "squinch" with a blink, followed by a short wave of activity which soon subsides. On repeated stimulation, the fetal-infant rapidly becomes impervious to sound. Inaction again supervenes. It is as though the action system were a toy with a weak spring which readily runs down. A mild jolt of the table on which the fetal-infant lies may also produce a small wave of activity which presently sinks into a drowsy quiescence [p. 112].

Tone is minimal; it is prevailingly limp and flaccid. But relaxation is not always bilaterally equal. When the palm of the hand is stimulated by insertion of the observer's finger, a barely perceptible grasp is evoked, stronger in the occipital than in the face hand.

Such tonal differences are highly characteristic of the early stage of fetal-infancy. The general body tone is not firmly consolidated. It never sinks beneath a low limiting level, but above this level it rises and falls and shifts, producing the phenomenon of meandering tonus. As tonus tires, it wanders from one region to another, not in a whimsical manner, but electing those regions where neuromotor functions are nascent. This is a lawful organizing process. Although the organism seems to react in a somewhat mosaic manner, it is still consolidating its growth gains as a unit [p. 113].

AT 32–36 WEEKS. His behavior, likewise, has more body. His reactions are more positive and sustained. His gross postural activity comes in definite and configured waves, rather than in small localized ripples. The basic level of muscle tonus has risen from a minimal to a moderate level and is less fluctuant than in the early stage. General tonus increases on manipulation, and rises to meet limited emergencies. The capacity to respond tonically gives added substance to the behavior. This increment of robustness is very important from a developmental standpoint. Although there have been no startling innovations in the behavior repertoire, there has been a definite gain in the texture and stamina of the motor activity. The organism seems more firmly integrated and, relatively speaking, more powerful [p. 117].

All things considered, the most important developmental advance achieved by the mid-stage fetal-infant is his capacity for brief periods of

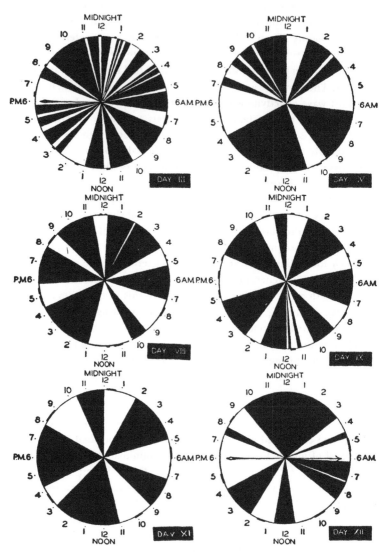

FIG. 13 Diurnal cycle of behavior for days 3, 4, 8, 9, 11, 12. (Gesell, A., *The Embryology of behavior.*)

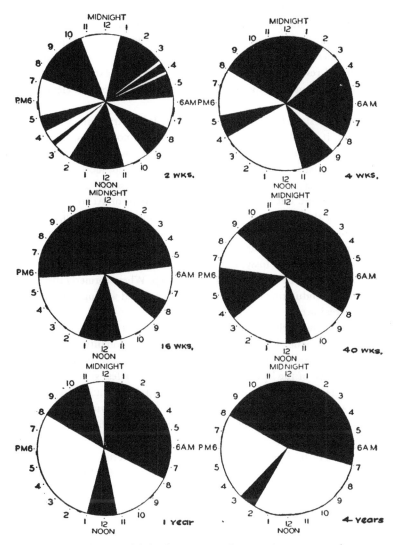

FIG. 14 Diurnal cycle of behavior at 2, 4, 16, 40 weeks, 1 year, and 4 years. (Gesell, A., *The embryology of behavior.*)

wakeful alertness. They are the growing germs which will elaborate into the complex cycle of diurnal wakefulness and sleep. The early-stage fetal-infant gives virtually no sign of this cycle because neither sleep nor alertness is discernible in his stage of amorphous dormancy [p. 121].

THE MATURE FETAL-INFANT (36–40 WEEKS). Patterns and rhythms of activity and rest are taking shape. He has been in an extrauterine world two months or more. Experience has made him an expert at elementary living.

Even his sleep behavior is more expert. It has structure. A month or more ago, it was shallow, variable, fluctuant, and not always distinguishable from wakefulness. The mature fetal-infant has caught the knack of sleeping. He falls off to sleep more decisively; he sleeps more profoundly; he clings to sleep more tenaciously. The depth of sleep varies from moment to moment, but he is rarely completely quiescent. At frequent intervals during the sleep, the eyelids part and flutter, the eyeballs roll, the corner of the mouth twitches, he smiles vacuously, he stirs and snuggles under the cover. He resists waking and is not easily aroused. Under the stress of waking, he is fussy; frequently he is at the same time both fussy and awake. Then he literally drops off to sleep. Where formerly there was a vague and undulating boundary between sleep and waking, there is now a steep precipice.

His feeding behavior likewise is decisive and competent. He can furrow his tongue, he sucks well; and the directionality of gastro-intestinal peristalsis is under good control. There is little regurgitation. The slightest touch of the lips tends to induce a more or less vigorous sucking response. He may announce hunger with a lusty cry. But sleep and feeding are still not completely differentiated. He may drowse during a feeding and fall asleep, too soundly for rousing [pp. 125–126].

The gradual evolution of distinctly wakeful and distinctly sleep reactions as well as feeding behavior is graphically shown in the accompanying figures reproduced from Dr. Gesell's book.

III. RANDOM BEHAVIOR IS TRANSITIONAL
J. W. Bowles, Jr.

Activity is characteristic of the newborn infant and of the fetus long before birth. Although the infant at birth may be lethargic or even stuporous owing to the effects of anesthesia and sedation, activity may be considered as characterizing living organisms. This, however, does not demand any assumptions of mystical "drives" or "urges" to be active but can be adequately handled as biological stimulus-response. The infant at birth is a living thing. Whatever modification of action may have taken place prior to birth is necessarily limited and restricted at most to reflex modification, as in fetal conditioned responses.

The "random activity" of the newborn child can be described in terms of organismic biology; responses on the part of the organism to various physical and chemical stimuli such as tissue needs for food, irritating conditions, and, as Ribble's [2] observations seem to indicate, lack of oxygen. These responses represent adaptations of the organism to its biological environment.

These actions are the basis of the needs of the infant for "psychological mothering" such as handling, rocking, patting, and bathing. The "needs" do not rest upon any inherent or instinctual basis but upon the fact that the newborn infant is an inadequate and poorly organized biological organism (Gesell [3]). Respiratory, circulatory, digestive, eliminative, and other biological actions are unorganized. "Psychological mothering" is important here in aiding biological adaptation. As Ribble has observed, these motherings aid in the organization and integration of such reflex actions. For example, patting and bathing stimulate the skin and thus aid circulation; handling and rocking stimulate deeper respiration, relieving oxygen deficiency; digestion and elimination are also improved by such attention. In sum, "psychological mothering" is conducive to biological well-being.

Ribble reports some cases of extreme reactions to inadequate mothering. Some infants were observed to show loss of appetite and even failure to assimilate food. Various muscle tensions were observed, at times accompanied by vomiting and violent screaming. Other infants showed less and less activity, finally reaching a stuporlike condition. A variety of biological disturbances occurred in these infants.

There is much more involved here, however, than sheer biological adaptation. In the infant's new complex surroundings,

---

[2] RIBBLE, MARGARET A. Infantile experience in relation to personality development, in HUNT, J. McV. *Personality and the behavior disorders,* Vol. II. New York: Ronald, 1944. Pp. 621–651.

[3] GESELL, A. *The embryology of behavior.* New York: Harper, 1945. Pp. 289.

there are a variety of psychological stimuli. The random action of the infant quickly becomes attached to many such stimuli, resulting in the origin of definite psychological activity. Although these responses on the part of the infant are uncoordinated and transitional, they show many of the characteristics of psychological phenomena.

Consider random-movement behavior in response to voices. The newborn child does not discriminate voices; at most, he demonstrates biological startle reflexes to sudden noises and other stimuli. However, through contacts with his parents, by being picked up, rocked, and talked and sung to, voices take on psychological stimulus functions related to the reinforced random movements that occur in the infant.

For another example, consider the infant's series of contacts with toys, such as a ring dangling over his crib. At first, although ring and infant are in close spatial relationship, no psychological response occurs. But through progressively more complex visual contacts, discrimination takes place, and soon the dangling object functions so as to call out random kicking, arm waving, and other movement reactions. Little by little these random adjustments show improvement. By the age of 3 months, the infant may succeed in approaching the ring with his hands, and in another month, he may readily reach and secure the ring. Soon the child and ring interact in many ways; the ring is transferred from one hand to the other, brought to the mouth, turned about, and inspected.

For a final example, let us consider vocal actions. Early in his infancy, the human organism reveals an extensive collection of random vocalizations, sufficient apparently to fit any language group in which he may live. From such random vocal adjustments develop language responses by selection and reinforcement from the child's language community.

With regard to the transitional character of random behaviors, note that parent-infant relationships are important for behavioral as well as biological reasons. The infant who receives a great deal of "attention," i.e., who is frequently held, rocked, talked to, and otherwise mothered, has more extensive and varied contacts with his surroundings than the less-mothered infant. Hence, the former may be expected to show more rapid acquisition of behavior. This is born out by Ribble's observations as well as by instances of extreme lack of "mothering" and other opportunities for stimulation as in the case of "cupboard children."

IV. COLOR DISCRIMINATIONS SHOW PROGRESSIVE ELABORATION
J. W. Bowles, Jr.

The discrimination of color properties of objects does not take place with newborn infants; it constitutes behavioral acquisition in the early stages of the reactional biography. The exact origins of color reactions are difficult to determine. Comparatively young infants may be observed to discriminate and adjust to a colored light moving in a field of different color, and perhaps the beginnings could be fixed here, although these actions are exceedingly simple when contrasted with the later discrimination of colors as definite properties of objects, matching objects on the basis of color characteristics, and the like. The latter are occasionally observed with children near the age of 2 years in play situations, but they are fleeting discoveries that may not be reperformed for long periods of time.

Except for chance observations, these reactions with colored objects are very difficult to investigate. Somewhat later the child comes into contact with colored objects under human surroundings, where a parent calls the child's attention to his *red* ball, *green* car, or *yellow* sweater. As a result, he builds up discriminatory responses to them so that he can select the appropriate object in response to the parent's directions. Here we find illustrated just how specific psychological events are. At first, although "red ball" may refer the child to a certain object, "red truck" does not necessarily refer him to a truck of any specific color. In other words, "red ball" functions as a label for a certain definite object. "Red truck," "red wagon," and "red block" labels may also get attached to specific objects so that eventually the child is referred to the color properties of objects as such, and builds up verbal (color-naming) responses to these properties.

So complex are adjustments of this latter sort that a long history with colored objects is essential for their development. In an exploratory study of color-naming responses and complex behaviors involving discrimination, Synolds and Pronko [4] found that in a small sample of 3-year-old children, none was successful in correctly naming the eight hues of the Dvorine Color Perception Test Charts. Only 25 per cent of their 4-year-old sample was successful with this task. However, this percentage jumped to approximately 80 per cent in a sample of 6-year-old first-grade children. These responses were rapidly acquired by most children under the formal training of the school situation.

With a more complex discriminational task, this rapid behavioral evolution did not occur. The Dvorine color plates contain one- and two-digit numbers of a given hue on a background of another hue. Here the subjects just either name the numbers or trace them. Since the younger children in the Synolds and Pronko sample had not acquired number-naming responses, the tracing technique was employed with them. With this task, the subjects showed a slower increase of successes with age, from zero successes at the 3-year level to approximately 80 per cent at the 8-year level.

This study raised many questions in regard to traditional beliefs about "color blindness." For one thing, no sex differences were discovered. Boys performed as well, or as poorly, as did girls. Further, the successful responses seemed highly specific. Red numbers might be accurately traced on a blue background, but blue numbers might be failed on a red field, and the same with many other color combinations. In addition, no "color-blind" versus "noncolor-blind" categories were found. By the test used, all the 3-year-olds could have been labeled "color blind." But successful performances above this age varied along a continuum. Also, the younger children appeared to have learned many color labels, but they had not yet attached them to specific colors of objects. These observations led to a more detailed study [5] which attempted to isolate some of the variables involved in such complex color perceptions.

Since the early school years appeared to be the crucial point

---

[4] SYNOLDS, D. L. & PRONKO, N. H. Exploratory study of color discrimination of children. *J. genet. Psychol.*, 1949, **74**, 17–21.

[5] PRONKO, N. H., BOWLES, J. W., JR., SNYDER, F. W., & SYNOLDS, D. L. An experiment in pursuit of color blindness. *J. genet. Psychol.*, 1949, **74**, 125–142.

in the color responses required by the Dvorine test, the second study was conducted with kindergarten, first-, second-, and third-grade children. An entire school population in these grades was employed to avoid selection. Further, the school sample that was chosen provided a rather homogeneous socioeconomic group. This was considered a rather important variable since a sampling of a children's home group with deprivational conditions in the children's histories was strikingly inferior to the Synolds and Pronko sample.

Altogether, 245 children made up the sample, 119 males and 126 females. These subjects were administered the nomenclature (color-naming) section and the 60 chart tests (colored digits on differently colored fields) of the Dvorine Color Perception Test. When the subject could not name all the digits, determined prior to administering the test, he was encouraged to trace them with a small brush.

The results of this experiment are treated here in some detail since they illuminate the highly complex, specific nature of color perceptions. First, the naming of the eight shades of the nomenclature section showed a sharp increase between kindergarten and first grade. Thereafter, these naming responses were almost universally correct. They could be described as comparatively simple discriminations and namings which become stabilized by the first grade as a result of formal school training. With tints, the story was different. A more progressive increase from kindergarten through the third grade was obtained, and the naming of tints was not universally correct in the oldest group. This seems to show differences in experience with shades and tints.

In color naming, no sex differences were found (Fig. 15). This is embarrassing to traditional color theory, which talks of sex-linked genes for color blindness. The only marked male-female difference was in naming the violet *tint.* No sex difference occurred with the violet *shade,* nor with red and blue tints, which, in terms of tradition, are the components of violet. "Sex-linked" educational differences would be a simpler alternative explanation of this finding, i.e., female contacts with dresses, hair ribbons, and other violet-tinted objects may be more frequent than the small boy's contacts with such colors. As in the Synolds and Pronko study, the younger children in this sample were observed to apply color labels indiscriminately to all the color patches; "color-blindness" is indeed rampant among kindergarten children.

With regard to the digit-naming responses to the color plates, kindergartners were extremely poor, first graders were markedly better, and a plateau was reached at the second- and third-grade levels with about 85 per cent of responses correct. No sex differences were found in these results, nor were differences discovered when the children's responses to individual plates were examined. No sex differences in percentages of successes were great, and, as a matter of fact, the largest that were found favored the males.

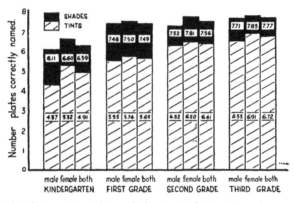

FIG. 15 Showing a comparison of the mean frequencies of correct color-naming responses for the light Dvorine shades and tints between the sex and grade groups.

"Color-blindness" as defined by the Dvorine test, namely missing one or more of the most diagnostic plates (Nos. 2, 3, and 4), was characteristic of the entire group. By such a definition 98 per cent of the kindergartners were "color-blind"; this figure was reduced only to 75 per cent in the case of the third graders. Here, however, we have the specificity principle illustrated. Approximately 75 per cent of the children *who failed* the diagnostic plates *passed* other plates of the *same* color combinations. In other words, these color perceptions were apparently exceedingly complex responses involving the interrelationships of colored *digits* and colored *backgrounds* and were not simple hue discriminations. Change the digit and you influence the perceptual response.

This was further demonstrated by comparing performances

where figure and ground colors were reversed. Discrepancies in levels of success were sometimes striking in these situations, e.g., a green "99" on a yellow field was passed by only 15 per cent of the children, while a yellow "62" on a green background was passed by 64 per cent. Again, the shape of the digits is a variable in addition to figure-ground reversal and changes in contrast.

The analysis in this experiment revealed a developmental trend in different sorts of color discriminations—color naming and colored-figure discrimination and naming. It further illuminated some of the complex field factors that condition color-seeing reactions; on the part of the object, the figure-ground relationships, possible brightness relationships, the shape of the figure, and color contrasts; on the side of the organism, the color-naming and digit-naming history, the variety of color contacts, and the association of color labels with color properties of objects. All of these were found to be important variables in the color-seeing responses that were observed.

V. MECHANISMS OF EARLY INFANT FEEDING
J. W. Bowles, Jr.

A large portion of the behavioral equipment of the infant is reflexive, including feeding responses. That feeding reflexes are highly complex organismic actions, however, and not the functioning of isolated parts of organisms is demonstrated in an experiment by Halverson.[6] His subjects were fourteen infants from whom feeding records were obtained. The age of the infants at the first recording varied from 8 hours to 2 weeks. Sucking movements were recorded by placing a small rubber capsule under the chin. This was connected by a closed air column to a recording tambour which recorded the sucking movements on a revolving kymograph. Respiration was similarly indicated on the kymograph by means of two light pneumographs, one around the chest and the other around the abdomen. A stethoscope held against the neck was used to observe the sound of the milk in transit through the pharynx. Thus, the interrelationships of breathing, sucking, and swallowing could be observed as the infant was fed.

---

[6] HALVERSON, H. M. Mechanisms of early infant feeding. *J. genet. Psychol.*, 1944, 64, 185–223. (Reproduced by permission of the author and the publisher.)

Although sucking, swallowing, and breathing were variously coordinated, the three activities functioned most smoothly when sucking occurred during the first half of the respiratory cycle, viz., during either inspiration, or the pause after inspiration, or both, and was followed by swallowing during the same pause. Three reasons may be advanced to explain why the best feeding performances took place under these conditions. In the first place, conditions were optimal for sucking. Secondly, swallowing occurred at a natural pause in breathing. Thirdly, both sucking and swallowing occurred at fixed points in the respiratory cycle with no appreciable pause between them. The last condition is important, since swallowing is closely linked with sucking and normally occurs as soon as the milk enters the mouth. The conditions as a whole appear to indicate that when sucking, swallowing, and breathing were well-coordinated, breathing was so regulated that sucking regularly occurred when the chest and abdomen were in positions at which they could expediently reinforce the sucking movements, and swallowing occurred naturally with reference to sucking at a natural pause in breathing [pp. 204–205].

The age at which coordination between breathing and sucking and swallowing was first exhibited varied from subject to subject. One subject, G, showed good coordination eight hours after birth at her first feeding. As soon as she was placed at the breast, she made three feeble sucks. From there on she proceeded as follows: rested two seconds, made five strong sucks in rapid succession; rested six seconds, and sucked four times. No coordination was shown up to this time. After a rest period of five seconds, she sucked more regularly once per respiration 13 times, showing coordination. From this point on, the sucks occurred regularly once per respiration in series of 12 to 21. Subjects F, K, and T showed coordination within the first three days, and eight other subjects exhibited coordination on one or more occasions at varying stages before the experiment was concluded. HE and WA consistently failed to maintain a steady temporal relationship between the breathing and food-taking activities, and subsequent tests at 24 weeks revealed no improvement in feeding performance [pp. 217–218].

Halverson's experiment throws much light on early infant feeding. The traditional view considered sucking as an "instinct" in which the tongue was thought to function automatically and without experience. An exceedingly oversimplified picture described it as the operation of an isolated set of structures. Halverson's work shows that that infant sucks best who *learns* to integrate his sucking and swallowing at certain fixed points in his own respiratory cycle. Individual differences showed up in the speed and ease with which these reactions were acquired. And, finally, this study shows that even such simple responses as feeding are really organismic, and not "part-reactions." Other things go on and affect sucking at the time the infant sucks.

VI. REACTIONS OF THE INFANT TO PINPRICK
J. W. Bowles, Jr.

McGraw [7] investigated the modification in the infant's responses to pinprick from birth to 4 years. Seventy-five infants served as subjects. They were pricked with a blunt sterile pin at repeated intervals on the head, trunk, and upper and lower extremities. Many of the observations were recorded on motion-picture film.

Considering first the postural adjustments to the pinprick, it was observed that some newborn infants showed no postural reactions to the pin, although with deeper pressure a response usually was elicited. Within a few days, however, infants were observed to respond characteristically with random movements, crying, and more circumscribed withdrawal responses. The reactions also became more vigorous during the first month.

Somewhat later, infants tended to show a decrease of random movements and withdrawal responses, and crying became the most characteristic action. This was followed by more deliberate and organized withdrawal postures or stances as well as conditioned responses to mere sight of the pin.

However, these complex visual perceptions were not observed for some weeks. As they first appeared, they were simple differentiations—the pin was discriminated, reached for, and played with as in the case of any object. With further visual experience, the perceptual reactions became more complex—they were followed by fussing, crying, withdrawal responses, frowning, or ducking. At other times the pin was not immediately perceived as "harmful." The child, on coming into visual contact with

---

[7] McGraw, Myrtle B. Neural maturation as exemplified in the changing reactions of the infant to pin prick. *Child Develpm.*, 1941, 12, 31–42. (Reproduced by permission of the author and the publisher.)

the object, might reach for it, perceive it as an unpleasant thing, and inhibit the reaching response.

With further contacts, this behavior situation became more complex. Children were observed to defend themselves vigorously, or accept the situation, or take the pin and playfully prick themselves.

Although we have treated these reactions to pinprick as modifications in behavior due to successive organism-object contacts, i.e., conditions of the reactional biography, it should be pointed out that McGraw does not interpret them in this way. She considers the changes in response to be indicative of progressive neural maturation.

As an alternate explanation, the concept of the reactional biography appears to be simpler and less speculative. Further, it avoids the common error of identifying behavior with neural happenings. Although the incomplete biological status of the newborn child prevents the performance of coordinated adjustments to any object, the evolution of complex, organized responses cannot be adequately explained in terms of general maturational processes, let alone neural maturation.

Thus, these infants had a highly complex history of tactual and visual contacts, not only with pins but with a multitude of other objects. Had this history been lacking, evidence (see, e.g., Riesen's study of chimpanzees reared in darkness) indicates that the children would not have performed the complex adjustments observed at the end of the study. In fact, had they had no visual contacts with objects, they would not, at the age of 4 years, have differentiated the pin from surrounding objects. Had all tactual contacts been prevented for 4 years, it is improbable that coordinated postural adjustments to pinpricks would be performed, though there would be no question of "maturity."

VII. USE OF THE STICK AS A TOOL
BY YOUNG CHIMPANZEES
J. W. Bowles, Jr.

Among the earliest acquired responses are discriminatory, manipulative, and other actions in which the sizes, lengths, weights, uses, colors, or relationships of objects are discovered. Some of the characteristics of these activities are illustrated in a chimpanzee learning situation contrived by Jackson.[8]

The experimental setup was composed of a cage with iron-bar grilles in two adjoining walls. Platforms were placed before the grilles to hold a food object and sticks of different lengths. Eight chimpanzees, ranging in age from 3 to approximately 7 years, served as subjects. Something of the past history of the animals was known. They had served as subjects in a variety of experiments but had not previously manipulated tools.

Two test situations were arranged. In the one-platform test, the subject had to reach for a stick with which he could then rake in food. This was complicated by requiring the chimpanzee to reach a stick, use it to drag in a larger stick, and then secure food with the larger one (two-stick test). In further complications, three- and four-stick tests were used. In the latter, the subject had successively to secure four sticks and employ the last (the longest) to drag in the food.

The two-platform test which followed required the subject to shuttle back and forth between platforms in securing the sticks in sequence. For example, stick No. 1 was in arm's reach on one platform. In the one-stick test, this stick was taken to the other platform and the food was secured. In the two-stick test, the subject used stick No. 1 to secure stick No. 2 on the second platform, and then returned to the first platform and secured food with stick No. 2.

Thus, the chimpanzees had to discriminate the various lengths of sticks, their relationships, and the stick of appropriate length for a tool to secure the food object.

The experiential nature of these reactions is revealed by the consistent superiority of the older animals. They more rapidly perceived the relationships between the sticks and the food object, and their manual adjustments were more adequate, smoother, and better coordinated. Further, they were more persistent and less easily upset, when compared with the younger chimps.

The older subjects showed "insight" learning; i.e., quick perceptions and permanent adaptations to the relationships existing between the various sticks and the food. On the other hand,

---

[8] JACKSON, T. A. Use of the stick as a tool by young chimpanzees. *J. comp. Psychol.*, 1942, 34, 223–235. (Reproduced by permission of the author, the American Psychological Association, and the Williams & Wilkins Company.)

the younger animals showed the variability of performance characteristic of trial-and-error behavior, as is shown in the accompanying figure. Bula was the younger chimpanzee and Kani the older.
General conditions of the reactional biography are extremely important here.

The evolution of the earliest activities of the reactional biography, showing the flexibility and adaptability of discoveries to
new situations, is especially well demonstrated in the case of Velt.

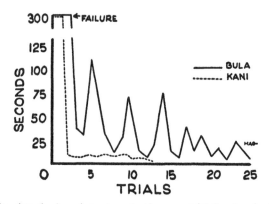

FIG. 16 Showing the learning curves in time per trial for the single-stick test
situation. The younger chimpanzee (Bula) showed "trial and error" learning
and accidental successes; the older chimpanzee (Kani), after the first trial,
promptly and effectively solved the problem. (Jackson, T. A., The use of the
stick as a tool by young chimpanzees.)

A young male chimpanzee, Velt, who had probably had no experience
in using sticks or other instruments, was given ten trials on the single-
stick, single platform test. He failed utterly, making no attempt to use the
stick to get the food. He was then allowed to play with a stick, in his living
quarters, for 28 hours (two hours per day for 14 days). During this "training" he used the stick to beat, hammer, pound, poke, and pry, but at no
time did he use it to get food or any other goal object. Following the
period of stick familiarization he was again given the stick test. After an
initial delay of about 300 seconds, he came forward, looked over the problem situation, and in a deliberate manner used the stick to draw in the
food. He manifested the skill of an animal that had used a stick dozens
of times. This performance was followed by three more trials in each of
which the stick was promptly taken and used to draw in the food. All were
accomplished in less than 10 seconds per trial [pp. 232–233].

5

BASIC PATTERNS OF BEHAVIOR

I. INTRODUCTION
N. H. Pronko

At birth and shortly after, the infant is a functioning biological organism. In this period, a great many reflex actions and movement sequences of a physiological sort have been studied and described. Very early in this period, too, specific behaviors begin to appear, i.e., the child begins to recognize and respond differently to persons and objects, to make approach actions toward certain things and withdrawal actions to others. Certain chance actions are repeated, with or without modifications. A great many of these differential ways of behaving are subtle and difficult to observe at this stage. Psychologists have been handicapped in the study of these early psychological activities because of the frequent practical difficulties in obtaining such young subjects for observation and study. Very frequently, it is difficult to observe the occurrence of these early behaviors outside of the intimacy of the home situation. However, an increasing number of studies of early basic patterns of behavior have been done. Following are some sample selections of studies of basic behavioral patterns in the early period of the psychological life history.

II. THE FAMILY AND PERSONALITY DEVELOPMENT [1]

Parents determine their offspring's biological inheritance simply and finally when their individual contributions merge at conception to form

---

[1] CAMERON, NORMAN. *The psychology of behavior disorders.* Boston: Houghton Mifflin, 1947. Pp. 622. (Reproduced by permission of the author and the publisher.)

the single cell whose product, the child, exhibits characteristics traceable to each. Parents are also instrumental in determining their child's cultural inheritance. Its conditions, however, are never simple and its effects may never be final. The conditions and the effects of cultural inheritance are complex and mutable because a child's two parents usually differ from each other in personality, and because they and he are always more or less affected by the cultural impact of the wider community. Moreover, these two parents are not just two human organisms that happen to be domiciled together for procreative ends. They are themselves a dynamic interacting unit, two biosocially different individuals who are functioning toward each other in a complementary relationship. Therefore, what the infant and child shall experience at their hands will be a resultant of interparental relationships, as well as the direct product of each parent's personal needs and wishes.

Human parenthood is always expectant for a long time before it finally becomes actual. This means that babies, whether they are welcome or not, are born into a psychologically prepared situation. The materials for this prepared situation include the diverse personalities of the two parents, each of whom brings his or her unique cultural contribution to the biosocial partnership. There is first the sex distinction. It is not always recognized that, even within a single family living together under the same roof, the customs, traditions, attitudes, and experiences of the male subculture usually differ markedly from those of the female subculture. This is a most important source of sex differences in perspective. In addition, husband and wife generally come from different family cultures as well, with their different social techniques, values, standards, and goals, and their different preconceptions in relation to children, how they should be reared and what exact function each parent should perform in the process. Their patterns of expectation with regard to each other, as husband and wife, may be widely different, depending upon the interparental patterns in their respective homes, and how each has reacted to them.

These and a great many other differences like them enter into the phase of marital readjustment that normally precedes a first child's advent. Many of them are commonly settled by compromise, many more by will or unwilling sacrifice and revision. Some are simply driven into concealment or disguise, but not eliminated as potential influences in the rearing of children. Some differences remain unconcealed and unsettled, as present or future sources of marital discord. Many of them can not or need not be resolved. They persist openly as accepted distinctions between the paternal and the maternal personality in a given household, and may have a reciprocal or balancing effect in parent-child relationships. The degree of acceptance that a child enjoys and his general treatment during infancy and childhood will be affected, not alone by the quality and character of interparental adjustment, but also by the specific personal needs, hopes, and expectations of each parent individually. Each may entertain in advance a definite preference as to the child's sex and hopes regarding its ultimate appearance and special abilities. Each may cherish expectations and harbor secret fears concerning the child's general temperament in relation to what they consider their spouse's or their own to be, or in relation to someone else on one side of the family or the other. Because marital partners very often do differ fundamentally in their interpersonal techniques, and because popular thinking ascribes an almost superstitious finality to biological heredity in the determination of personality trends, this pre-occupation is much deeper and more widespread than the facts warrant. None the less, the expectations or fears of a parent, to the extent that they enter into his overt interactions with the child and the other parent, may play a decisive part in shaping the child's social behavior patterns [pp. 31–32].

III. SPEECH PATTERNS AND CULTURAL CONDITIONS

Inappropriate or unadaptive reactions, such as stuttering behavior, commonly have their origin in the basic stage of the reactional biography. These are activities that are directly conditioned by human (primarily parental) influences. Therefore, it is to be expected that parental attitudes toward, and training methods for, the child's speech are critical factors in the development or nondevelopment of stuttering. These domestic conditions are referred to by Johnson [2] as the child's semantic environment, which he otherwise defines as "those aspects of the total environment that are least important to a dog or an oyster."

Under family conditions which are rather typical throughout the United States, one finds parents who are overconcerned with their children's speech, who interpret ordinary hesitations and

2 JOHNSON, W. The Indians have no word for it. *Etc.: A Review of General Semantics*, 1944–1945, **2**, 65–81. (Reproduced by permission of the author and the publisher.)

stumblings as defective or abnormal, and who subject the child to increasing pressures and tensions, providing him with emotional stimuli for eventually serious stuttering problems. With strikingly different basic family conditions for speech evolution, no such problems develop, as Johnson indicates, in the case of North American Indians.

The significance of semantic environment in relation to stuttering is further suggested by certain experiences that the writer has had in attempting to investigate stuttering among North American Indians. A few years ago one of his students, Miss Harriett Hayes, became a teacher on an Indian reservation in Idaho. She carried with her a set of detailed instructions for making a study of the stutterers among the Bannock and Shoshone Indians, with whom she was to work. At the end of the school year, however, she returned with the highly interesting information that *she had been unable to find any stuttering Indians*. Moreover, the superintendent of the school and the other teachers, many of whom had been in close association with Indians for as long as 25 years, had reported to Miss Hayes that they had never seen any stuttering Indians. Since then we have received reports, from unknown original sources, of one stuttering Indian in the state of Maine and two in the Rocky Mountain area. It has not been possible, however, to verify these reports. Over a 25-year period there have come to the University of Iowa Speech Clinic one half-breed Indian from South Dakota, who had lived almost entirely among white men, and one strange case of a full-blooded Indian, also from South Dakota, who had been educated in a mission school . . . [p. 65].

A year or so after Miss Hayes had made her preliminary study of the Indians in Idaho, the writer arranged with another of his students, John Snidecor, who was then located in that region, to continue the investigation. Professor Snidecor was to make special note of two things; the language of the Indians, and their policies and standards concerning the care and training of their children. He made a thorough investigation, interviewing several hundred Indians. He was also granted permission to appear before the chiefs and members of the tribal councils.

He learned in the main two things. First, these Indians had *no word for stuttering* in their language. In fact, when he asked whether there were any stutterers in the tribes, he had to demonstrate stuttering for the chiefs and the council members before they could understand what he was talking about. They were intensely amused by his demonstration. Second, their standards of child care and training appeared to be extraordinarily lax in comparison with our own. With respect to speech in particular, it seemed to be the case that every Indian child was regarded as a satisfactory or normal speaker, regardless of the manner in which the child spoke. Speech defects were simply not recognized. The Indian children were not criticized or evaluated on the basis of their speech, no comments were made about it, no issue was made of it. In their semantic environments there appeared to be no speech anxieties or tensions for the Indian children to interiorize, to adopt as their own. This, together with the absence of a word for stuttering in the Indians' language, constitutes the only basis on which the writer can at this time suggest an explanation for the fact that there were no stutterers among these Indians . . . [pp. 66–67].

In the preceding quotation, only speech behavior was studied. In passing, it should be mentioned that similar sets of conditions operate in the child's acquisition of responses of fear, anger, superstitions, and beliefs, and in his attitudes toward things, people, and situations in his surroundings.

IV. THE DEVELOPMENT OF HANDEDNESS PATTERNS IN YOUNG CHILDREN [3]

In the past, handedness has allegedly referred to some entity, usually considered to be inherent, which was somehow characteristic of an individual. That is, a person was said to be "naturally" right-handed or left-handed or, occasionally, ambidextrous. The following selection, quoted from a study by Hildreth, shows "handednesses," i.e., characteristic ways of performing *specific* actions with the hands, to be built up early in the individual's reactional biography.

Although the development of handedness in young children is a matter of considerable importance to parents and nursery school workers, little research on the topic has been done in the early age levels. Since hand usage habits are largely formed during the nursery years, observations during this early growth period would have the most significance for all who are responsible for early childhood training.

Most surveys of the incidence of right- and left-handedness have been based on school populations over five years of age. The results reveal

[3] HILDRETH, GERTRUDE. Manual dominance in nursery school children. *J. genet. Psychol.*, 1948, 72, 29–45. (Reproduced by permission of the author and the publisher.)

little about developmental tendencies in hand dominance, for by school age manual habits for the most frequently repeated usages are well-established. The few studies that have been made of nursery school children report observations of isolated individuals, lump together data from several age levels, or tend to report results of limited testing and observation. Sometimes preconceptions as to the origin of handedness have tended to limit observations and to bias conclusions.

Until recent years, it is true, young children have scarcely been accessible in substantial numbers for research on this subject, but with nursery schools everywhere prevalent today it is possible to undertake more comprehensive and better controlled studies.

DEGREES OF HAND DOMINANCE. Anyone who observes young children even casually realizes that there are not two distinct categories, right- and left-handedness, but that manual dominance is a matter of degree. This fact has been recognized in the studies of Durost, Heinlein, Koch, and many others. Every normal child is two-handed to some degree. In fact, most strongly right-handed people use the left more often for seldom practiced usages than they themselves realize.

"NATURAL" VERSUS "LEARNED" HANDEDNESS. Through all the years that handedness tendencies have been reported in scientific literature, the common assumption has been made that hand dominance is hereditary, a recessive trait; some people are born right-handed, some left-handed, and some are ambidextrous. Specialists in this field have admitted the difficulty of explaining "stubborn" or "fixed" left-handedness in any other way. Most of the data on which the assumption of hereditary handedness has been made have been obtained from clinical cases and older subjects with long-established hand habits.

In child training, parents and teachers, following the dictate of the experts, have tended to wait for "natural" hand dominance to appear, and then to train accordingly, encouraging right- or left-handedness, whichever seemed to be the most natural for the child. It is assumed that unless the child's "natural" dominance is discovered early and encouraged, nervous conditions and speech disorders commonly attributed to confusion from "changing-over" may arise. The belief is certainly widespread that handedness is a fixed and definite trait.

Furthermore, many persons have the impression that training, for example in eating, imposes an artificial or unnatural dominance on "natural" left-handedness. The common viewpoint is that many naturally left-handed persons become right-handed for some activities through the training they receive.

Within recent years, chiefly due to greater interest in the pre-school child, increasing evidence has suggested that handedness is a developmental trait, and that social conditioning involving many complex factors largely accounts for the emergence of hand dominance. What the child inherits is capacity to achieve dominant skill in either hand; [4] but since a right-handed bias prevails everywhere in our civilization today, the majority of people become right-handed.

All young children in infancy and the early years show considerable tendency toward both right- and left-handedness. Between seven and nine months right-handedness begins to prevail but only to a slight degree. Through the years right-handedness gains the ascendency, and left-handedness is gradually eliminated until by adulthood not more than three or four per cent of the population are left-handed for skills such as eating and writing.

Between birth and age four, manual habits are still largely in the formative stage and dominance can scarcely be considered a fixed trait.

The popular attitude toward handedness was summed up by one parent who said, "We don't believe in interfering with a three-year-old's natural handedness. Since it is largely a physical matter, we always consult our physician in these matters." Some parents guard and defend the child's first indications of left-handedness with religious zeal, considering the tendency an "Act of God" or an inborn handicap. "If you try to influence handedness you upset the child's brain," is a common belief. Parents commented of one lively infant, "She shows signs of becoming a left-hander." The idea of training the child's handedness comparable to training children to overcome their fears, to like squash, or enunciate words more distinctly is seldom entertained. Yet there is mounting evidence that children drift into handedness largely "hit and miss," and that the chance direction once taken is confirmed as a habit with continued practice. Of course, preference tends not to be shown until the child begins to gain more refined skill in the use of both his hands [pp. 29–31].

Observations were made by Hildreth on forty-four normal nursery-school children between the ages of 2 and 4 years. Behaviors observed were such as the following: eating, drinking, throwing, picking up, pulling, pushing, scratching, and so on.

---

[4] We would prefer a simpler statement here. Since the infant comes equipped with two hands, he may build up either right- or left-handed ways of doing things, depending upon his life circumstances. Does the statement, "capacity to achieve dominant skill in either hand," say anything other than that the child *does* achieve dominant skill in either hand?

These were observed so that an adequate behavior sample over 5 or 6 successive days was obtained for each child. Indices of handedness were computed on a continuous scale of +1.0 through zero to −1.0. A high positive score indicated a strong right-hand dominance; a high negative score indicated a strong left-hand dominance, and a score of, or approaching, zero indicated ambidexterity or no distinctive dominance. By this method small steps of *degree in hand dominance* could be ascertained. Among Hildreth's conclusions on the effects of training on handedness are the following:

> In all the observations that were made, those acts that are most strongly influenced by the child's parents or teachers tended to show right-handed indices. These acts were eating with spoon and fork, writing or crayoning, and to some extent throwing. Young children tend to be right-handed in the trained things, either handed in the untrained. Right-handedness appears to be learned behavior, initiated largely through the use of eating implements. Children who get an early start in right-handed eating tend to become right-handed. There tends to be more right-handedness in acts that are subject to social censure when performed with the left hand. In acts that would seem to demand comparable dexterity, for example, eating with a spoon and putting pegs in a board, young children tend to be right-handed in the former, but ambidextrous in the latter chiefly because the first is taught, the second is not . . . [p. 43].

Although all the staff of the nursery school appeared to be committed to a "hands off" policy in matters of hand dominance, certain direct and indirect training influences appeared to be at work right along. Some of the younger children had scarcely used silverware before entering the school. Teachers tended to place the spoons for the two-year-olds to the right of the bowl or within the bowl on the right side. The three- and four-year-olds found the spoon or fork on the right hand side of the plate or dish. The drinking cup and glass tended to be placed to the right or to be handed to the child toward his right side oftener than toward the left. Teachers sometimes gave uncertain children or poor eaters help by lifting the right arm, or placing the spoon in the right hand. There was never any emotional disturbance over this matter because the teachers made the suggestions in calm, matter-of-fact tones. No child was ever observed corrected for left-handed "finger feeding" though they were sometimes cautioned to use fork or spoon instead of fingers. New, incoming children sat alongside the others and watched how the others ate.

They seemed to want to imitate the teacher and to eat the right way, so as to merit approval from the teacher and other children. The social conditioning appeared to be a strong element in the whole training program . . . [p. 44].

We must point out that not all psychologists are agreed that handedness is strictly determined during the individual's life history. Some still believe in a hereditary determination or basis for handedness.

V. CHILDREN WHO WALK ON ALL FOURS

According to popular psychology, walking is just "natural." When any thought whatsoever is given to this behavior, it is assumed to be either hereditary or believed to "mature" in a manner similar to a person's "growing up." As a matter of fact, some contemporary psychologists hold this maturational view of walking.

In this connection, we present some field observations gleaned by Hrdlička,[5] an American anthropologist. The letters included are representative of the scores that were sent him from all over the United States and other lands once people knew that he was interested in this problem. Many also sent pictures of the sort shown in the figure.

In our opinion, these observations show that the particular mode of locomotion that a child develops is related to his specific life circumstances. In some instances, apparently, a child through his own individual efforts acquires a manner of locomoting on all fours. Judging from Hrdlička's book, this is more common than we have been led to believe. That humans do not continue to walk around on hands and feet as adults is undoubtedly due to the interference of parents and guardians who see to it that a more conventional manner of locomotion gets established. However, the case of Miss K. S. shows that running on all fours or "walking up" trees can occur in a rather basic manner *simultaneously with* upright locomotion (see Fig. 17). Miss K. S., 11 years old, can still, when she is so inclined, run on all fours, and climbs by "walking up the trees" [p. 69].

---

[5] HRDLIČKA, A. *Children who run on all fours.* New York: Whittlesey, 1931. Pp. 418. (Reproduced by permission of the publisher.)

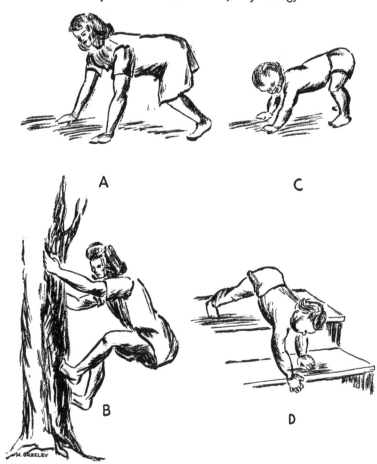

FIG. 17   Children who run on all fours. (Artist's sketch suggested by photos in Hrdlička's book by that title.) A and B show the expert quadrupedal loco-motion of Miss K. S. both on the ground and in "walking up" trees. C and D illustrate similar locomotion in infants. Walking on the level and down or upstairs is accomplished with hands flat on the ground, fingers extended, and the legs straight. Note that this is not the same as walking on hands and *knees.* (Drawn after Hrdlička, A. *Children who run on all fours.*)

The youngest child, a girl, was (and she is!) extremely active. She climbed steps, ladders, bars on doors, chairs, anything in fact before she made any effort to walk. She has gone up small trees and posts by literally walking up them ever since she was a small child. . . .

(My husband said, on reading your last note, tell him "the child climbs a tree as the Philippines go up coconut trees"; but thinking a picture better than all descriptions I am inclosing two I took of her as she climbed a tree)—M. K. S.; girl, between ten and eleven now, a former runner on all fours [p. 71].

January 28, 1928

Dear Dr. Hrdlička:

In the *Journal of the American Medical Association* of Jan. 21 I read your note regarding Children Who Run on All Fours. A nephew of my wife did this until he was about five or six years old, although he had begun to walk perfectly well at about one year of age. It was a source of considerable amusement to his family and it became a sort of game with him. I have seen him travel as much as a quarter or half a mile on all fours when he was about five years old. The sequence of hands and feet was sometimes a trot and sometimes it was much like a fox trot. I can not give many details.

I give such facts regarding the performance as are at my command: (1) race, white; (2) nationality, American for at least seven or eight generations on all sides, he is a great-grandson of Edward Hitchcock, the geologist, also a great-great-nephew of John Randolf; (3) male; (4) always healthy and robust, now 24 years old, over six feet tall, 210 pounds, powerful and active; (5) second child; (6) the gait was sometimes a square trot, sometimes a running walk or fox trot. When he was four or five years old, he would cover ground at a rate somewhat faster than a man would ordinarily walk; he never seemed to tire; (7) the hands are fully open, but I do not remember whether the whole hand touched the ground or only the fingers. I am not sure of the position of the head, but believe it was kept raised.

Yours truly,
Dr. J. B. B. [p. 143].

6

SOCIAL BEHAVIOR

I. THE SOCIAL PSYCHOLOGICAL RESPONSE
John Bucklew, Jr.

Current writers on social psychology regard it as the study of the individual living in groups or as the influence of groups upon the development of the individual. Sometimes social behavior is considered as responses made to other *people* or in a social setting. Although these conceptions satisfy the ordinary use of the word "social," they fail to isolate a distinctive subject matter for the science of social psychology. Consequently, the data usually included in the subject seem heterogeneous and badly organized. Basic to this confusion is the lingering idea, itself a reflection of popular thought, that psychology can divide behavior into hereditary and environmental categories. Thus, social psychology, as the study of the latter, has come increasingly to include a vast collection of data garnered from several fields of psychology, such as developmental and abnormal psychology, and from neighboring sciences such as sociology, anthropology, and ethnology.

It is axiomatic in science that orders of data must be distinguished as well as related. For the distinction of social psychology from its neighbors, we thus require the isolation of some type of behavior which can be studied and related to other things. As psychologists, we should keep our attention centered upon specific behavior of organisms, and as *social* psychologists, we should note how such behavior is related to those aspects of living which we call "social." If we consider psychology as an objective study of certain events occurring in nature, there exist two criteria by means of which we can isolate a subject matter for social psychology. On the side of the organism, we note whether or not the response function being performed is essentially the same as we can see other people making; in other words, whether the behavior being observed is shared by sets of people. For example, if we watch men removing their hats upon entering an elevator we may be sure we are observing conventional, or social psychological, behavior. Sets of people can be observed performing such actions, but not everyone performs them.

The second of our criteria is obtained by shifting our attention to the action of the stimulus instead of the action of the responding organism. Here we note whether or not the stimulus functions in the same way for groups of people. If so, we have isolated the counterpart of the conventional response or the conventional stimulus function. A mouse running through the living room will stimulate strong feelings of aversion, disgust, and fear among the seated company because mice have been endowed with that stimulus function in our society. A dog in the living room will not elicit comparable reactions. People have learned to accept one as a pet, but not the other, thus the two animals represent different types of institutional stimuli.

The difference between the two criteria stated above is one of emphasis only. In one case, we single out the action of the organism, in the other, the action of the stimulus. It depends upon which we are most interested in at the moment—the psychological institutions which exist at any given time or the groups of people who share certain conventional actions. Stimuli and responses, of course, are integral parts of unitary events and are separated from one another only for the purposes of convenience.

It is not possible to classify the entire behavior of the individual as social psychological in origin. Individuals may evolve personal ways of responding to things which they do not necessarily share with someone else. The behavior has not been taken over from others and, therefore, is not social psychological. Individualistic contributions of painters, writers, and others illustrate such distinctive ways of responding. Beethoven's *Fifth Symphony* is a unique affair.

The following social psychological test may serve to clarify the distinctions outlined above and at the same time will illustrate some of the outstanding characteristics of social psychological behavior. Other characteristics will be illustrated in the selections which follow. It is only because the reader possesses conventional

ways of responding to various stimuli that he is able to complete
any of the phrases or sentences listed below.

A Social Psychological Test

See if you can complete the following phrases or sentences:
1. Haste makes ———.
2. Neither rhyme nor ———.
3. You have hit the ——— on the ———.
4. I escaped by the ——— of my teeth.
5. Into each life some ——— ——— ———.
6. Revenge is ———.
7. The flower of our young ———.
8. Fools rush in where angels ——— ——— ———.
9. When a rich man becomes poor, he becomes a ———.
10. No one teaches a cat how ——— ———.

[The answers can be found at the end of this chapter, p. 159.]

The first eight of the above phrases are products of Western
European culture, and it is by virtue of membership in this cultural tradition that one is able to complete them. The last two
come, respectively, from China and Africa, and it will be only
very rarely that anyone living in this country can complete them.
The phrases are mostly artificial metaphors, but to the person
knowing them they possess a "natural," familiar sound. Some of
them are quite old, and others are comparatively recent in origin,
although the individual usually cannot tell either where or when
they originated, or at what time in his life he came into possession
of them.

All this is generally true of social psychological behavior. It
seems natural, almost inevitable, and its origin or distribution
over the world is unknown to the individual performing it unless
he is educated in such matters. Insight into the conventional nature of his behavior comes only when the individual becomes
aware of other possible ways of behaving which various groups
possess. For this reason, the study of social psychology is closely
related to, although distinct from, cultural anthropology, a science
which has undertaken the study of *groups* as such living throughout the world. The following three selections are taken from the
writings of a well-known anthropologist. They will serve to illustrate still other characteristics of conventional behavior.

II. CULTURE [1]
R. H. Lowie

If you saw a man spitting at another, you would infer that he was expressing contempt for the victim. Well, that would hold in France, but you would be all wrong if it happened in East Africa among the Jagga Negroes. There spitting is a kind of blessing in critical situations, and a medicine-man will spit four times on a patient or a newborn babe. In other words, it is not "natural" for human beings to expectorate in order to show loathing. Such symbolism is purely conventional. Raise a Frenchman in Jaggaland, and only as a well-wisher will he spit on a fellow man. Bring up a Jagga in France, and he will not dream of spitting on a baby. His behavior will depend, so far as spitting goes, on the company he keeps.

Most of us harbor the comfortable delusion that *our* way of doing things is the only sensible if not the only possible one. What is more obvious than eating three meals a day or sleeping at night? Well, in Bolivia there are Indians who think otherwise; they sleep for a few hours, get up to eat a snack, lie down for a second rest, rise for another collation, and so forth; and whenever they feel like it they do not scruple to sleep in the daytime. *We* drive on the right-hand side of the road; and what is more logical for right-handed folk? But the custom of England, Sweden, and Austria is precisely the reverse, though left-handedness is no more common there than elsewhere. But surely it is natural to point with the index finger? It is not. Many American Indians do so by pouting their lips. Again, there is nothing eternally fit about weaning a baby at nine months; among the East Africans and the Navaho of Arizona, a boy of four or five will come running to take his mother's breast.

In short, there is only one way of finding out whether any particular idea or custom is natural or only conventional, to wit, experience; and that means not our limited experience in Ottumwa, Iowa, or the United States, or even in Western civilization as a whole, but among all the peoples the world over.

Human beings generally act and think as they do for no other reason than that they have picked up such behavior and thoughts from some social group of theirs, whether family, gang, church, party, or nation. Every newborn unit of this sort is bound to invent some little tricks, badges, songs, and what not of its own. How, otherwise, would one college

---

[1] From LOWIE, R. H. *Are we civilized.* New York: Harcourt, 1929. Pp. 306. (Reproduced by permission of the author and the publisher.)

fraternity stand out from its neighbors? It's the particular Greek letters, and the pin, and the ingeniously unique way of hazing the novice, that give it individuality. Every human being belongs to a number of such social groups, some important, some trivial, from a philosophical point of view. Each group has somehow developed its peculiar style of thought and behavior and thrives on adding to its quips and cranks. Accordingly, every one of us does a vast number of things that are imposed upon him as a member of some group. The way he eats, courts, loves, fights, worships, is not his individual invention, and it is largely independent of his mental make-up. All we have to do is to place him in a new setting, and at once he follows new rules for the game of living in society. An American Negro does not speak Bantu or Sudanese, but English; he does not pray to the spirits of his dead ancestors, but takes communion in the Baptist Church. Indeed, standards change even without a change of residence. What a difference between England under Queen Bess and under Cromwell! Or, to come nearer home, what a difference between our generation and its immediate predecessor! Thirty years ago American women wore long skirts and called legs "limbs"; it is no secret that they have become less fastidious [pp. 3–5].

III. FOOD: THE STORY OF COFFEE [2]

The story of coffee is no less entertaining. The tree is indigenous to Abyssinia. The Arabs used the beverage in the fifteenth century of our era and began to spread it. However, even from Constantinople it is not reported until the following century. It reached Marseilles in 1644, but except for a few of the larger cities, France for several decades remained immune to temptation. Although Levantines and Armenians dispensed it in little shops where patrons could smoke and play cards, even Parisians failed to be interested until the Turkish ambassador who arrived in 1669 made it popular at private parties. The more pretentious cafes of modern type did not spring up until the latter part of the century. Then they rapidly turned into favorite haunts of all the upper classes of society—officers, men of letters, fine ladies and gentlemen, newsmongers, and soldiers of fortune. About the same time the coffee house became an established institution in London—an exchange for news and political opinions.

By the eighteenth century coffee was a fixture in Germany, but violent protests were heard against the new habit. Husbands complained

---

[2] *Ibid.*, pp. 36–37.

that their wives were reducing them to beggary and that many women would willingly forgo paradise if coffee were served in purgatory. At Hildesheim, a Government ordinance of 1780 admonished the people to abandon the novelty and to revert to the tried custom of their forebears: "Your fathers, German men, drank brandy and, like Frederick, the Great, were raised on beer; they were merry and of good cheer. That is what we also desire. . . . All pots, elegant cups, and common bowls . . . in short, everything that admits the epithet 'coffee,' shall be destroyed and smashed, so that its memory shall be annihilated among our fellows. Whoever shall sell (coffee) beans, shall have his whole supply confiscated. . . ."

Evidently prohibition is not an invention of the twentieth century and may be leveled against other than spirituous beverages.

IV. DRESS AND FASHION: WHITE MAN'S FASHIONS [3]

The white man's fashions are as whimsical as the Polynesian's or the Negro's. Even when a change is rational, it is dictated by chance rather than reason. In the early nineteenth century, Galton tells us, no Briton was supposed to wear a mustache unless he were a cavalry officer; otherwise "it was atrociously bad style." But during the winter of the Crimean War it would have been a hardship to make the soldiers shave every day, so their beards grew and when they returned to England the custom changed through their influence. The beard now became a token of manliness, and at last even the clergy yielded "and forthwith hair began to sprout in a thousand pulpits where it had never appeared before within the memory of man."

The eighteenth century bristles with examples of what Caucasians will do in periods of superlative refinement. Under Marie Antoinette French ladies wore headdresses so high that a short woman's chin was exactly midway between her toes and her crest. No carriages could conveniently accommodate these towers of gauze, flowers, and plumage. When the Queen added to the height of her panache in 1776, its uppermost tier had to be removed as she entered her coach and replaced when she alighted. Ladies of the court knelt on the floor of the carriage, thrusting their heads out of the window. In dancing they were always afraid of bumping into the chandeliers. The heavily powdered and padded pyramids worn on the head came to teem with vermin. Discomfort was intense,

---

[3] *Ibid.*, pp. 83–85.

but Western European genius did not abolish the fashion. Instead it invented an ivory-hooked rod and made it good taste to jab at the itching spots with it. Many American tribes forbid menstruating women to scratch themselves with their fingers; they have to use a special stick for the purpose. Thus, the powerful intellect of *Homo sapiens* succeeded in twice inventing a headscratcher. With Indians it formed part of the sacred setting of an adolescence ritual. In eighteenth century France the device was sensible enough if it proved effective—granted that powdered headdresses were indispensable. As a matter of fact, the remedy failed, but the vogue persisted. Were the French ladies more rational than their Indian sisters?

Europe had a counterpart to feminine folly. For some time past the men had been wearing wigs. Of course these would not stay on in active movement, so tennis and all violent exercises ceased to be genteel pasttimes. Wigs started as a sign of distinction. At one time it was said in England that a doctor would as soon forgo his fee as his wig. But soon the lower ranks of society began to imitate their betters. Still there were differences in style and cost, and a man of quality had a varied assortment for different occasions. Pepys in 1663 bought perukes at two and three pounds sterling, but a dress wig came to cost up to sixty. No wonder English wig manufacturers were alarmed when about 1765 smart folk began to wear their own hair again.

We are now in a position to summarize some of the prominent features of conventional behavior. These are not all the possible features that could be named, nor does every specific example display all the characteristics enumerated. But all conventional behavior will exhibit some of them.

1. The responses are distributive. They can be found in definite geographical regions. Even in so restricted a region as that represented by a small town, not all of the conventional behavior will be shared by all. Instead, there are innumerable groupings and cleavages.

2. The responses are diffusive. They may spread from one individual to another and from one region to another. The custom of coffee drinking is an example.

3. The responses are historical in origin. They arise at some definite time and place and ofttimes seem to be perpetuated by mere chance.

4. The responses are often correlated with one another. Head

scratchers were an adjunct to huge headdresses in France, and to the menstruation rituals in Indian tribes. This is one characteristic which makes conventional behavior seem so important and indispensable to the person performing it. He cannot conceive of one action being changed without changing many others, too. Whether the whole conglomerate is essential to his life usually falls beyond the scope of his understanding.

5. The responses are powerful. They tend to remain as permanent features of the individual's equipment and to resist change or modification. Consequently, changes, when they do come about, are usually accomplished in a protracted series of small steps. Resistance gives way to partial tolerance, and finally to acceptance.

6. The responses are nonrational. The person possessing them has not "thought them out" or compared them to any objective standards.

Social psychological behavior is an important item in the study of human behavior. This type of behavior can be encountered in any of the general categories of psychology, such as perceiving, feeling, reasoning, recalling, and so forth. Social psychology really cuts across the other branches of psychological science, and a proper orientation in it is essential to an adequate study of almost all other topics.

The following studies are mainly social psychological in character.

V. SUPERSTITIONS OF SCHOOL CHILDREN [4]
Rosalind M. Zapf

One of the most readily accepted objectives of science teaching today is the elimination of false beliefs and the development of scientific attitudes. In working toward this objective, it is obviously necessary to determine the degree of superstitiousness existing in a given group of pupils as well as to measure growth away from these false beliefs at a later time. Within a classroom a paper-and-pencil test is usually resorted to. The question as to whether a superstition paper-and-pencil test is a valid measure of

---

[4] ZAPF, ROSALIND M. Comparison of responses to superstitions on a written test and in actual situations. *J. educ. Res.*, 1945–1946, 39, 13–25. (Reproduced by permission of the author and the publisher.)

superstitiousness arose from the observation that an actual situation involving a superstition seemed to arouse much more emotion in a superstitious individual than did a discussion concerning the same occurrence. When responding to the situation in written form, an individual might deny belief in it while actually believing in it very strongly. It was noted that even the word, "superstition," spoken during the time that a paper-and-pencil test was being given sometimes caused a decided decrease in the number of superstitions marked as true. The realization that the statements are superstitions, which many pupils know are laughed at, had a bearing on the answers made.

Thus, it seemed possible that what the paper-and-pencil technique measured might not be the same thing as would be revealed by confronting the subjects with the situations described in it. It was for the purpose of determining the degree of consistency that might prevail between the two types of responses that this restricted study was carried out.

The *Superstition Test,* constructed by the writer, contained 140 items, 100 common superstitions, and 40 neutral items which were inserted between the superstitions. The latter had no bearing on the study and no further reference will be made to them. The term *superstition* was defined in this study as follows: "1. A disposition or tendency to ascribe phenomena which admit of a natural explanation to occult or supernatural causes. 2. An accepted belief whose falsity has been scientifically demonstrated." [5]

In order to compare paper-and-pencil responses and responses to actual situations, it was necessary to choose from the Superstition Test such superstitions as could be converted into actual situations suitable for presentation. Only the following twelve proved to be of such a nature:

1. Three is a lucky number.
2. Opening an umbrella indoors is bad luck.
3. If you spill salt, you must throw a pinch of it over your left shoulder or you will quarrel with a friend.
4. Always put your right shoe on before your left shoe, or you will have bad luck.
5. Walking under a ladder will bring bad luck.
6. See a pin, pick it up,
   All day long have good luck;
   See a pin and let it lie
   Before evening you will cry.

---

[5] WARREN, HOWARD C. *Dictionary of psychology.* Boston: Houghton Mifflin, 1934. Pp. 372. (Reproduced by permission of the author and the publisher.)

7. Horse hairs will turn into horse hair worms if put in water.
8. Breaking a mirror will bring bad luck.
9. Number 7 is a lucky number.
10. A rabbit's foot will bring good luck.
11. Make a wish while breaking a wishbone with a friend. If you get the larger piece, your wish will come true.
12. Thirteen is an unlucky number.

PUPILS STUDIED. The individuals selected for this comparative study were drawn from groups of 9A pupils tested with the written superstition test in the Cleveland Intermediate School of Detroit between September, 1938, and November, 1939. Thirty-two pupils who claimed on the written test to have no belief in the 12 superstitions listed above constituted Group I. Nineteen pupils who claimed belief in 7 or more of these superstitions made up Group II.[6] The testing was carried on at three different periods, one each semester, the experiment in actual situations following the written testing in every case by no less than one and no more than two weeks.

PROCEDURE. The rooms used for observation were two small workrooms with which the pupils were very familiar. These two rooms were connected by a door, the upper half of which was glass. This was covered by fine mesh copper screening that had been sprayed with aluminum paint, which permitted the experimenter to observe the subjects without being seen. The pupils entered the observation room from the library. While each was in the library an assistant gave the following written directions:

Go into the little room off the library. Sit down at the table. On the table is a row of boxes, each one numbered. Open each of these, starting with number 1. Read the directions on the outside and inside cover of each box. You will be all alone in the room. No one can see you at all. If the directions tell you to do anything which you do not really care to do, that is all right. Just don't do it. But do those that you don't mind doing. You will have ten minutes in which to do all that is asked of you. Watch your time. When you have finished come out the same door you went in and give your paper, without your name, to the person who gave it to you.

Each pupil was sent individually into the observation room. Upon entering he seated himself at a table set at such an angle that the observer could see clearly all that took place. On the table were 13 candy boxes,

---

[6] It was impossible to find an equal number of pupils showing belief in *all* 12 of the superstitions.

some one-pound and some two-pound size, numbered from 1 to 13 in red numerals. In addition there were on the table an umbrella, a hammer, and a dish of water. Near the table was a folding type ladder such as is used in any home.

The pupil then proceeded to open the boxes. Box 1 contained a sheet of paper on which were typed the same directions given previous to his coming into the room. The other 12 involved the 12 superstitions listed earlier. The directions printed on the inside of the cover of each of these were as follows:

BOX 2.   Many people believe that the number 3 is a lucky number. In this box is a set of 3 figures fastened together and also a set of 2 figures fastened together. If you think 3 is a lucky number, pin the set of 3 figures on your clothes and wear them while you are in this room. If you do not believe that 3 is a lucky number, wear the set of 2 figures.

The box contained a set of three small china figures of animals tied together with a red ribbon fastened to a safety pin, and a set of 2 figures fastened in the same manner to a white ribbon.

BOX 3.   There is a belief that if you open an umbrella indoors, bad luck will come to you. If you do not think this is true, open the umbrella that is on the table. If you think it is true, do not open it.

BOX. 4.   Directions on the outside of the box: Turn this box over and then open it. Directions on the inside of the box: There is a belief that if you spill salt you will have a quarrel with a friend unless you throw some of it over your left shoulder. When you opened this box you spilled some salt. If you think you may now have a quarrel with a friend because of this, throw a bit of salt over your left shoulder. If you do not believe this, close the box and go on to the next box.

The box was so arranged that in turning it over, a salt cellar, fastened to the inside of the cover of the box, poured out some of the salt which it contained.

BOX 5.   Directions on the outside of the box: Before opening this box take off your shoes. Directions on the inside of the box: There is a belief that it is bad luck to put your left shoe on first. If you do not believe this, put your left shoe on first. If you feel that this might be true, put your right shoe on first.

BOX 6.   Many people believe that if you walk under a ladder, bad luck will come to you. If you do not believe this, walk under the ladder that is in the room. If you would rather not do this, don't bother. Go on to the next box.

BOX 7.   The following verse is believed by a great many people:

See a pin and pick it up,
All day long have good luck;
See a pin and let it lie,
Before evening you will cry.

If you think this is true, pick up the pins that are on the floor at the right side of your chair and pin them on your clothes. If you don't think this is true, don't pick them up.

BOX 8. It is said that horse hairs will turn into worms if they are put in water. Here are some pieces of horse hair. If you think that they might turn into worms, try it by placing a piece in the water in the dish. If you do not think this will happen, leave the hair in the box.

BOX 9. Breaking a mirror is said to bring bad luck. If you don't believe this, take the hammer and break the mirror that is in this box. If you would rather not do this, put the mirror back in the box.

BOX 10. The number 7 is said to be a lucky number. If you think this is true, find the number 7 in this bunch of numbers and put it in your pocket for a day. If you do not think 7 is any better than any other number, take some other number.

Small pieces of cardboard on which were printed a variety of numbers were in the box. Among them were several printed with the number 7. These were on red cardboard in order to make it easier to find them.

BOX 11. A rabbit's foot is said to give you good luck. If you think this is true, hold the rabbit's foot in one hand while you write a wish on the piece of paper. If you do not think this is true, leave the rabbit's foot in the box and write the wish without holding it.

The box contained a rabbit's foot, a pencil, and a piece of paper.

BOX 12. It is said that if two people make wishes while breaking a wishbone, the one who gets the longer piece will have his wish come true. If you think this is true, take one of these wishbones with you and wish with one of your friends. If you do not think this is true, leave it in the box.

BOX 13. This is the thirteenth box. If you feel that 13 might be unlucky, do not open this box. If you do not think that 13 is unlucky open the box and follow the directions inside. If you do not open the box take your paper into the library and give it to the teacher who gave it to you.

The directions inside the box merely repeated those given on the outside concerning leaving the room.

At the time the pupil entered the observation room he was given a list of questions which he was to answer as he proceeded from box to box.

He was directed not to put his name on the sheet, thus leaving him free to answer as he wished but giving an added incentive for doing what was asked of him. Records were kept, however, by numbers so that each pupil could be identified. This pupil record sheet read as follows:

Box 2. Did you pin on the 3 figures or the 2 figures? ————.
Box 3. Did you open the umbrella? ————.
Box 4. Did you throw salt over your left shoulder? ————.
Box 5. Did you put your left or right shoe on first? ————.
Box 6. Did you walk under the ladder? ————.
Box 7. Did you pick up the pins? ————.
Box 8. Did you put the horse hairs in the water? ————.
Box 9. Did you break the mirror? ————.
Box 10. What number did you take? ————.
Box 11. Did you hold the rabbit's foot while writing your wish? ————.
Box 12. Are you taking a wishbone with you? ————.
Box 13. Did you open the thirteenth box? ————.

The observer kept a separate record sheet for each pupil on which were recorded all reactions that could be observed for every superstition tested.

Observation of the reactions of these pupils proved to be most interesting and enlightening, not to say amusing at times. None showed any awareness of being watched. A quick glance around the familiar room sufficed in most cases. None came near the screened doorway, nor in any way gave indications of suspicion in that direction. In some cases the reactions to situations were very emphatic. These were sometimes in the form of gestures, sometimes in words and sometimes in facial expressions. Any number of individuals picked up the hammer to break the mirror, apparently toyed with the idea, but finally put it down again without completing the action. One boy did not go under the ladder although he sat and looked at it for some time. Then, several minutes later, he suddenly jumped to his feet, hurried around the table, ducked under the ladder and upon coming back to his seat said, "Boy!" Another did not hold the rabbit's foot while making a wish, but walked away with it at the end of the experiment.

In some cases indecision was the most outstanding characteristic. In one case a girl took from Box 2 neither the two nor the three charms, although hesitating for some time. After Box 7, she went back and put on the three charms. After Box 8, she changed this to the two charms. A few minutes later, she took these off and finished the experiment without either. Still another wore the three charms throughout, but wrote on his paper, "Took none. I don't believe it." In some cases individuals showed great amusement at different situations. An outstanding case was a Negro boy who, upon coming to the rabbit's foot, laughed aloud, slapped his knees and clapped his hands, then took the rabbit's foot and kissed it and held it tightly in his left hand while writing his wish.

In a few instances, it was felt that interpretations of reactions by the observer were justified. In one instance, a boy, after much hesitation and handling of the umbrella, finally opened it but held it far from him, keeping his head turned away and his eyes shut. Another, upon choosing a number, quickly took the 7 and put it in his pocket, patting the pocket several times. Near the end of the experiment he stopped, then took the 7 out of his pocket, looked at it, and put it slowly back in the box. Still another wrote no wish, but held the rabbit's foot tightly to her and sat quietly for a moment with her eyes closed. In cases such as these, the interpretation was made that these pupils reacted superstitiously even though, strictly speaking, they did not respond exactly as other superstitious individuals had.

Table 2

Percentage of Pupils Responding in Various Ways to Actual
Superstitious Situations

Item	Did Not Touch			Superstitious Reaction			Nonsuperstitious Reaction		
	Group I *	Group II	Total	Group I	Group II	Total	Group I	Group II	Total
2. Number 3	21.88	10.53	17.65	12.50	52.63	27.45	65.63	36.84	54.90
3. Umbrella	0.0	0.0	0.0	12.50	63.16	31.37	87.50	36.84	68.63
4. Salt	0.0	0.0	0.0	0.0	47.37	17.65	100.00	52.63	82.35
5. Right shoe	71.88	42.11	60.78	9.38	26.32	15.69	18.75	31.58	23.53
6. Ladder	0.0	0.0	0.0	28.13	78.95	47.06	71.88	21.05	52.94
7. Pins	0.0	0.0	0.0	6.25	63.16	27.45	93.75	36.84	72.55
8. Horsehairs	0.0	0.0	0.0	21.88	47.37	31.37	78.13	52.63	68.63
9. Mirror	0.0	0.0	0.0	75.00	84.21	78.43	25.00	15.79	21.57
10. Number 7	0.0	0.0	0.0	12.50	57.89	29.41	87.50	42.10	70.59
11. Rabbit's foot	6.25	0.0	3.92	12.50	94.74	43.14	81.25	5.26	52.94
12. Wishbone	0.0	0.0	0.0	0.0	57.89	21.57	100.00	42.11	78.43
13. Number 13	3.13	5.26	3.92	6.25	15.79	9.80	90.63	78.95	86.27

* Group I, 32 pupils who claimed on the written test to have no belief in the 12 superstitions; Group II, 19 pupils who claimed belief in seven or more.

RESULTS. An examination of the responses made to the twelve situations showed that not all were equally satisfactory as measures of response to actual situations. As can be seen in Table [2], which is a summary of the observed reactions for each group, responses to items 5 and 13 are distinctly different from the rest. Item 5, the belief that it is bad luck to put your left shoe on first, was completely ignored by 60.78 percent of the pupils. They did not bother to remove their shoes at all. Item 13, the belief that the number 13 is unlucky was ignored by 3.92 percent of the pupils. In these cases the boxes were opened without even a glance at the directions on the outside of them. In addition to this, there was a non-superstitious reaction by 86.27 percent. Thus, it was felt that these two items were definitely so artificially set up that they contained practically no stimulus value and were therefore dropped in an interpretation of the results. Thus all results are on the basis of the 10 remaining superstitions. It must be acknowledged, of course, that none of the situations was natural, but they were attempts to approximate reality in an artificial setting.

An examination of the columns giving total results in Table [2] indicates that in all but one item a greater percentage of pupils showed non-superstitious reactions when facing actual situations than showed superstitious reactions. As a partial explanation of this, it must be taken into consideration that over three-fifths of the pupils had stated their disbelief in the situations involved on the paper-and-pencil test, and would therefore be expected to show fewer superstitious reactions than those who had stated that they believed them. The totals would therefore be expected to be overbalanced by those claiming not to believe these specific superstitions. A comparison of the responses of Group I and Group II on individual items proves this to be true. Group II, claiming belief in the superstitions on paper shows a much higher percentage of superstitious reactions than Group I, which claimed no belief. Conversely, under the heading, *Non-Superstitious Reactions,* Group I, claiming no belief on paper, showed a far higher percentage of non-superstitious reactions than Group II.

An interesting fact is to be noted in the column headed *Superstitious Reactions* of Group I. The superstitions causing the greatest change in response from no belief on paper to evidence of belief in actual situations, were 6, 8, and 9. In superstition 6, which is the belief that it is bad luck to walk under a ladder, 28.13 percent of the pupils did not go under the ladder despite the fact that all had claimed no belief whatever in this statement. Superstition 8, the belief that horse hairs turn into worms drew more superstitious response in the actual handling of the object than were admitted on the paper-and-pencil test, 21.88 percent, trying it out. An element of curiosity may perhaps have accounted for some of this as well as superstitiousness, however. The belief that it is bad luck to break a mirror, item 9, was by far the most stimulating of all the superstitions. In this it was found that 75.0 percent of the pupils refused to break a mirror even though they had claimed that they did not believe the superstition. It was effective as well in Group II since it is seen that 84.21 percent reacted superstitiously to it. There is the possibility that the situation was too artificial for some, accidental breakage being the real test of the superstition. For others the fear of breaking school property may have prevented them from responding as they wished. In Group II this super-stitious reaction was exceeded by item 11, the belief in the luck involved in a rabbit's foot.

The coefficient of correlation between the scores for the ten super-stitions tested by the paper-and-pencil method and the scores in actual situations was found to be .79 ± .03. Thus a fairly close relationship existed between the two types of scores.

Table 3

Distribution of 51 Pupils with Respect to Consistency of Response to Superstitions on Paper-and-Pencil Tests in Actual Situations

Percentage of Consistency	Group-I Frequency	Group-II Frequency	Total Frequency
100	2	0	2
90	14	3	17
80	9	1	10
70	3	6	9
60	2	5	7
50	2	2	4
40	0	1	1
30	0	1	1
Mean percent	81.56	65.26	75.49
Standard Deviation	11.99	15.68	15.88

A comparison was then made of the consistency between the responses made with paper and pencil and the responses made when pupils faced these same superstitions in actual situations. Table [3] presents a sum-mary of these data. The results are given in terms of percentage of con-sistency between the two types of response, that is, for example, two pupils in Group I gave the same responses in all ten situations, both on the paper-and-pencil test and in the experimental room, thus showing 100 percent consistency; 14 gave the same responses in nine situations, re-sulting in 90 percent consistency.

The range of consistency for the entire group of 51 pupils was from

30 percent to 100 percent, the mean falling at 75.49 percent, with a standard deviation of 15.88. Group I, those stating their *disbelief* on paper, showed a mean of 81.56 percent with a standard deviation of 11.99, while Group II, those stating *belief* in 7 or more of the 10 superstitions, showed a mean consistency of 65.26 percent with a standard deviation of 15.68. Thus it would seem that, within limits, the pupils expressing no belief in certain superstitions acted more in accordance with their statements than those claiming to believe in them.

A further examination of the responses of pupils who had indicated belief in 7 or more items on the paper-and-pencil test indicates an interesting point, however. The mean consistency in responses to those superstitions in which these pupils had stated *no belief* on paper, was 47.37 percent as compared with 68.15 percent consistency on items in which they had stated *belief* on paper. Among these more superstitious pupils, therefore, statements of *no belief* on paper were not as reliable as the statements of *belief*.

It must be remembered throughout this phase of the study that Groups I and II were not only small, but not equal in numbers, nor were they equated with respect to such factors as intelligence or age, although all of the pupils were in grade 9A. However, results indicate that, for the pupils tested, less consistency in response existed among pupils who claimed to believe a larger number of superstitions. Any shift in response by these pupils to the same superstition presented in two different ways may perhaps be accounted for by the greater tendency toward suggestibility existing in the superstitious group. As a result of other work on belief in superstitions, the writer found a correlation of $.50 \pm .02$ between belief in superstitions and suggestibility. Because of this it would seem reasonable to expect that on reacting to a superstition on a paper-and-pencil test, the more suggestible pupil might say that he believed it, whereas upon meeting it in an actual situation the response might easily not be the same. The reverse could be true as well, that the superstitiously inclined pupil might claim on paper not to believe a superstition, but upon meeting it in an actual situation, would, again due to his tendency to be influenced by the suggestion, react superstitiously.

A comparison was also made of the answers to the list of questions each pupil responded to before leaving the observation room with the overt responses he had actually made. Since the individual did not sign his name, he was free to answer the questions either in accord with what he had actually done, or with what he thought others would consider commendable. The result obtained by checking the sheets against the records of the observer are recorded in Table [4].

Table 4

Denials of Superstitious Actions Made by 51 Pupils on Unsigned Questionnaire

Number of Denials Made	Group-I Frequency	Group-II Frequency	Total Frequency
0	18	6	24
1	11	3	14
2	3	7	10
3	0	3	3
Total	17	26	43

From this it can be seen that 24 pupils made no denials while 27 pupils refused to admit that they had made superstitious responses, although the observer's records showed that they had. In addition, one pupil omitted answers to 5 items to which he had reacted in a superstitious manner. No one said that he had made a superstitious response when none had actually been made. It is to be expected that Group I would have a smaller number of denials since this group was the less superstitious. The conclusion might be drawn from these results that an individual, behaving superstitiously, frequently is conscious of the fact that his behavior is not entirely approved by others, and denies such behavior. This is in full accord with the ordinary reactions of individuals when the question of superstition is brought up. Among otherwise intelligent adults it is not hard to find one who claims he is not superstitious, but who secretly carries a coin when he feels it to be a lucky piece, tosses a bit of salt over his shoulder when no one is looking or "outsmarts" the black cat by turning around!

CONCLUSIONS. The responses to superstitions on a paper-and-pencil test and the responses made to the same superstitions in actual situations were consistent to the extent of 75.49 percent. Since the coefficient of correlation between the scores for the two types of response was found to be .79±.03, it would seem to indicate that the paper-and-pencil testing method is reasonably valid as a measure of superstitiousness, although it is not possible to say that it is as good a measurement in actual situations. The situation method, however, is quite impossible to use in testing any large number of pupils, nor can it be applied to more than a few superstitions. Further, it can not be made at any time stimulating enough to be anything but an artificial substitute. It would seem, from these results, therefore, that the paper-and-pencil method may be used as a measure of superstitious tendencies despite the fact that it is not completely accurate in the case of every specific superstition [pp. 13–24].

VI. VOODOO DEATH [7]
Walter B. Cannon

Anthropologists and others who have lived among primitives frequently report the death of natives who have been placed under some spell of sorcery or "black magic." Such cases have been reported from natives in South America, Africa, Australia, New Zealand, and Haiti. This phenomenon seems extraordinary and bizarre to us. The author therefore proposes to inquire whether reports of such deaths are trustworthy and, if so, to look for a possible explanation for them in terms of acceptable psychological and physiological principles.

Some of the testimony follows.

Leonard (1906) [8]

I have seen more than one hardened old Haussa soldier dying steadily and by inches because he believed himself to be bewitched; no nourishment or medicines that were given to him had the slightest effect either to check the mischief or to improve his condition in any way, and nothing was able to divert him from a fate which he considered inevitable. In the same way, and under very similar conditions, I have seen Kru-men and others die in spite of every effort that was made to save them, simply because they had made up their minds, not (as we thought at the time) to die, but that being in the clutch of malignant demons they were bound to die.

According to Tregear [9] (1890) the taboo among the Maoris of New Zealand is an awful weapon. "I have seen a strong young man die," he declares, "the same day he was tabooed; the victims die under it as though their strength ran out as water."

Dr. S. H. Lambert wrote in a letter the following report of a medical

---

[7] Adapted from CANNON, WALTER B. Voodoo death. *Amer. Anthrop.*, 1942, **44,** 169–181. (Reproduced by permission of the author and the publisher.)

[8] Adapted from LEONARD, A. G. *The lower Niger and its tribes.* London: 1906.

[9] Adapted from TREGEAR, E. *Journal of the Anthropological Institute,* 1890, **19,** 100. (Reproduced by permission of the publisher.)

doctor working on the sugar plantation of North Queensland. One day a young member of the Kanaka tribes came to him and reported that a spell had been placed on him and he would soon die. The doctor examined the man thoroughly, including an examination of the stool and the urine. Everything was normal. He was put to bed but gradually grew weaker. The next morning he died. A postmortem examination revealed nothing that could account for the fatal outcome.

In this case at least the possibility that witch doctors actually kill their victims by poisoning or some other means would seem to be ruled out.

Dr. J. B. Cleland, Professor of Pathology, at the University of Adelaide, Australia, reports on a robust native tribesman who was injured in the thigh by a spear on which a spell had been cast. The man slowly pined away and died, although the wound was only in the fleshy part of the thigh and there were no surgical complications. Cleland believes that poisoning the victim is highly improbable because the natives evidently know nothing of poisons and there are few such plants in that region.

Dr. Herbert Basedow [10] (1925) in his book, *The Australian Aboriginal,* wrote the following account of the curse placed on victims by pointing a bone at them.

The man who discovers that he is being boned by any enemy is, indeed, a pitiable sight. He stands aghast, with his eyes staring at the treacherous pointer, and with his hands lifted as though to ward off the lethal medium, which he imagines is pouring into his body. His cheeks blanch and his eyes become glassy and the expression of his face becomes horribly distorted; . . . From this time onwards he sickens and frets, refusing to eat and keeping aloof from the daily affairs of the tribe. Unless help is forthcoming in the shape of a counter-charm . . . his death is only a matter of a comparatively short time.

In general ethnologists have tended to consider it probable, on the basis of reports from many parts of the earth, that being placed under a spell may result in the death of the victim. Physiologists and physicians have tended to discredit it.

In order to evaluate the probabilities accurately, it is necessary to have some conception of what it means to a primitive to be placed under a spell. The aborigines are more ignorant and have more superstitions

---

[10] BASEDOW, H. *The Australian aboriginal.* Adelaide: 1925. (Reproduced by permission of the author and the publisher.)

than most people in our culture do. Instead of dispassionate knowledge they have fertile imaginations which fill their environment with evil forces and powers. Their fear of surroundings is partly overcome by community living. If they have the fixed assurance that some specific action, such as pointing a bone at them, will certainly result in death, and if their fellows regard them as doomed when this happens, the effect can be very profound. In some cases the victim is completely avoided by his fellows, even his relatives, and is left alone with his overpowering fear of mishap.

The question at stake is whether a prolonged state of fear can lead to death. It has been well established that emotional states can violently disrupt the ordinary workings of the organism and result in sickness. Cannon demonstrated that in decorticate cats, when the sympathico-adrenal system becomes active during "sham rage" the cat may die after four or five hours. During such activity of the sympathico-adrenal system the hair stands on end, heart rate may double, blood pressure increases, and sugar concentration in blood increases three times the normal. Various other studies indicate that a persistent and profound emotional state may induce a disastrous fall of blood pressure which results in death. Lack of food and water will help this outcome.

During war surgeons report cases of surgical shock when the soldier may die from apparently trivial wounds because of the terrifying experience connected with being wounded. One famous American surgeon even refused to operate on civilian patients who expressed a fear of the outcome, so afraid was he of the important factor of surgical shock.

Cannon suggests that "voodoo death" may be a real phenomenon explainable as due to shocking emotional stress. The known physiological changes occurring during surgical shock could be used as a check. If the victim of the voodoo spell were dying because of emotional shock the following symptoms should be present: pulse towards the end would be rapid and "thready"; skin would be cool and moist; red blood corpuscle count would be high; blood pressure would be low; blood sugar would be increased. Perhaps some witness of a "voodoo" death may some day be able to check on these changes before the victim dies.

VII. SEXUAL BEHAVIOR AND SOCIAL LEVEL [11]

Humans are members of large numbers of social groups, such as family, neighborhood, school, occupational, religious, and club groups. Within these groupings smaller sociopsychological units can be isolated, some of them involving only two individuals. Units of this sort can be isolated when two or more individuals perform a certain action in the same way, as when a father and son share a dislike for carrots, a fraternity shares certain attitudes toward a rival organization, or a squadron responds to the command, "Present arms." Clearly, a particular individual shares behaviors with a very large number of other individuals and groups.

In spite of the fact that a person has membership in such a diversity of sociopsychological units, tendencies can be demonstrated for the sharing of responses or performance of similar reactions in such general group classifications as educational level and occupational class. Kinsey, Pomeroy, and Martin have found this to be true in the case of sexual responses in the human male.

FINDINGS OF THE KINSEY STUDY WHEN GROUPS ARE CRUDELY ISOLATED ON THE BASIS OF EDUCATION OR OCCUPATION

1. TOTAL SEXUAL OUTLET. (The term "total outlet" refers to the sum of orgasms derived from various forms of sexual behavior.)

Earlier investigations have suggested possibilities for striking differences in the frequency with which sexual responses are performed between different social groups. In his sample of American males, Kinsey found that those belonging to the college level, even though not yet of college age, performed fewest sexual responses. Such differences could not be due to school conditions, since they existed at early adolescent ages when the students were in contact with members of all educational groups. To explain such differences one would have to look to the students' membership in other social groups, particularly the family.

2. FORMS OF SEXUAL OUTLET. Educational group differences also are found with reference to different forms of sexual behavior. Although Kinsey found masturbation appearing in nearly all male

---

[11] KINSEY, A. C., POMEROY, W. B., & MARTIN, C. E. *Sexual behavior in the human male.* Philadelphia: Saunders, 1948. Pp. 804. (Reproduced by permission of the authors and the publisher.)

histories, it was reported most often by college-level males and least frequently by males not going beyond the eighth grade (see Figure 18). Similar but more striking differences were found with regard to nocturnal emissions (differences in imaginative behavior and in the range of objects that operate as sexual stimuli probably are involved here) and to heterosexual petting. The results obtained for educational groups were consistent with a

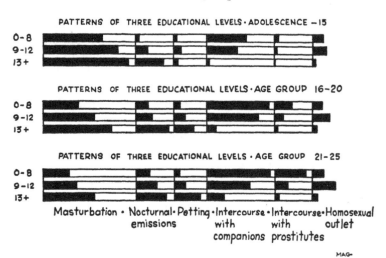

PATTERNS OF THREE EDUCATIONAL LEVELS·ADOLESCENCE —15

0-8
9-12
13+

PATTERNS OF THREE EDUCATIONAL LEVELS·AGE GROUP 16-20

0-8
9-12
13+

PATTERNS OF THREE EDUCATIONAL LEVELS·AGE GROUP 21-25

0-8
9-12
13+

Masturbation · Nocturnal· Petting ·Intercourse · Intercourse·Homosexual
emissions   with   with   outlet
                    companions prostitutes

MAG·

FIG. 18 Patterns of sexual behavior at three educational levels, among single males for 3 age groups. Each horizontal line extending across the page summarizes the pattern for one of the educational levels. Relative lengths of bars in each outlet show average mean frequencies for the group. The scales vary for different sources of outlet, but there is an approximate indication of the relative importance of each source in total outlet. (Kinsey, A. C. & Pomeroy, W. B. & Martin, C. E., *Sexual behavior in the human male.*)

distribution of the subjects on the basis of occupational level. Masturbation, for example, occurred most often in the professional group.

The frequencies with which different educational and occupational groups of males engage in premarital intercourse differs markedly from the above. Such forms of behavior are infrequently performed by members of the college group and by upper occupational groups. About 85 per cent of the grade-school sample (age 16 to 20 years) report this behavior, and it constitutes about 60 per cent of their total sexual outlet, while only about 40 per cent of the college group engage in premarital intercourse, and usually this occurs infrequently, accounting for only 11 per cent of the total sexual outlet of this group. Apparently, differences in ideals or moral standards as absorbed from their respective groups accounts for this behavioral difference.

These findings suggest striking differences in the culturalization to be found with regard to sexual responses, and they are consistent with the discovery that in the early adult years extramarital intercourse occurs with relative infrequency among the higher occupational- and educational-group males as compared with the lower groups.

Rather marked educational-group differences were found concerning homosexual responses. These responses were found most frequently among single males in the high-school group, approximately 55 per cent of the sample reporting one or more homosexual experiences, while such behaviors accounted for 10 to 25 per cent of the total sexual outlet of the group. In contrast, only 40 per cent of single males in the college group reported such experiences, and these were rarely more than occasional contacts, accounting for very little of the total sexual outlet of the group.

It has long been known that sexual contacts occur between human and infrahuman animals. Occasional enterprises of this sort are conventional in some adolescent groups. Further, the attitudes of different societies toward this sort of sexual behavior have varied greatly. For example, in thirteenth-century Sweden, it appears that animal contacts were regarded as offenses against the owners of the animals, and the owners were entitled to compensation. In other groups, it has been ridiculed, and the person committing the act has been viewed as unable to compete with other males for the favors of the women of the community. In still other societies, no discrimination may be made between human and infrahuman sex partners.

For obvious reasons, animal contacts in the United States are most frequently found in rural areas. Only rarely, however, are these more than occasional contacts. Among none of the educational groups does animal contact account for an appreciable amount of total sexual outlet.

3. STIMULI FOR SEXUAL RESPONSES. The objects and conditions which operate as sexual stimuli vary with different educational groups, e.g., males of the upper educational levels are most fre-

quently stimulated sexually through daydreaming or imagination, by visual contacts with females, burlesque shows and pictures, by obscene stories, by erotic literature and love stories in "good literature," by movies, and by animals in coitus. The reading of erotic literature is limited principally to the upper educational groups. Clearly, sexual responses in these groups have become conditioned to many and diverse stimuli.

Such a range of sexual stimuli is less common with males of the lower educational groups. Actual contact is the most prominent sexual stimulus for these males. The basic development of these different culturalizations in sexual behaviors lies primarily in the complexities of behavioral evolution in the family situation.

4. ATTITUDES CONCERNING SEX. The artificial and arbitrary characteristics of cultural actions are excellently exemplified by the variety of attitudes found toward sex.

Consider masturbation. Attitudes toward this form of sexual behavior vary among cultural groups from the one extreme of considering it immoral, abnormal, and conducive to deterioration and insanity to the other extreme of considering it a desirable form of sexual activity. For instance, among some human groups over the world as well as certain sociopsychological units in the United States, masturbation of the infant is used as a form of play or to sooth the infant, while among other groups such activities would not be tolerated.

Kissing shows many cultural differences. In some ethnic groups it is unknown, in others it is regarded as disgusting, while in some groups kissing is elaborate and extensive. In some groups one finds in place of kissing the biting of the neck, lips, cheeks, or eyelashes. Within the United States extreme variation in kissing is also found. Note that members of upper educational levels may be disgusted by the common drinking cup but consider certain forms of kissing an essential part of their sexual behavior. Individuals from "across the tracks" may not be disturbed by the unsanitary nature of the common drinking cup but may be shocked and revolted by such kissing. As a matter of fact, kissing (in any form) may be considered improper. Nowhere is the arbitrary nature of conventional behavior better illustrated than here.

Attitudes toward premarital intercourse also tend to differ with various educational groups. Moral objections are rather infrequent among males of lower educational groups but are offered by more than half the males of the college-level group in the Kinsey report. Also more males of upper educational levels tend to be fearful of public opinion regarding premarital relations. Attitudes with regard to nudity and manual and oral stimulation also tend to differ with educational levels.

Although a sociological grouping on the basis of educational level or occupational class is extremely rough and individuals may be members of many sociopsychological units in various levels, it is apparent that the way of behaving sexually that an individual acquires is primarily a function of the persons which whom he is reared. This is illustrated in Fig. 18 summarizing some of the findings here discussed from the Kinsey report.

VIII. CULTURAL FACTORS IN GESTURE

Efron [12] has been interested in discovering possible differences in the gestures of people belonging to different cultural groups. More specifically, he made a comparative study of Eastern Jewish and Southern Italian immigrants and their descendants in New York City. Thus, he had "traditional" Jews and Italians on the one hand and "assimilated" or Americanized Jews and Italians on the other.

The study utilized direct observations of people in spontaneous everyday situations, 2,000 sketches of gestures by an artist, a count of the number and kinds of gestures per unit time, and an analysis of approximately 5,000 feet of motion-picture film, through observations and judgments of naïve observers, and through graphs and charts derived from projecting the separate frames on coordinate paper. The subjects observed consisted of 850 traditional Jews, 700 traditional Italians, 600 assimilated Jews, and 400 assimilated Italians. None of the subjects realized that he was being observed.

The observations were made at the following places: traditional Jews in the lower East Side parks, markets, streets, synagogues, restaurants, homes, and social meetings; traditional Italians in the parks, markets, restaurants, homes, social meetings, and public games of "Little Italy" and Southern Italian meetings at the Teatro Venezia. Assimilated Jews were observed in the sum-

[12] EFRON, D. *Gesture and environment.* New York: Columbia University Press, 1944. Pp. 184. (Reproduced by permission of the author and the publisher.)

mer resorts of the Adirondacks and Catskills, Saratoga race track and hotels, Columbia University (both faculty and students), Temple Emanu-El, other schools, homes, and social and political gatherings. Assimilated Italians were studied at Columbia University, Casa Italiana, gatherings of Italian-American societies, homes, and fraternity and political meetings.

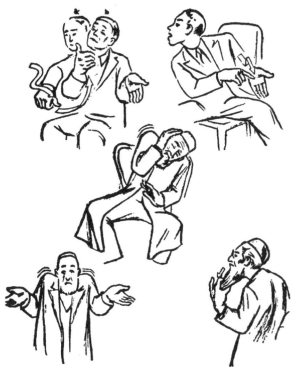

FIG. 19   Characteristic gestures of Ghetto Jews. (Efron, D., *Gesture and environment.*)

RESULTS

TRADITIONAL JEWS. The "Ghetto Jews" showed a type of gesture that was much more restricted in radius than that of Southern Italians. The gestures of the former seemed to take place within the immediate area of the speaker's chest and face, hardly ever going beyond the limit of head or hips. Nor was the upper arm of the Jew very active in gesturing, being mostly rigid and attached to the side with the axis of gestural motion centering at the elbow or wrist. In general, Jewish gestures were more complex than those of other groups, showing sudden changes in direction or plane. Head gestures, too, which were common here, were almost absent among Italians. Another distinctive characteristic showed itself in group conversations during which traditional Jews tended to huddle in compact groups. This, as well as simultaneous gesturing of two or more individuals and gesturing with objects, was not in evidence among traditional Italians (see illustrations).

"FAMILIARITY" WITH THE PHYSICAL PERSON OF THE INTERLOCUTOR. "Traditional" Eastern Jews quite often touch the body of their conversational partner. This is done either as a means of interrupting his discourse, or in the way of capturing his attention. In the course of our exploration of the swarming streets of the lower East Side, we soon became accustomed to the idea of seeing a person firmly grasping the coat lapel of his companion with one hand, while the other was describing all kinds of arabesques in the immediate vicinity of his nose. No less frequent was the spectacle of an individual seizing the wrist of his opponent, or boring with the index finger through the buttonhole of his coat. Pulling or shaking the body of the conversational adversary are also habitual procedures in the gesture technique of the ghetto Jew.

The most current phenomenon is that of grasping the arm of the interlocutor, and its extreme case makes itself apparent, in a rather ludicrous way, when the two participants in the gestural fencing become clamped to each other's hands or coat lapels, and fight out the battle by means of head motions only. One of the most curious examples of what one might call gestural "promiscuity" in conversation is a case in which the speaker (or to be exact, *one* of the speakers, for the two interlocutors were enthusiastically talking and gesturing at the same time), not only grasped the arm of his impatient opponent, but *actually gesticulated with it!* The latter was admonishing the former, who seemed to be quite annoyed by the didactic gesture of his friend. The victim tried a few times to stop his movement by doing the same thing, but apparently to no avail. Finally, he seized the other's wrist, and started admonishing him back with his own (the companion's) hand. This situation is illustrated by figure [20c].

We have never seen anything of the kind in the American (whether Anglo-Saxon or Jewish) or the Italian (whether "traditional" or "as-

similated"). The latter, for example, when wishing to attract the attention of his opponent, very rarely takes possession of his wearing apparel or his hand, but is likely to raise his index finger in front of his
face or chest, or make some other sign of notice [p. 65].

"TRADITIONAL" ITALIANS. The spatial confinement of the Jewish gesture was not observed in the gesticulating of immigrant
Italians, whose motions were of wide amplitude extending from
above the head to down below the knees in a sweep that coincided
with the full stretch of the arm. Occasionally, the body would be
bent so as to supplement the extent of the gesture. Thus, Italians
take in all the space at their command.

Elbow and wrist movements were seen only rarely. Instead,
the majority of gestural motions was performed with the shoulder
as the axis. Furthermore, Italian gestures were less complex in
form than those of the ghetto Jew. Broad elliptical and arched
gestures were preponderant, as compared with the Jewish restricted sinuous ones. In contrast to ghetto Jews, traditional Italians tended to bring both arms into simultaneous play (twin
gestures), showed a more even and rhythmic tempo as if accentu-
ating their speech, and failed to show "familiarity" with the person of the listener, the dual gestural monologues of Jews, and their
huddling or "turtlelike" head gestures. When broad gestures occurred, they were performed "solo" and there was a goodly space
between.

AMERICANIZED JEWS AND ITALIANS. These can be treated together because they resemble each other in that they both showed
a similarity to the gestures "characteristic of the average American,
namely, expository, indicative, and pictorial patterns of movement, using them with great freedom and abandon" [p. 110].
There was little similarity to gestures of their corresponding traditional groups.

For example, in describing the gestures of "Jewish" students
at Temple Emanu-El who have only a denominational identification with other Jewish groups and who show a high degree of as-
similation to their American environment, Efron writes:

Their gestural behavior, or rather, its absence, appears to be a
reflection of their socio-economic status. None of the tendencies found
among ghetto Jews have been observed by us among the Temple
Emanu-El youngsters. In fact, *they just do not gesticulate*. Only once in

a while one of them may be seen performing a restrained, expository, or didactical gesture, ceremonious in its form and somehow "conceited" in its quality. The general impression we have drawn from our observations and interrogations is that their conversational gestures are in-

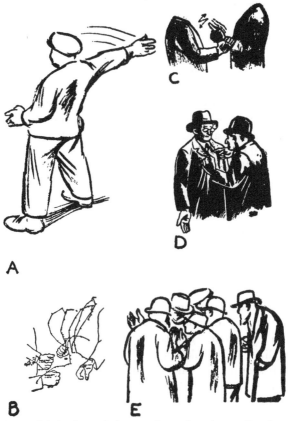

FIG. 20 Gestural behaviors of the members of various cultural groups. A, Traditional Italian: wide gestural radius; movement from shoulder. B, C, and D, Ghetto Jews: observed on Rivington Street, lower East Side, New York. Gesticulation with the arm of the interlocutor. E, Ghetto Jews crowding in conversation. (Efron, D., *Gesture and environment*.)

hibited by the social norms of their "good society." In this, we think, they do not differ much from any of the other "elites" in America (whether of Anglo-Saxon, Jewish, or any other origin) among whom gesture is considered a "bad habit" of "common people," and is controlled by education and social censure [p. 124].

The difference between the gestural behavior of ghetto Jews and that of the above mentioned Americanized Jewish individuals (in this case, almost complete absence of movement) raises a great doubt as to the validity of the theory, according to which Jews are "racially" inclined to gestural movement in conversation [p. 125].

Efron made one other interesting observation to the effect that some individuals gesticulated with combinations of gestural elements common to both American and traditional Italian or Jewish groups. These were people who had only partially broken away from the mores of the corresponding "traditional" groups. Efron called this a "hybrid" gesture.

SIGNIFICANCE OF EFRON'S STUDY. In our opinion, this study shows clearly that an individual's gestural behavior is very definitely related to that of the group in which he is reared. Efron believes that it disproves the alleged inbornness of reactions which are coming to be more and more attributed to culturalization. It appears that an individual reared in the ghetto or Southern Italy is psychologically different from one reared in America, or, more specifically, New York.

IX. *FOLIE À DEUX*

By this time the student must realize that an individual learns to chew gum or smoke opium as the result of a psychological membership in a particular group. He acquires the language, praying behavior, likes and dislikes, and beliefs of his associates.

When groups are widely distributed in the manner of English-speaking, Mohammedan, Christian, or Buddhist communities, the individual within that group performs behavior which adapts him to a widely disseminated environment. But culturalization may be restricted to minority groups such as nudist colonies or societies of conscientious objectors. In such cases, the resulting uniform behavior of the minority group is at variance with the action approved by the larger group and may lead to conflict. Separationists and dissenters who start their own schools or religious organizations are examples.

Still smaller cultural bodies may develop behaviors which are so peculiar and specific that no one else can accommodate himself to them, or vice versa. "Twin language" illustrates the point well.

Twins that play intimately in isolation from others sometimes develop a highly individualistic language, imaginative behavior, and other reactions. However, not only twins but any two individuals may evolve behaviors in common, i.e., shared reactions.

Just as a mother on a lonely farm may culturalize an only child to behave like others of the group which culturalized her, so may pathological individuals cause others to acquire delusions and hallucinations which, in this case, only the two persons share in common. Nevertheless, the technique is essentially that of culturalization in which one person succeeds in getting another to act like himself. Some authors have named this situation *imposed* or *communicated psychosis*. The French name, *folie à deux*, is particularly appropriate inasmuch as it suggests that just as one may have tea-for-two, so one may also have insanity-for-two. Of course, there are also *folie à trois, quatre, cinq,* and so on. The following cases are mostly of the *folie à deux* variety.

REPORT OF CASES [13]

CASES 1 AND 2—E. S. AND H. S. Two sisters who present an identical psychosis. Little information has been obtained concerning their early life except that they were always said to have been peculiar. There is a difference of about 10 years in their ages, the older being about 50 years of age. Not much is known concerning their conduct before admission to a state hospital except that the janitress in the house in which they lived said she had known them six years, that they never visited with other tenants in the house and scarcely answered their greetings of the day. They dressed in a very fantastic manner, and at times talked about their imaginary ideas. They were admitted to a state hospital in 1923 and were found to have a very bizarre trend of thought to which they have constantly adhered during their hospital residence since that time. They believed they were made by a machine which they referred to sometimes as "it" and sometimes as "he." Each one said that neither she nor her sister were ever born, but that both had lived for thousands of years. They felt very sure that all their activities were controlled by this machine and that they would never die. Their only explanation for admission to the hospital was that they lost contact with the machine for some reason which was unknown to them, but when they re-established contact with it their difficulties would be solved.

---

[13] GROVER, M. M. A study of cases of *folie à deux. Amer. J. Psychiat.*, 1937, 93, 1045-1062. (Reproduced by permission of the author and the publisher.)

During all these years they have both clung very tenaciously to the ideas expressed. When any attempt was made to obtain any information from them concerning their past life, they invariably reverted to their ideas about the machine as given above. They spent a large part of their time doing art work in the occupational therapy class and when not thus engaged sat together conversing in a very low tone of voice, always making sure that no one around them heard what they said. When interviewed together, the older sister took the lead in the conversation, the younger quickly agreeing to her statements. When interviewed separately, they expressed the same trends.

These patients were separated in the institution at times, but were so much depressed by separation and the one seemed to depend to such a great extent on the other that separation was not continued. During the periods that they were apart, there was no change in either as regards the false beliefs which they held. The older, more dominant, sister died about a year ago. Since that time there has been no change whatsoever in the younger sister. She sticks very tenaciously to the ideas she expressed when they were together. She insists the sister is not dead but that she has gone away.

It is interesting to note that the dominant sister was more masculine in her physical development than the other. Her pelvis was narrower and she had a much lower pitched voice. In fact if one did not see her one could well imagine her voice to be that of a man.

CASES 3 AND 4—TWO SISTERS C. R. AND E. R., AGES 50 AND 55. They have been together practically all their lives, there being only short periods in which they were separated. In these patients there was a very strong hereditary background for mental disease [?]. There was a history that the mother had a mental breakdown on two occasions and an older sister is now in a mental institution. In these cases there was considerable difference in their personality make-up. The elder sister was a very sensitive stubborn person, making few friends and living within herself. At no time was she a good mixer. The younger more dominant sister, though very sensitive and easily offended, was a well-liked girl, good mixer, is said to have had many friends and admirers, was happy, cheerful, and optimistic. There has always been a very strong attachment between these two sisters. The one has depended very largely on the other and they are much grieved when separated. Both had good educational opportunities but were not of the studious type and neither secured a good education. The younger sister was admitted to a sanitarium in 1919 where she remained about six weeks and made a temporary improvement. The physician in charge of the sanitarium said that at the time of the younger sister's residence in the institution, he saw the older sister who was also definitely abnormal and under the influence of the younger's delusional trend; that she was the weaker of the two and of a much more submissive personality make-up. He further says: "I am not surprised that they are both in an institution, a typical example of insanity in two." These patients did not get along well with their relatives, and soon after the death of the mother brought suit against the executors of the estate. During the litigation it was discovered that they were definitely abnormal with paranoid trends. They both developed paranoid ideas against the judge and also against several attorneys whom they secured to take charge of the litigation. They became very annoying to the judge and called him frequently on the telephone and went frequently to his office. Not much is known concerning them after this litigation until they came to New York City in the fall of 1929 where their conduct at the hotel was considered devilish. They complained to the manager that they feared someone was trying to harm them. They were, at times, heard to make peculiar moans and groans in their room.

On admission to the hospital they talked about their troubles in the courts for the past ten years and that a certain lawyer in Louisville, Kentucky, had taken advantage of them and was trying to steal their money. They thought the physicians were their enemies and were constantly harping about persecution they received at the hands of lawyers in Louisville and also the judge. At times both of them have expressed ideas concerning interference with their minds. One sister said that the judge hypnotized her and kissed her while under his influence. They remained very suspicious and very guarded in their statements.

Observers of cases of *folie à deux* have expressed the opinion that a younger person is more likely to accept the delusions of the older one than for the reverse to occur. However, in the above cases it is evident that the older sister was dominated by the younger and took up the delusional ideas of the younger sister.

CASES 5 AND 6—TWO SISTERS, N. B. AND E. L.   Not much is known concerning their family history or early personal history. There is a difference in their ages of two years, the younger being 65 and the older 67. They came to this country from Ireland 46 years ago and apparently have rarely been separated since that time. The younger sister was married about 30 years ago and lived with her husband for a number of years, but the older sister to whom she is very much attached lived with her during that period. The younger sister is the more dominant one and is apparently the one who has transmitted her psychotic trends to the older sister. The first information we have concerning them is that they were sent to the magistrate's court for non-payment of rent. They were said to be well-known in the Municipal Lodging House and had attacked a physician there.

On admission the younger sister expressed numerous delusions of persecution and auditory hallucinations which had apparently controlled her behavior for the last 15 years. She admitted hearing voices and said they sounded like angel voices. She expressed other persecutory ideas and ideas of a religious character which were fantastic and absurd. The older sister, who was the less dominant one, expressed many persecutory ideas which, while not exactly the same, were very similar to those of the younger, more dominant, sister. The impression the physician received who examined her on admission to a state hospital was that her ideas originated with the other sister whose delusions of persecution she very largely accepted. These patients spent much time together. The younger sister was more aggressive and domineering. While interviewed separately, the older sister did not express as many absurd ideas as the other. However, when they were together, the older sister acquiesced in what the younger said and agreed with everything.

As in the other cases, the younger sister was the more dominant one and is apparently the one who transmitted her psychotic trends to the older sister.

CASES 7, 8, AND 9—M. MK., R. M. MK., AND M. MK.   In these cases we have a mother and two daughters who came to the hospital at the same time. The mother's age is 70, the elder daughter 29 and the younger 26. Little is known concerning the family history. The mother has been a widow for seven years and during that time the daughters have lived with her. The mother has always held aloof from others. When the daughters were children, she refused to allow them to play with other children and as they grew up she kept them very close to home. The mother apparently exercised a strong influence over them, was in constant touch with them, and did not want them out of her sight. The daughters were never interested in the opposite sex and made no social contacts.

All three developed the idea that the mother's brother did not interest himself in them because of the influence of his wife. Later they developed the idea that her brother's wife was bothering them because she was jealous of them. They thought that she would ring the bell of their apartment and would look through the keyhole and was often around their home. They finally had the wife of the mother's brother arrested, but the judge gave them a lecture and threw the case out of court. The morning before they were sent to the hospital, they got up at 3 o'clock, saying the house had been electrified and that someone was going to kill them. *All three shared this belief.* The younger daughter expressed the most active trends and hallucinations which were later taken up by the mother and sister. This same sister began to say that she could hear Rudy Vallee, Mary Pickford, and other movie stars performing over some kind of machine, either radio or dictaphone. The next day the other daughter began to say she could hear the same voices quite distinctly. The mother accepted the belief and when interviewed says, "Of course I believe it. There is no doubt about it." She admitted that on one or two occasions she heard a voice through a machine but was unable to tell just what it said. The mother and elder daughter say they have not actually heard voices since coming to the hospital but the other daughter continues to hear them. They both believe that they heard voices before coming here and can see nothing absurd in the fact that the voices came through the air over some invisible machine.

We have in these cases, a mother and two daughters who have lived together intimately, having excluded practically all outside interests. Psychotic ideas developed at practically the same time. The younger daughter was a little more actively psychotic but her delusional ideas and hallucinations were at once taken up by the mother and sister [pp. 1046–1049].

X. CONTINGENTIAL RESPONSES
John Bucklew, Jr.

Of the behavioral forms characteristic of the societal or mature stage of behavioral acquisition, the contingential response stands in decided contrast to the idiosyncratic and social psychological responses. With the first of these, it shares the characteristic of being noncultural; it differs from both by being a temporary adjustment which forms no permanent part of the individual's behavior. The momentary nature of contingential action derives principally from the fact that it is above all a product of unique, complex stimulus situations for which the individual has no suitable behavioral equipment. If the person is going to adapt at all, it must be through some novel mode of behaving which he has never performed before. This does not mean that the adjustment of the response will be completely novel or different, for few responses would be of that nature, but it does mean that the total behavioral segment contains elements which cause it to vary decidedly from previous responses.

The existence and character of these adaptations depend mainly upon the intricate circumstances with which the person is more or less suddenly faced. In describing them, the emphasis must be placed upon the stimulus situation of the moment rather than the reactional equipment which the individual possesses. This feature, along with their temporary character, distinguishes them from the idiosyncratic response. Probably all complex stimulus situations contain an element of novelty in them, since the circumstances of living rarely repeat themselves exactly, and so, in a sense, all behavior displays some contingentiality. However, in the majority of cases, the individual's behavioral equipment is quite adequate to the occasion. It is only when the element of novelty is large that the necessity for contingential behavior emerges.

Contingential behavior can be illustrated from nearly all areas of life. The quality of "spontaneity" which we notice in our friends consists largely of contingential action. In various sports, contingential behavior may be observed most strikingly. No matter how thoroughly the athlete may have built up his reactional equipment, he cannot expect to be prepared for all the emergencies of athletic contests. In the heat of the fray, he may even "surprise himself" in the adroitness with which he solves some emergency of the game. The intricate interplay of conversational art furnishes another example of contingential adaptations. We are delighted with the wit of the guest whose remarks are uniquely derived from the circumstances of the moment, and perhaps equally bored with the individual whose humor is the repetition of conventional jokes or remarks. In the practical affairs of life, we may be amazed at the cleverness of the mechanic who can devise novel methods of repairing a faltering engine.

The give and take of life requires that all organisms be able to perform contingential action; otherwise, they could hardly survive. Nevertheless, it is sometimes difficult to do so. Idiosyncratic and contingential behavior both thrive best when the person is not too dominated by conventional modes of responding. We all tend to cherish the notion that we are capable of acting individually and uniquely if the occasion requires, but the history of human behavior indicates that this is not so true as we might want to think. The accompanying photograph illustrates one such occasion in which Americans evidently were unable to behave in new ways, although the process of removing the coconut husk, once observed, is relatively simple to repeat.

XI. IDIOSYNCRATIC BEHAVIOR
N. H. Pronko

The preceding article on contingential responses indicates that the organism is not merely a mirror image of *all* the responses performed by members of his group. Behavioral development and the conditions of behavioral performance are so complex for each individual that, psychologically speaking, he may stray from his culture.

As a matter of fact, everybody shows development of reactions which no one else in his group shares with him. Many of one's likes and dislikes and attitudes toward others or himself (such as the so-called "inferiority complex") are not acquired in the same way as are his language, manners, customs, or dress behaviors, inasmuch as the former are built up as the result of the individual's *own* contact with such stimulus objects.

The reader will recall that cultural reactions always originate from contact with another person or persons; not so with idiosyncratic behaviors. On the contrary, these responses evolve in the individual's *solitary* experience with things. While on a walk through the desert, *A* handles a Gila monster and learns more effectively than he would through social instruction that such animals are to be avoided if one is to escape the discomfort of their bite. Creative behavior of all sorts also comes under this class of action.

The highest degree of idiosyncracy may be illustrated by such a composition as a poem, novel, painting, symphony, or invention. Note that not one other person in the world has contrived

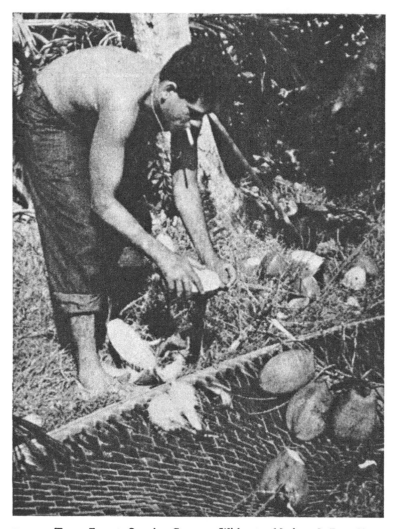

FIG. 21   To an Expert, Opening Coconuts Without a Machete Is Easy. Navy annals record cases of wartime castaways going hungry because they did not know the simple technique demonstrated here. Goniske pries off the tough husk in strips by thrusting the nut downward against a hard sharpened stick anchored in the ground. Courtesy of the National Geographic Magazine.

this same arrangement, so highly individualistic is the behavior involved in its creation. While it is true that inventions or theories may have been announced by individuals in different parts of the world simultaneously, nevertheless this is no exception to the rule that these are solitarily developed. The formulations of the theory of evolution by Darwin and Wallace simultaneously but *independently* is a case in point.

Nor must we be confused by the fact that the component reactions out of which idiosyncratic responses evolve are culturally derived. Obviously, Beethoven was instructed to read and to combine notes in accordance with the instruction prevalent in his culture. Undoubtedly, without such culturalization there would not have been a *Fifth Symphony,* but the important point is that no one instructed him how to write this composition. It resulted only from his individual, *solitary* interactions with paper, pen, musical instruments, and so on.

Pathological reactions are an attention-compelling form of idiosyncratic response, although it is true that these personality characteristics may be group-acquired, as illustrated by the cases of *folie à deux* discussed in this chapter. Many, however, are individually acquired; for instance, such beliefs as that of the patient who thinks he has a glass stomach or that his brain is decaying fall in this category. Included here is the strange ritual which another patient practices. The gestural activity and posturing of still another also belong under the class of idiosyncratic action. When the person becomes very desocialized, he often develops individualistic modes of speaking (neologisms) which are *unique* to the patient and, therefore, cease to function in a communicative way to the hearer.

Answers to Social Psychological Test

1. Haste makes waste (English proverb).
2. Neither rhyme nor reason (Shakespeare, *As You Like It*).
3. You have hit the nail on the head (Rabelais, 1495–1553).
4. I escaped by the skin of my teeth (The Bible).
5. Into each life some rain must fall (Longfellow, 1807–1882).
6. Revenge is sweet (Byron, 1788–1824).
7. The flower of our young manhood (Sophocles, 496–406 b.c.).
8. Fools rush in where angels fear to tread (Pope, 1688–1744).
9. When a rich man becomes poor, he becomes a teacher (Chinese proverb).
10. No one teaches a cat how to steal (Proverb of the Ashanti tribe).

7

PERSONALITY

I. WHAT IS PERSONALITY?
N. H. Pronko

Through the ages, personality has been elusive and difficult to define. Even today, psychologists are not in complete agreement on their interpretation of personality. We shall here consider some of the main types of definition.

PERSONALITY AS AN EFFECT ON OTHERS. One class of personality explanations is in terms of the way people affect others, i.e., their social stimulus value. Obviously, according to such a definition, a person would have as many personalities as he had different effects on people. Conversely, the hermit living alone and affecting no one would, by this criterion, have no personality, which reduces to an absurdity.

POPULAR PSYCHOLOGY'S NOTION OF PERSONALITY. Personality is even more fuzzy and evanescent according to popular psychology which conceives it to be some sort of mystical, inner entity. The person is thought to have within him an entity of some sort that effuses "charm," "perversity," "magnetism," and so on. According to such theories, personality is a will-o'-the-wisp—an imaginary quality or aspect of people—something allegedly apart from behavior yet somehow determining it. It is hardly necessary to point out that such theories, rather than facilitating the understanding of personality, actually succeed in obscuring it.

PERSONALITY AS ACTION. The writer would suggest that, from a psychological viewpoint, the term "personality" can only refer to behavior or stimulus-response units because that is all that there is to study. "That's all there is; there is no more." But how many of these reactions shall we include? It must be apparent that we cannot stop short of the inclusion of all—every single reaction belonging to a given individual.

PERSONALITY MUST BE DATED. At this point, the reader may intrude to ask how could we possibly list all of an individual's responses since the performance of behavior goes on to the moment of death? The answer is that a personality inventory in the terms framed here would be a never-ending job. No sooner have you listed the last behavior that you observed than you have more to list that occurred during your listing. So let it be. However, there is no theoretical difficulty in such a procedure, only a practical one. These facts also show the dynamic character of personality as viewed from the framework suggested here. Apparently, personality is a "going concern"; it must, therefore, be *dated.* Thus, it follows that John Doe's personality as of June 6 is not the same as it is June 8. How striking such "personality changes" may be is illustrated by instances of religious conversion, the ethical and moral shifts of the soldier (compared before induction, during the war, and after his return to peaceful pursuits), and the behavioral changes in individuals under stress. The time element in personality study is of utmost importance, then, and we must take it into account in our interpretational scheme. Consequently, it is scientifically crude to refer to the dynamic, changing patterns of behavior constituting personality by such conventional labels as Jane Doe. Although from a social, legal, or even anatomic viewpoint an individual may be treated as identical with himself over long stretches of time, this does not follow in a psychological study where such notations as the following are more appropriate: Jane Doe$_x$, Tuesday, 10:25 A.M.; Jane Doe$_y$, Tuesday, 6:30 P.M., and so forth.

PERSONALITY AS A SYSTEM OF REACTIONS. Another aspect of personality soon looms up in our study, namely, that the total series of reactions that constitute the individual's behavioral equipment is not helter-skelter or hodgepodge. On the contrary, each person's behaviors constitute a certain organization, coherence, or order. They fall into some sort of pattern or system.

The term "system" is just as applicable to personality as it is to the solar system, a bookkeeping system, irrigation system, or nervous system. Let us call attention to a fact about the interrelationship of the behavior composing the personality of a particular individual. It is not chaotic. A person does not ordinarily dance one moment, then pray, eat, jump, swear, or cry during succeeding moments. He does not speak English through a part of a sentence, then shift into German, French, or Chinese through subsequent parts of it. There is a homogeneity in the successive behavior segments which shows an orderly interrelationship among them.

As a matter of fact, even when we have so-called behavior "disorganization" as in the psychoses or neuroses, we may still observe organization, for note that the ravings of the maniac are related to his past behavioral development. They are in the language that he acquired and are about things which he has encountered in his past psychological history. Even the "insanities" permit a classification (i.e., systematization) of the behavior included under that term, so that personality reactions may be grouped under such principles as schizophrenic, paranoiac, hysteric, and compulsive and may be dealt with accordingly.

EVERY PERSONALITY IS UNIQUE. Uniqueness constitutes one other general characteristic that pertains to personality. Thus, each individual's personality is different in its details from that of every other individual. This is an illustration of the fundamental law of individual differences in psychology and, translated into personality terms, calls attention to the fact that component reactions differ from one individual to another. One person excels in mechanical skills, another in arts or crafts, a third in cooking or sewing. Thus, the uniqueness of personality is not evanescent but can be pinned down to the number, varieties, and ways of performing all of the constituent reactions organized into a personality system.

The definition of personality suggested above, in terms of reactions which include all the behavior pertaining to a single individual, their organization or systematization, and their uniqueness for each individual, appears to us a profitable framework for more detailed analysis.

HOW SHALL WE UNDERSTAND THE HOMOGENEITY AND UNIQUENESS OF PERSONALITY? The fact of the individual's acquisition of personality at all is not in need of explanation since everybody has observed himself, infants, and others during the actual process of building up piano playing, machine operating, dancing, skating, and other behaviors. We need only stress that this acquisition applies to every last behavioral segment. Popular psychology has gone along most of the way but excludes certain behaviors (e.g., mathematical activity or musical creativity), thus employing a dual explanation. In effect, it says: Almost all behaviors are acquired but a few, although they must be built up (obviously), also must have a basis about which nothing much may be said except to *call it* an "ability," "capacity," or "tendency." According to the view expounded here, we do not require a dual set of principles to explain personality. Acquisition of behavior from a zero point is adequate for explaining all personality reactions alike, complex or simple.

How shall we understand the homogeneity or system shown in personality? Why is there an orderly interrelationship of the stimulus-response units composing it? We believe that the answer comes from an examination of the conditions under which these reactions are built up, for note how stable these conditions may be for a given individual. He lives in the same community over long periods of time and is a member of the same social, economic, family, occupational, religious, political, and other groups. As a matter of fact, these conditions may be common to large numbers of people, thus accounting for the uniform personality reactions of individuals composing such groups as Mohammedans, "Holy Rollers," plumbers, physicians, criminals, and artists, among others.

As a matter of fact, the stability of conditions is shown even in the constancy of the atmospheric envelope. Imagine what personalities might be like under rapid and serious fluctuations of the oxygen content of the air or of surrounding temperatures. Fortunately, these and other conditions are relatively stable, and, therefore, the resulting personality reflects stability; but change them (as in war or political or economic crises) and you get personality change. Here, for example, is a peace-loving benevolent physician in Germany with a certain, stable personality. A Hitler takes over; political, social, economic, and legal conditions change; and our physician's personality changes dramatically. Now he builds up behavior which appears to be even contradictory to his previous personality make-up. Now he is an underground worker, carries a gun, and shoots to kill, dynamites defense plants, wears filthy clothes, talks cruelly and vulgarly, and has lost his professional manner. Had conditions remained stable, the personality would have continued stable, too. It is apparent, then, that personality reactions are definitely related to the specific conditions under which they evolve. When setting factors are homogeneous, personality is, too; when they are chaotic, so is personality.

MULTIPLE OR SPLIT PERSONALITY. Since an individual's psychological history is complex, it could hardly be uniform and consistent. Life circumstances are not that repetitive. As a matter of fact, the kind of reactions that a horse trader evolves as a horse trader do not comport with the personality reactions that he builds up as a member of a church congregation, nor are his reactions at the poker table consonant with those that he performs toward his children at home.

When behavioral circumstances are quite contradictory or inconsistent, there may be whole blocks of personality reactions that become organized in a similar fashion. For example, a young lady, Loretta B., was reared under extremely strict religious observance so that prayer, fasting, and church attendance were the order of the day—day in, day out. At school, she had a series of traumatic experiences in which she was initiated into sexual orgies and use of alcohol and drugs, over which she built up serious guilt reactions. On a trip to a relative, the father and mother were horribly mangled in an automobile accident. Now Loretta's behavior shows a striking alternation with respect to whole blocks of personality reactions. On certain days, she rises early, fasts, and attends church, praying devoutly both at church and at home and is altogether a pious person; at other times, there are behavioral phases which show an incompatibility or contradictoriness with the reactions listed above, for she now rages and swears, talks obscenely, makes frequent sexual allusions and proposals to others, and drinks heavily.

To one who has followed her personality development under the two radically different sets of conditions surrounding her, there is nothing unusual about this alternation of personality. On the contrary, what else than a "saint-sinner" formula would one expect? After all, "saint reactions" are more likely to be performed with other "saint reactions" and "sinner" ones with others of the same sort than a fluctuation back and forth. In the same way, our horse trader performs a host of reactions related to his horse trading and another set which relate to his church, his home, and his club stimuli. In the same fashion, do we all show some degree of shift in our personality reactions. In pathological degrees, these are the cases of the "Dr. Jekyll and Mr. Hyde" variety. More widely disseminated ones include you and me as we shift our activity from one to another sphere of interest.

PSEUDOPERSONALITY. Because stressing the important temporal aspects of personality will bring into focus its dynamic characteristics, we wish to discuss briefly a datum that might be called "pseudopersonality."

An individual wishing to impress others may temporarily assume certain personality reactions which we do not see him perform when we have extended our observations of him over longer periods of time.

For example, a person affecting a Harvard accent or an unschooled person who inappropriately interspersed the phrase, "No doubt," throughout his statements when talking to people in a higher socioeconomic group would fall into this class. We should also include here the nonperformance of reactions that are habitually performed; people who refrain from acting in certain ways when the minister comes to dinner and parents who fail to swear or tell risqué stories as soon as their children appear on the scene are examples of the latter sort.

The essential characteristic of pseudopersonality is either the performance of reactions under certain circumstances that are not habitually or characteristically performed, or the converse, namely, the nonperformance of habitual reaction systems. Actors assuming various roles to the extent of wearing hair or beard styles not previously worn, or accent or a language not a part of that individual's past or future behavioral equipment, are a final example of the former, and the lovers in the first blush of love illustrate the latter. Both show the fluidity of the operation of the reactions that go to make up personality and stress the importance of the temporal factors.

II. NORMAL AND ABNORMAL PERSONALITY [1]

Neuroses and psychoses are often referred to as disorders of personality because in them the disturbance in one's interpersonal relationships is so fundamental. The distinction between normal and abnormal person-

---

[1] CAMERON, NORMAN. *The psychology of behavior disorders.* Boston: Houghton Mifflin, 1947. Pp. 622. (Reproduced by permission of the author and the publisher.)

ality, from our point of view, must rest upon the relative adequacy of a given individual's performance, in comparison with his previous level and with the cultural norms that are current in his society for persons of his status. One further distinction must be made. Normal personalities are not the same as ideal or perfect personalities. The latter do not exist; the former are on every hand. Everyone behaves in an irregular or un-predictable way now and then, but this does not automatically place him outside the broad range of normality.

We would speak of personality as abnormal, for example, if at any age an individual who was otherwise in good health grew seriously or progressively ineffectual as a social person. We would call it abnormal if, in order to carry on ordinary activities, he were obliged to expend disproportionate effort in comparison with his previous level and with others of his age, physique, intelligence, and training. We would speak of abnormal personality if an individual proved incapable of organizing and maintaining socially adequate relationships with other persons, if he proved unable to derive personal satisfactions from these, or if his behavior became socially inappropriate in terms of the prevailing cultural norms.

This rough criterion of normal and abnormal personality—the relative adequacy of performance, now and in the foreseeable future—is not peculiar to the field of behavior pathology. We use the same yardstick when we judge whether or not one of our internal organs is normal. We use it, moreover, to judge the normality of a machine, a factory, or a whole industry, of a community, a nation, or a family of nations. For example, we call that kidney normal which excretes competently and shows no serious signs of oncoming incompetence. But the normal kidney is never an ideal or perfect kidney. Like the normal person, it too may now and then do irregular and unexpected things. When it does, we look for an explanation in its intricate relationships with other organs, with food intake, water balance, body temperature, blood stream or urinary tract infection, and the like. Sometimes the explanation eludes us and we chalk it up to renal complexity and our own ignorance. From the same standpoint, a normal industry or a normal community is never ideal or perfect. We say it is normal if it carries on its own affairs with reasonable competence, maintains an economical balance with other related organizations, and shows no serious signs of heading progressively into trouble or of deteriorating.

As every close observer of human action knows, it is sometimes quite impossible to account for a person's odd conduct or unexpected attitude.

Neither he nor anybody else can understand it. From this some draw the immediate conclusion that therefore we must introduce an unnatural, unknowable factor or some other-worldly influence to fill the gap. That is giving in to the challenge of ignorance without a struggle. In our present state of knowledge we should expect to find human behavior often unintelligible. We should expect chance factors to play a larger role than in simpler dynamic systems. Consider for a moment how enormously complex our relationships with our fellows are, how meaning-laden are the countless cultural objects and symbols that saturate our daily life. Consider how many half-digested, unassimilated, contradictory attitudes we all carry along in our personality organizations.

In behavior pathology we must expect very often to face too many unanalyzed and uncontrolled variables for our present stage of development in scientific knowledge and technique. The cure for this deficiency, however, lies not in retreating to something less clear and certain, but in advancing to meet the challenge with better formulations of our problems, with better recognition of what we could but do not know, with new and better techniques, with more objective studies of behavior pathology and its precursors [pp. 7–9].

III. A CASE OF WAR NEUROSIS
John Bucklew, Jr.

The following case history was reconstructed chronologically and recorded after the soldier's release from a military hospital following personality breakdown during stress of combat.

John M., the 25-year-old son of immigrant parents, was born and reared in a small city in the southeastern part of the United States. He was the third child in a rather large family. The father was a molder in a local foundry.

In school, John did not do very well, requiring 9 years to finish six grades. He explains this by saying he was too distracted by the quarrels and fighting at home, and that in school he was picked on by the schoolmaster for some inapparent reason. He would get the blame for anything that happened. When pressed to explain why this was so, John said that the girls in the classroom would report him to the teacher in order to tease him.

The home situation was unstable owing to the fluctuating

moods of the father. He was strict with the children and used to punish them by rapping them over the head with his knuckles, or even with a hammer. The patient states he often experienced severe headaches following a fatherly blow with the hammer. The father was a heavy drinker and had an eye for other women. John's relations with his father were often cordial but subject to change on short notice. Because of the remarks and actions of the father around girls, the patient was often embarrassed when girls came to the home to see him or the family.

The mother took good care of the children and was a hard worker. Often, she took the boy's part in family quarrels. His relationship to her was close, and her death was a hard blow to him.

The patient had had many kinds of jobs after leaving school, including farm work, semiskilled laboring and carpentering jobs, handyman in garages and filling stations, and molder in a foundry. This last was his main occupation at which he worked intermittently for several years in the same foundry as his father. The work was hard, and he quit on several occasions because he could not stand the gas fumes from the burning crude oil in the foundry. The work required much standing and lifting of heavy molds, and John often experienced exhaustion and weakness in the legs and arms.

John states that he has always been popular with girls but will have nothing to do with them. He disclaims sexual experience and says he will refrain until he is married, although he says many girls have been interested in him. He attributes his popularity to his shyness and to the fact that he never played around with women. He first masturbated while quite young and before he realized the significance of the act. At about the age of 13, he learned more about it from other boys. He has a strong religious compunction against the act, and in support of his attitude quotes the Bible reference condemning it. He strongly denies any homosexual activity and states that he detests individuals of that sort. He claims he has often been approached by them.

For about the past 7 years, the patient has experienced pains in his arms and legs which have been getting worse. In the army, he seemed to make a reasonable adjustment, although he has one absence without leave against him in his service record. For this, he was fined part of his pay and reduced to the rank of private.

He expresses resentment against this and claims other fellows who went AWOL at the same time received much less punishment than he did. He spent several months in active combat in a special combat force. Finally, he developed bad headaches and excessive pains in the legs. During battle, he became badly confused, suffered from shaking spells, and was often paralyzed with fear. He was finally evacuated and placed on limited assignment.

The patient's chief complaints at the time of the interview were headaches and extreme pains in the back part of the calf and thighs. He often props his legs above the level of his head at night in order to ease the pain.

His speech is rapid, dramatic, and not too well organized. During interview, it is difficult to control the conversation and to elicit desired information. There is a strong religious cast to his thinking; he has always been closely attached to his church and desires to be a minister. He has had frequent dreams and nightmares during his life, especially after his mother died. Many of the dreams are of annihilation, the world coming to an end according to the Book of Revelation, dreams of accidents, of babies being killed, auto wrecks, and earthquakes. He has also dreamed of being a minister, standing on a balcony in a church, surveying the crowd gathered below him, and telling them their sins and wrongdoings.

His attitude toward his family is ambivalent. At times, he speaks of them as looking up to him as a model person, as seeking his advice. At other times, he expresses hatred for his father and some of his brothers and sisters. He says he feels that one of his sisters hates him because he always tried to point out her wrongs to her and to set her right again. One brother-in-law he dislikes intensely and claims he caught him in an affair with another woman. He also claims he has often cooperated with the police in tracking down thieves and "guys who take girls out in autos and rape them."

According to him, he had an intuition of his mother's approaching death 3 months ahead of time and consulted a minister about it. He describes in great detail the events of the day on which his mother died. She died suddenly at home while he was at work. The patient says his father was the only person in the house at the time and he strongly suspects his mother did not "die a natural death." He at first claimed the doctor could assign no reason for her death, but a few minutes later stated that it was diagnosed as heart failure.

The patient speaks of a girl friend in California whom he thinks he will marry although he has never written her. He has known her for some time but feels that he must "investigate her background" before he marries her.

In the army, he suspected that one soldier contrived to harm him because he was popular with everyone and the soldier was envious. He has often felt that everyone was watching him when he walked down the street, and used to smoke cigarettes incessantly when out in public because this made him so nervous. He feels he doesn't want to return home after the war and wants to notify his family of this in a "blue" envelope (a special form of noncensored communication reserved by the army for special circumstances). He is suspicious about the conduct of his father and about the activities of other members of his family group. He claims that a lot of things have gone on behind his back about which he is going to find out some day. In his own estimation, he has always been well liked by friends and neighbors, but, on the other hand, he states that he has often left social groups because he felt he was not wanted.

ANALYSIS OF CASE. The soldier's sleep difficulties, battle dreams, headaches, and somatic disturbances were mostly precipitated by combat experience and have been diagnosed as psychoneurotic in nature. The leg and arm pains antedate military life and are associated with his working conditions as a molder. The picture is typically that of disorganized behavior following the tensions and stress of combat experience.

In addition, the soldier displays a nonsystematic paranoia derived from the instability of his background and his fluctuating relationship to his father and other people. His family and social relations have never been firm enough to permit an organized development of the reactional biography. As a result, he exhibits bizarre, uncritical inferences concerning the behavior of others, displays alternate moods of affection and hatred toward individuals, suspicion, false ideas of reference, and delusions of grandeur associated with religion and morality. Apparently, he has never been violent toward others, but on the contrary he is apt to faint, in true psychoneurotic fashion, at the sight of accidents or violence.

IV. "BODY TYPE" AND PERSONALITY
D. W. Fiske

Everyone likes to have complex things reduced to a simple basis. Small wonder that people, through the ages, have searched for such anatomic features as blondness, eyes wide apart, large foreheads, and so on, which could be related to temperament, intelligence, and other personality characteristics.

A modern system of this sort is Sheldon's [2] classification of physiques according to relative degrees of the following somatotypes (body types).

1. Endomorphy—relative predominance of soft roundness throughout the body.
2. Mesomorphy—relative predominance of muscle and bone. This physique is heavy, hard, and rectangular.
3. Ectomorphy—relative predominance of linearity and fragility.

A given individual's body type, or somatotype, is designated by three numbers which show the relative strength of the above three components on a seven-point scale.

The following summary of Fiske's [3] study shows the results of an attempt to relate physique to various personality characteristics.

A group of private school boys (N = 133 to 176) were somatotyped according to Sheldon's procedure for the classification of physiques. They were then grouped on the basis of similarity of physique into 9 to 22 groups. The analysis of variance was used to test whether the variables employed in this study were related to somatotype group.

Several intelligence tests and also scholastic averages were found to be unrelated to this classification of physique. Four scales of the Bernreuter Personality Inventory showed a similar lack of relationship.

Out of 40 variables used to score responses to a series of inkblots, 3 showed a significant relationship to somatotype group; these were the percentage and also the absolute number of Vista responses, and the number of Human Movement Responses. These were associated not

---

[2] SHELDON, W. H. *The varieties of human physique.* New York: Harper, 1940. Pp. 347.

[3] FISKE, D. W. A study of relationships to somatotypes. *J. appl. Psychol.*, 1944, **28**, 504–519. (Reproduced by permission of the author and the American Psychological Association.)

with components of physique but rather with patterns of component dominance. Pure Color Responses showed a low correlation with Ectomorphy.

Ratings on good adjustment and possession of a "good personality" showed no relationship to somatotype group. Measures of motor speed, precision, and point pressure also produced no statistically significant findings. Electroencephalograms were analyzed to determine the relative energy at the different frequencies; the resulting energy patterns were unrelated to somatotype groupings. Although basal metabolic rate, variability of metabolic rate, and number of inspirations per minute during the determination of basal metabolic rate were unrelated to physique, the mean height of inspiration proved to be slightly associated with the Mesomorphic component of physique. Blood group and somatotype group were uncorrelated.

The number of significant findings in this study of adolescent boys is not greater than chance expectancy. The use of Sheldon's improved procedure for classifying physique yielded the same paucity of significant relationships to physique that has been found in earlier studies [pp. 516–517].

Since, in objective psychology, behavior is studied as it evolves from the beginning of each individual's life history, there is no felt need for finding some touchstone to the understanding of personality. Because personality is not the functioning of anatomic structures but the sum total of reactions involving an organism and its stimuli in a series of contacts, personality is studied operationally as it develops and changes in a dynamic system. The study reviewed here stresses the problems raised by the traditional view.

V. THE ROLE OF TESTING IN PERSONALITY STUDY

The following selection of quotations from an article by Hunt [4] indicates the role of psychological tests in the study of personality structure.

───────────

[4] HUNT, W. A. The future of diagnostic testing in clinical psychology. *J. clin. Psychol.*, 1946, **2**, 311–317. (Reproduced by permission of the author and the publisher.)

The main contribution of the psychological test is that it offers an opportunity of sampling a subject's behavior in a standard situation.

The main contribution of the individual test (as opposed to the group test) is that it offers the tester an opportunity personally to observe such behavior as it takes place.

It follows from the first premise that the primary datum offered by the psychological test is the subject's raw behavior in the test situation. The mathematical symbols into which this behavior can be translated are secondary instruments of convenience and should not be allowed to conceal the primary datum, the actual behavior [p. 311].

Many individual clinicians do not overlook such data. They are not content to base their judgment upon the mere test score or profile of scores but carry their interpretation back to the subject's original performance. This is done somewhat shamefacedly, and is referred to apologetically as the exercise of "clinical judgment" or even more apologetically as "clinical intuition." This is not intuition in the mystical sense. It is the same sort of intellectual process of judgment that ensues when a psychologist considers a test score in the light of the known validity and reliability of the test used before making an interpretation, and in many cases the mathematical data upon which such an interpretation is based are no more reliable than the observational data upon which we base our clinical "intuitions" [p. 312].

The foregoing selection from the pages of a technical journal are included to counteract the notion so widely prevalent among laymen and students of psychology that a personality test is comparable to a thermometer which immediately tells the tester all about the person being tested.

Actually, Hunt is saying, a test is only a situation which is contrived to observe a sample of the testee's behavior. Stress is on the personality available for study before one, the test itself taking a subordinate role. In the past, there has frequently been greater concern shown in regard to the score on the test than to the individual's behavior in the test situation.

Again, as with body typing, the implication seems to be that there is no shortcut to understanding of personality. To know personality, there seems to be no way but to study personality directly.

VI. SOME TECHNIQUES FOR PERSONALITY STUDY
J. W. Bowles, Jr.

The techniques for the study of personality reactions to which we wish to call attention may be roughly grouped into the three categories: situation tests, paper-and-pencil tests, and "projective" techniques.

1. SITUATION TESTS. Situation tests consist of controlled situations in which the subject is unobtrusively observed. For example, cheating behavior may be studied by contriving a situation, unknown to the subject, which permits such actions to occur. Introvert reactions might be studied by observing the subject in a variety of social situations such as classrooms, groups of friends, of strangers, work groups, and the like. Here we have the observation of personality reactions as they happen. There is, of course, no implication that cheating as it is observed here will occur in all sorts of situations. Emphasis is on the behavior of the individual in specific situations.

2. PAPER-AND-PENCIL TESTS. Paper-and-pencil tests, such as the *California Test of Personality* or Bernreuter *Personality Inventory* are indirect approaches to the investigation of personality reactions. A modification of this technique is the *Minnesota Multiphasic Test*. In these tests, the subject is asked to report his own reactions, e.g., to tell whether or not he ever walked across the street to avoid meeting someone. With regard to our example of cheating reactions, the subject would be asked directly or indirectly whether he had ever cheated. Such question-answer tests attempt to study introvert behavior by asking such questions as: "Do you ever feel alone in a crowd?" "Are you ever the life of a party?" "Do you take the lead in starting conversations with strangers?" and the like. The source of error in this type of test is obvious. A subject may deliberately or unwittingly give a false report of his behavior. Validation of these tests is usually on a group level, consisting of statistical comparisons of control groups and others, such as samples from mental hospitals or mental hygiene clinics.

3. "PROJECTIVE" TECHNIQUES. Projective tests represent a somewhat indirect method of personality study. Although they vary as to details, most tests under this label have certain general features in common. Some behavior is observed in the testing situ-

ation, and the investigator then makes *inferences* about the "personality structure" of his subject.

One group of such tests, for example, brings the subject into visual contact with vague objects like cloud pictures or ink blots, and the subject is asked what he sees. The nature of his verbal response is then analyzed and inferences are made. Sometimes these take the form of analogizing. Thus, if a subject attends to many details of the pictures, it may be concluded that he is preoccupied with the petty details of everyday life. The label "projective technique" deserves some attention. Although defined in different ways, in essence the term "projective" implies that some "thing" called personality is "cast out" upon the picture or ink blot, or, when other methods are used, this "thing" is illuminated by what the subject says or does, as when he performs "free-association" responses to word stimuli. The term hardly achieves refined description of observable facts.

Since the tests subsumed under this heading are varied, a few of the recent ones are briefly described:

1. THE RORSCHACH TEST. The Rorschach test consists of a series of ten ink blots, some in black and white, some with additional colors. The subject is asked to tell what the blots look like. Objectively speaking, the blots serve as a set of substitute stimuli, and the reactions performed are a function of the subject's behavioral history. Utilizing the sorts of reactions given, to whole blots and parts of blots, whether colors are important in the responses, whether objects are described as moving, and so forth, the examiner attempts to make generalizations that would apply to many areas of behavior. It is a justifiable criticism that "interpretation by analogy" is extremely common here.

2. THE THEMATIC APPERCEPTION TEST. In the Thematic Apperception Test, the subject is given a series of pictures illustrating people in action. Like the Rorschach test, the actions in which the people are engaged are somewhat vague. Hence, the pictures operate principally as substitute stimuli. The subject may be asked to make up a story including the picture as a scene in that story. It is hoped that the story will be autobiographical and will reveal significant features of the subject's past experiences.

3. THE MIRA MYO KINETIC PSYCHODIAGNOSIS. In the Mira Myo Kinetic Psychodiagnosis, unlike the preceding tests, the subject makes a series of different sorts of marks with a pencil while

the paper is hidden from view. These lines are drawn in various planes. In one trial, the subject attempts to draw ten parallel lines, each 5 centimeters long from left to right, then ten more in the opposite direction. Similar drawings are made with the other hand. Drawings of controls and various clinical groups have been compared. Analogizing seems to be an important feature of diagnosis, e.g., if a right-handed person makes drawings with the left hand that move *downward*, it is inferred that he is a "constitutional depressive" [*sic*].

4. FINGER PAINTING. A subject may be asked to paint anything he likes with his fingers. A variety of colored paints is provided. From what he draws and the colors that he uses, the investigator attempts to draw conclusions about the personality reactions of his subject. In one case, an investigator asserted that use of brown represented a thwarted desire to play with fecal matter.

The preceding description of personality tests includes but a few of the thousands that psychologists have evolved as an aid in the study of the complex problem of personality. The student is urged to be critical in their evaluation, with the hint that the closer one adheres to direct observation of behavior or personality, the more valid will the resulting interpretations be. Surely, such a conservative approach is not to be easily dismissed.

One final comment on the topic of personality—this pervasive subject matter will not permit one to confine it within the bounds of a single chapter. As a matter of fact, it has not been shut out from any chapter of this book. The subjects of attention, perception, and intelligence, as well as the early chapters on behavioral acquisition and social behavior, involve themselves in personality consideration, also. The present chapter simply stresses and focuses upon certain problems which have traditionally been placed under the heading of personality.

𝟪

INTELLIGENCE

I. THE ELABORATION OF "INTELLIGENCE"
N. H. Pronko

According to the hypothesis of the reactional biography, behavior can originate in only one way, i.e., through a very specific history involving an organism and stimulus objects. Obviously, this should hold for those reactions that are usually lumped together and labeled "intelligence."

It is possible to start with behavior as such even in the infant and to trace out the origin and growing complexity of intelligence reactions without once resorting to traditional phrases such as "innate I.Q.," "native capacity," "inborn tendency," and so on. After all, the proof of the pudding is in actually understanding, predicting, or controlling the class of events observed.

Examination of the infant at birth would show little of the behaviors which will develop very quickly. It has been shown that psychological classes of events emerge out of animal action. At first, the infant is simply a locus of reflexes and random movements. The former are structure-function mechanisms—reactions of a portion of the organism (mostly) put into function by an adequate stimulus. Earlier psychologists attributed all of the organism's behavior to the conditioning of his original stock of reflexes.

While we agree that these are raw materials for behavioral development, we must not overlook another important source in the infant's random movements. Touch an infant on any portion or pinch, chill, or shock him, and he "reacts" with a miscellaneous assortment of turnings, twistings, wrigglings, kicking of legs and slashing of arms and hands, and jerking of head in all directions.

This is a diffuse, widespread, amorphous series of movements, but, once out of the isolating uterine environment, the infant comes into contact with a wide variety of stimulus objects and situations. Now will begin the reinforcement of certain of these reactions with the continued reappearance of the correlated stimulus objects. The end result of this gradual evolution is a series of definitely configured reactions that are related to very specific stimulus objects. Note how quickly the infant performs a relatively "short-circuited" turning of the head sideways to a bottle (present or absent) in place of the widespread unorganized, "total response" which it formerly gave. Here is definitely organized and genuine behavioral activity.

In principle, the same description applies to later stages of behavioral evolution. Reaching, manipulating, grasping, stepping, creeping, crawling, walking, jumping, hopping, skipping, dancing, bicycle riding, drawing, writing, designing, painting, sculping, sewing, shooting, babbling, talking, singing, operating picks, shovels, locomotives, automobiles, planes—all of these simply show more complex reactions integrated with one another out of simpler action and all having an origin out of random movement.

We may safely predict that if a given infant shows a total absence of the sorts of animal action here discussed, he will inevitably be feeble-minded. That is to say, he will stay at or near a psychological zero point as compared with infants who will evolve behavior out of such actions if they are present. Biological defectiveness of a less extensive sort will permit correspondingly limited behavioral development, although we must call attention to the compensatory effect of heroic efforts during the individual's reactional biography, as the case of Helen Keller eloquently demonstrates.

Now, we are ready for handling "intelligence." Our best procedure is to take intelligence tests already at hand which intelligence testers have worked out empirically. For the purposes for which they have been designed, investigators have assembled items that work about as well as might be expected in a general assessment of a given child's behavioral development. Next, let us examine the kind of reactions that are expected in infants of various ages.

The Cattell [1] Infant Intelligence test will serve our purpose. The first point is to note that there are no test items to be administered at birth, or at the 1-week or even the 1-month stage of development. Apparently, the reason for beginning the bottom of the test at the 2-month level is that there are no significant or stable "index behaviors" before this age—only meager and haphazard beginnings. At birth, the only resort is to enumerate the reflexes and minimal wrigglings, but there has been an unwitting realization that these are not "intelligence." What is, then?

The items at the second-month level of the Cattell test are informative. If the child *attends to the examiner's voice, inspects its environment, follows a ring horizontally, follows a moving person, or babbles,* it is considered "normal" for its age. Under somewhat standard conditions obtaining in the homes in our culture, most children attain this stage of organization of movements into reactions that have been generally recognized as psychological. Of course, they are elementary and rather intimately connected with the biological maturation of the infant.

Both through behavioral evolution as well as continued biological development, the infant's psychological status expands and changes constantly. As a result, more complex coordinations and integrations of previously elaborated movement reactions are made possible. These may involve leg and foot or head action, arm, hand, finger, and vocal-cord movements, or combinations of them. Whatever the details of the response, the important point is that we now have behavioral events in which the organism's activity occurs in relation to a stimulus object as a result of their mutual interaction historically. It is these rather simple but genuine psychological acts that have been incorporated into infant intelligence tests. This *is* "intelligence." (The following list illustrates the ever more complex integration of behavioral action out of random movements.)

Selected Items from Cattell Infant Intelligence Test

2 months—attends to voice
           inspects environment
           follows ring horizontally

---

[1] Cattell, Psyche. *The measurement of intelligence of infants and young children.* New York: Psychological Corp., 1947. Pp. 274. (Reproduced by permission of the author and the publisher.)

follows moving person
babbles
3 months—follows ring in circular motion
anticipates feeding
regards cube
regards spoon
inspects fingers
4 months—manipulates fingers in play
keeps hands open
follows ball rolled in front of him
turns to voice
increases activity at sight of toy
turns to bell
obtains ring
5 months—transfers object from hand to hand
regards pellet (looks or gets it)
picks up spoon
6 months—secures cube on sight
lifts cup
fingers own reflection in mirror
reaches unilaterally
reaches persistently
7 months—attempts to pick up pellet
pats and smiles at reflection in mirror
inspects ring
secures two cubes
exploits paper (crumples or swings it)
8 months—attains ring by pulling string
manipulates string
combines two syllables in vocal play
secures pellet
inspects details of bell
9 months—seizes pellet with scissorlike grasp
looks for spoon
rings bell
adjusts to gesture (pat-a-cake, bye-bye)
adjusts to words (where's clock, kitty)
10 months—uncovers toy
combines cup and cube
attempts to take third cube after holding **two**
hits cup with spoon
pokes fingers in holes of pegboard
12 months—beats two spoons together
places one cube in cup

marks with pencil
rattles spoon in cup
speaking vocabulary—two words
16 months—places round block in form board
speaking vocabulary—five words
puts beads in box
solves pellet and bottle problem
closes round box
20 months—builds tower of three cubes
places square in form board
attains toy with stick
attempts to follow directions
points to parts of doll
24 months—*identifies* object by name from Stanford-Binet
attempts to fold paper
recognizes incomplete watch
Stanford-Binet simple commands
give me the kitty
put the spoon in the cup
put the thimble on the block
naming objects from Stanford-Binet test
27 months—makes train of cubes in imitation of examiner
motor coordination test (operates toy egg beater)
imitates drawing vertical line
picture vocabulary
identifies pictures from name
30 months—builds block bridge
imitates drawing lines and circles
three-hole form-board test in reverse
folds paper
identifies objects by use

By referring to the items at the higher age levels of the Cattell test, it will be noted that there is increasing complexity. Of course, alongside those behaviors which the test samples, things are going on that do not appear there. All this time, the child is developing language behavior of the type usually called "comprehension." Soon he also speaks. The reader will note that the infant is expected to have a one-word speaking vocabulary at the eleven-month level. From here on, successive items become more and more infiltrated with language or derived from it (e.g., at 24 and 27 months). Eventually, items beyond this, for which we must go to the Stanford-Binet, involve numbers and complex vocabulary and implicit responses. By comparison with the early movement reactions, these behaviors are radically complex although, in the case of each individual, they can be traced out of the former.

It should be obvious, though, that presence or absence of language and other complex forms of stimulation count for much more in these later stages of the development of the reactional biography than in the earliest months. Perhaps that is why performance in the first few months prognosticates future success so poorly. Foundation behavior requiring only elaboration of motor-coordination responses cannot be predictive of action dependent upon conditions heavily loaded with cultural factors. In the following quotation, Cattell warns psychologists of evaluating or prognosticating infant behavior on the basis of a so-called "intelligence test."

The emphasis that has been placed on the caution with which these intelligence tests should be used applies not only to these tests but to all tests for infants, and with only a little less force to those for children of pre-school and school ages. There is no age from birth to maturity at which it is safe to base an important decision on the results of intelligence tests alone. The intelligence quotients obtained from these tests should always be interpreted in the light of other relevant information such as behavior during the examination, home environment, premature birth, serious illnesses, etc. [pp. 59–60].

It seems to us that Cattell is saying that a behavioral appraisal of an infant must be a highly specific affair because the tests as set up are founded on a statistical basis, i.e., on averages for *groups* of infants. When we examine how the items were standardized, we are informed for example, that

Those items placed at fourteen months were passed by a larger proportion of the twelve- and eighteen-month-old children than were those placed at sixteen. The percentage of twelve-month-old children passing each of the fourteen- and sixteen-month items varied from eleven to forty-three and from zero to thirty, respectively, and for the eighteen-month-old children from ninety-one to ninety-eight and eighty-three to ninety, respectively. The placement of other items between the age groups tested were estimated in a similar manner [p. 29].

One thing is obvious from a consideration of Cattell's statements, namely that these intelligence tests do not distinguish very sharply between groups of infants of widely varying ages. How, then, can they have significance in a comparison of children of the same age group? Note the unpredictableness in the intelligence-test performance of Cattell's Case 198.

This child had an obtained I.Q. of 73 at three months and one near 90 at both six and nine months. At one year and at each six month interval thereafter up to the end of the third year, she showed a com-

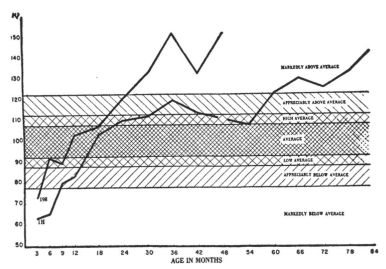

FIG. 22 Individual IQ curves for cases 198 and 1H. That for 198 starts at three months with an IQ of 73, which is bordering on "feeblemindedness" but goes progressively up to 150 ("genius") at four years of age. Development for 1H is somewhat similar but spread over a longer time period. (Cattell, Psyche, *The measurement of intelligence of infants and young children.*)

paratively steady gain. Between three and thirty-six months, eight examinations were made, and, with one exception, where there was a decrease of two I.Q. points, each test resulted in a higher I.Q. than the previous test. The mother, a patrolman's wife, selected the child's college at the time of her birth. At twelve months the pediatrician who examined the baby regretted that the mother was probably doomed to disappointment. The pediatrician's prediction was in line with mental test ratings obtained at that time, but at three years she informed the examiner that she was animate.

Case 1H . . . shows a somewhat similar rise in I.Q., though less regular and spread over a longer period [pp. 60–62].

Such extreme variations as the above are explained as the "result of changes in the tempo of development rather than the inadequacy of tests" [p. 60]. Implicit in this statement is the belief in some essential (apparently inborn) static quality of a person which simply manifests itself in a peculiar way by somehow speeding up or slowing down development. In our view, intelligence reactions are built up during the individual's life history, and their rate of development is only a function of the individual's developmental condition. Therefore, by manipulating the latter, intelligence can be prevented in a pretty total fashion, it can be accelerated, or, under somewhat standard conditions, it will be somewhat standard. Perhaps the "somewhat" should receive greater stress than heretofore. Since one cannot guess what an individual's future life history may be, then how can he predict what the future intelligence level of that person can be? In objective psychology, this becomes a risky business, and such cases as those discussed above are adequate proof.

SUMMARY.   An attempt has been made to account for intelligence reactions. These have been traced out as they are elaborated from the infant's original stock of diffuse, unorganized reactions to those of progressively more complex form. These reactions are then correlated with objects, situations, and persons in the infant's surroundings instead of with indifferent or internal and general stimulation, as occurred earlier. However, there is, at first, a heavy dependence on the infant's biological make-up which, if defective, may seriously interfere with the evolution of "intelligence" but the normality of which gives no guarantee of elaboration of intelligence reactions.

Later intelligence stages are less dependent upon biological constitution than upon cultural factors such as language. Perhaps that is the reason why investigators have been puzzled over their failure to prognosticate the infant's later development from his performance on the earlier index items. Since a new set of factors comes in later, then obviously items in the early months that do not involve such variables can hardly be expected to prognosticate subsequent behavior which is enmeshed with them. Within such a framework, intelligence is not an evanescent quality of an organism; it is an over-all evaluation of an organism's behavior empirically determined in terms of certain index reactions expected of groups of individuals of various ages, the latter also being empirically determined. As such, it may be expected to show acceleration, retardation, or "normality" in the same individual, depending on his developmental conditions. It is the framework that we have developed above which we hope will guide the reading of the following series of articles on "intelligence," although we must point out that not all psychologists agree with the above interpretation. Many psychologists still believe that, to some degree or other, there is an inherited basis for intelligence which sets the limits for its development.

II. ON THE "MEASUREMENT OF INTELLIGENCE"

The preceding article has indicated that there is no "entity," inherent or otherwise, to which the label "intelligence" can be attached. "Measuring intelligence" is more factually described as sampling in a limited way the complex behavioral equipment of the child or adult. Using some test as a tool, the examiner tests for the presence or absence of certain reactions. Such a testing device may be described as a set of standard stimuli.

An example of such a test is the 1937 revision of the Stanford-Binet.[2] This test was constructed by administering a large number of items to 3,184 rural and urban children of preschool and school ages in the North, East, South, and West of the United States. All children were American born and belonged to the white race. From these data, items were selected which best discriminated between children of different age levels (but not between sexes) and were combined to make two forms of the test (Form L and Form M).

The 1937 Standford-Binet tests for presence or absence of such reactions as the following selections taken at random from Form L:

1. Building a bridge of three blocks (Year III).
2. Answering questions, as: *"Why do we have houses* (Year IV)?"

---

[2] TERMAN, L. M. & MERRILL, MAUD A. *Measuring intelligence.* Boston: Houghton Mifflin, 1937. Pp. 461.

3. Counting four blocks, beads, and pennies (Year V).
4. Giving a similarity between two objects, as wood and coal (Year VII).
5. Detecting the absurdity of such statements as: *"Bill Jones' feet are so big he has to pull his trousers on over his head* (Year IX)."
6. Repeating digits forward or backward (several age levels).
7. Spatial orientation: *"Which direction would you have to face so that your left hand would be toward the east* (Year XIV)?"
8. Constructing sentences using three words, as: *civility, requirement, employee* (Superior Adult I).
9. Opposite analogies, as: *A debt is a liability, an income is. . . . .* (Superior Adult III).
10. Defining words, as: *orange, tap, haste, regard, stave, mosaic, incrustation, parterre.*

Regarding the vocabulary item, Terman has this to say: "We have found the vocabulary test to be the most valuable single test in the scale" [p. 302].

What evidence can be found in the vocabulary test or any of the above items for innate intellectual capacities? There is only a series of highly specific reactions to stimuli. Even a test maker, believing as he may that his test tasks "tap" such a capacity, is forced to agree that the responses required by his test stimuli are acquired through experience.

How, then, are innate capacities arrived at? Only by violation of certain rules of scientific procedure. First, the rule of parsimony is ignored. This rule states that when two theories are available, both of which are adequate to handle the facts, the simpler theory is to be preferred. In dealing with intelligence reactions, a stimulus-response theory covers the facts, but the "psychohereditarian" utilizes a stimulus-response explanation (to handle the obviously learned responses to test items) *plus* a hereditary capacity. He agrees that specific reactions cannot be inherent, but he alleges that innate general capacities make possible such specific acquisitions of behavior.

Further, the "psychohereditarian" is guilty of the logical fallacy of *circular reasoning.* The only facts available to him are the observable behaviors—the responses to test stimuli. If a subject performs poorly, thus obtaining a low I.Q., the holder of this viewpoint claims that he did so because of low innate capacity. *The low capacity explains the low test performance.* If it is then asked how he knows that the subject has low innate capacity, he may claim that the inferior test performance *proves* the existence of the low capacity. *The low test performance proves the low capacity.* The subject's performance is inferior because he has low capacity, and he has low capacity because his performance is inferior. This reasoning goes around and around.

Following the administration of a test, the correct responses are usually combined to form a total score. As the illustrative items indicate, the Stanford-Binet is an "age scale." Items are grouped at age levels. The scoring of this test begins by taking the highest age level at which the subject passed all the items, labeled the "basal age," and adding extra credits for each item passed above this level. For example, if a child passed all items at year VII, his basal age would be 7 years. If he correctly answered three of the six items at year VIII he would obtain ½ year's credit, or 6 months. Two of the six items passed at year IX would add 4 months, and one success at year X would add 2 additional months of credit. If all items above year X were failed, the subject would have a score of 8 years (8–0). This is referred to as his test age or *mental age* (M.A.) *on this test.*

To obtain a ratio between the child's test performance and his actual or chronological age, a test quotient or *intelligence quotient* (I.Q.) is computed by dividing the test-age score by the chronological age and multiplying the ratio by 100. If the child in our example were exactly 7 years old, his I.Q. on this test at this time would be 8–0/7–0 times 100, or 114. At best, this I.Q. is a highly abstract number comparing the subject with an even more abstract average of the group upon which the test was standardized.

The computation of the I.Q. raises the question of why a correlation should be expected between behavioral development and chronological age? Owing to varying life circumstances, some individuals have accelerated reactional biographies, while others are retarded. No two are identical. There may also be acceleration in certain behavioral areas and retardation in others. It might be suggested that, from a clinical standpoint, a detailed study of behavioral elaboration is considerably more meaningful than the extraction of any number of I.Q.'s.

Psychologists have worked out scales for the various ranges of I.Q. scores, of which the following is an example:

Class	Range of I.Q.'s	Class	Range of I.Q.'s
Very superior	140 and above	Borderline	70–80
Superior	120–140	Moron	50–70
Above average	110–120	Imbecile	25–50
Average	90–110	Idiot	0–25
Below average	80–90		

The lowest three groups including I.Q.'s 0–70 are designated feeble-minded. Thus, a 10-year-old child whose mental age was 7 years or less would be classified as feeble-minded, according to this scale. It would be more precise, however, to state that the subject's performance on this test at this time was within a certain class. An I.Q. level does not hold for all eternity nor for all tests. It is a not uncommon clinical finding for I.Q.'s for different tests given the same subject to range from feeble-minded categories through average or even superior levels. Seventy-five or more points difference in I.Q.'s between two tests given one subject have been recorded. The case of the idiot-savant discussed elsewhere in this chapter illustrates such striking differences in behavioral equipment in various areas of activity.

In addition, superior, average, or inferior performance at a certain time is no guarantee that the same level of test performance will obtain a week, a month, 1 year, or 5 years later, contrary to beliefs in the "constancy of the I.Q.," and contrary to the relatively high test-retest correlations of some tests. Rates of behavioral acquisition vary with changing life circumstances, and test performances vary accordingly.

Special training techniques are not, however, absolute necessities for I.Q. change. Figure 23, from Woodworth and Marquis [3] [p. 50], illustrates a study of 25 children who had the same level of test performance at the beginning of the study. But note the wide range in test scores 4 years later. Such variations under ordinary life conditions suggest that change is the only thing constant about the I.Q.

---

[3] WOODWORTH, R. S. & MARQUIS, D. G. *Psychology,* 5th ed. New York: Holt, 1948. Pp. 677.

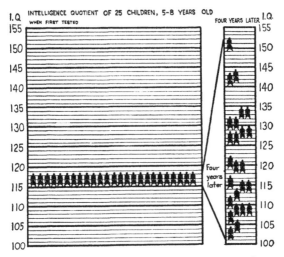

FIG. 23 Changes in IQ of 25 children whose IQ was 115 on first test. During four years in these stimulating schools, the IQ of some of these children went up, while the IQ of others went down. The changes were not large in comparison with the whole IQ range of 0–200. The *average* change was a gain of 5 points. (Data from the psychological records of the Horace Mann and Lincoln Schools of Teachers College, Columbia University and reproduced by their permission.)

III. INTELLIGENCE INTERACTIONS ARE INTERMESHED WITH, AND AFFECTED BY, OTHER BEHAVIORAL EVENTS

Behaviors called intelligent, informational, problem-solving, conceiving, and others, do not occur "in vacuums," but are inextricably interrelated with other behaviors, such as feelings and attitudes. Therefore, it is not surprising that such studies as that by Jolles reveal that severe behavioral lack ("feeble-mindedness") is conditioned by the other personality aspects of children. In the present study, Jolles [4] investigated 66 children, 10 through 15 years of age, who had Binet or Wechsler intelligence quotients below 80. These children had been referred to the psychologist for certification for placement in a special class for retarded children.

---

4 JOLLES, J. The diagnostic implications of Rorschach's test in case studies of mental defectives. *Genet. Psychol. Monogr.*, 1947, **36**, 91–197. (Reproduced by permission of the author and the publisher.)

From his investigations, which made use of the Rorschach test and case-history data, he came to the following conclusions regarding the complex conditions of the reactional history which may effectively prohibit the acquisition of intelligence responses.

The case history material gathered on the 66 subjects in this study reveals broken homes, inadequate parents, unstable and promiscuous parents, foster home situations, illegitimacy, and unwholesome parent-child relationships. In a few instances there are cultural and religious conflicts. In others there are racial conflicts. In most of the cases the children come from homes of a low socio-economic status. A great many have been known to relief agencies. However, the upper classes are not immune to mental deficiency of the familial and undifferentiated types. Approximately one-third of the children who make up this study come from homes of an average or better than average socio-economic status. The primary factors which were discovered in those cases were broken homes and poor parent-child relationships. The clinical data reveal rather forcefully the importance of the family background in the development of mental deficiency. Certainly it is not surprising to find personality maladjustments in these children in view of the family and social milieu from which they come.

From a clinical standpoint it might be rather difficult to place the mental defective in a clinical entity such as psychoneurosis, psychosis, schizoid personality, etc. As a matter of fact, we may continue to classify them as mentally deficient, but on the basis of the information which we have from this study our concept of mental deficiency may have to change. It is essential that we consider regarding mental deficiency as something that may be treated through the usual psychotherapeutic techniques. We must realize that merely providing special educational facilities will not solve the problem of mental deficiency and that institutionalization is often a mere evasion of the problem. . . . Finally, in the diagnosis of mental deficiency we should take into consideration, not so much the I.Q. of the child, but the total personality picture which is provided by his behavior, the case history material, and the results of projective techniques such as the Rorschach test.

There will be instances in which institutionalization of the mentally deficient will be necessary. However, this should not mean routine custodial care. The institution for the feeble-minded must resemble very closely our best institutions for the mentally ill. All forms of psychotherapy, diagnostic techniques, social case work, medical care, and educational facilities should be provided the subnormal in the hope that many may return to a more normal way of life, not only in a social and emotional sense, but in intellectual adjustment as well [p. 192].

IV. AN INTERESTING CASE OF CONGENITAL HYDROCEPHALY [5]

It is common knowledge that lack of proper fetal development may produce a "monstrosity." The degree to which he is crippled determines the difficulty that such a defective organism will experience in developing intelligence.

The following case history of congenital hydrocephaly is significant because it shows that, despite incapacitating defects, this child showed an above-average I.Q. By way of explanation, the word "congenital," as used here, refers to the fact that the condition was not inherited but *acquired* during the child's embryologic development. This must be stressed because students commonly misuse the word "congenital" for "hereditary."

Hydrocephaly is a condition marked by an excessive amount of pressure of the cerebrospinal fluid in the head region. As a result, the skull is pushed up and out and gives a bulging appearance to the head. Obviously, if the pressure is great, the brain tissue itself will be damaged. The fact that R. has been prevented from making complex movements would indicate such damage to the brain.

When R. was brought to the psychological clinic, he was 6 years, 7 months of age. He was an extremely pleasant, apparently well-adjusted child. He was unable to walk, and could sit upright only when supported by a leather and steel brace. At this time his head measured 28½ inches. (Normal children of his age average around 20 inches.) Except for his extremely large head, he seemed normal as to size and weight, his weight being somewhat more than average for his height. The overweight might be accounted for by his inactivity, exercise to any extent being impossible.

He was given the Revised Stanford-Binet, Form L. His M.A. was 7 years, 5 months, giving him an I.Q. of 113. His intelligence was no doubt somewhat higher, for several items were missed because of his physical

[5] TESKA, P. T. The mentality of hydrocephalics and a description of an interesting case. *J. Psychol.*, 1947, 23, 197–203. (Reproduced by permission of the author and the publisher.)

handicaps. He had had no school experience, so, although his parents had encouraged other children to play with him and to be with him, his social experience would be considerably different from an ordinary child's at 6½ years.

It was recommended that he be put into a crippled children's group and that he be taught to read. He has learned to read with good success, and his reading proficiency equals, if not exceeds, that of the average first grader with a similar amount of formal training.

He has some difficulty in coordinate use of his hands, which may be because of some vision impairment. He has had, at present, no vision tests. He is well adjusted in his group, takes part with great delight in school activities, and responds with eagerness to school situations.

Through the courtesy of Dr. Clifton T. Morris of Baton Rouge, Louisiana, the following medical history is included:

There is no history of family or hereditary disease. His parents on both sides are from healthy stock. There have been no other cases of hydrocephaly or any other malformations in the family.

His was a normal birth with no unusual birth difficulties. The examination following birth showed a well-developed infant with these measurements:

Head—14 inches in circumference

Chest—13 inches

Abdomen—13 inches

Body—20½ inches long

At six weeks of age it was noted that his head was increasing in circumference. Measurement showed a 2-inch increase. The reflexes were normal. . . . One month later (at 2½ months of age) the head circumference had increased to 18 inches. At this time spinal fluid showed increased pressure. . . .

X-ray treatment was applied over the temporal and occipital areas. In spite of the treatments, the skull continued to increase, and at the age of six months was 27 inches in circumference.

From the age of six months to the present, the head circumference has increased only 1½ inches. Radiographs of the skull show a typical hydrocephalic skull. There has been no eye examination. There is possibility of some damage to the optic nerve. Except for the contracted tendon of Achilles, which a minor operation would relieve, there is no physical reason save the extreme head size to prevent walking. R. has had no illnesses of any seriousness and no contagious diseases [pp. 201–202].

V. THE HOME AND FAMILY BACKGROUND OF OTTAWA PUBLIC SCHOOL CHILDREN IN RELATION TO THEIR I.Q.'S [6]

John S. Robbins

Dominion Bureau of Statistics, Ottawa

Dr. Robbins secured the I.Q.'s of Ottawa public-school children in Grade IV over a 10-year period and related them to the subjects' home and family circumstances by using information secured from the census.

Table [5] divides the 9,956 children into four broad I.Q. groups and gives certain items of information on homes, mothers, and fathers for each. The grouping was determined by reference to the mid-point in the distribution of I.Q.'s which, as Miss Dunlop has explained, was 109. Two groups were made to include twenty points each, one above and one below the median (110–129 and 90–109), and two others to include respectively 130 and over and under 90.

Contrasts in homes and families between the high and low groups are striking. Of the 913 children with the highest I.Q.'s (130 or over) 44.3 p.c. lived in homes owned by their parents, with an average value of $5,448; of the 1,250 with lowest I.Q.'s (under 90) only 22.9 p.c. lived in homes owned by their parents, and the average value was $3,700. The average monthly rental paid on the other homes of the high-testing group was $38.10; for the low-testing group, $24.10.

The homes of the more-favoured group averaged almost one room larger, although there were decidedly smaller families to live in them. The actual number of persons in the homes was not tabulated for the purpose of this study, but instead the number of children that had been born to the mothers, and this provides an indication of the relative size of household. The mothers of the high I.Q. group had had an average of 3.2 children each and were 42.7 years of age; the mothers of the low group had had 5.3 children and were 43.5 years of age.

Judging by the father's earnings there was nearly three times the annual income per person in the families of the children with high I.Q.'s. The year's earnings of the fathers (at least those on salary or wage, and

[6] ROBBINS, JOHN S. The home and family background of Ottawa public school children in relation to their I.Q.'s. *Canad. J. Psychol.*, 1948, 2, 35–41. (Reproduced by permission of the author and the publisher.)

these included three-fourths) averaged $2,512 for the five-member families of the high-testing children, or something like $500 per person; the corresponding earnings of the fathers in the seven-member families of children with low I.Q.'s were $1,244, or about $175 per person. Rather more of the mothers in the latter group were adding to the fathers' earnings (6.5 p.c. were gainfully occupied as compared with 4.3 p.c. in the former group), but their average earnings were lower.

Table 5 *

Home Conditions of Ottawa Public School Children Classified According to I.Q. Groups

	I.Q. under 90	I.Q. 90– 109	I.Q. 110– 129	I.Q. 130 and Over	All Groups
Number of children	1250	3944	3849	913	9956
In homes owned by parents p.c.	22.9	26.3	34.2	44.3	30.7
Median value of owned homes	$3700	$4475	$5116	$5448	$4916
In rented homes ....p.c.	77.1	73.7	65.8	55.7	69.3
Median monthly rental	$24.10	$27.40	$32.60	$38.10	$29.30
Median number of rooms in all homes	6.4	6.5	6.8	7.2	6.6
Living with:					
Both parents ....p.c.	80.7	82.1	86.6	89.4	84.4
One parent ....p.c.	17.1	15.8	12.4	9.4	14.0
Neither parent ....p.c.	2.2	2.1	1.0	1.2	1.6
Mothers:					
Median number of children born	5.3	4.3	3.6	3.2	3.9
Median age	43.5	42.0	41.9	42.7	42.2
Median years of schooling	8.3	9.3	10.0	11.1	9.6
Gainfully employed ....p.c.	6.5	6.5	5.8	4.3	6.0
Fathers:					
Median annual earnings	$1244	$1442	$1806	$2512	$1650
Median years of schooling	8.3	9.2	10.2	11.3	9.7
Occupations:					
Labourers ....p.c.	24.6	15.8	7.7	2.7	12.3
Operatives ....p.c.	20.0	16.0	11.4	5.3	13.6
Craftsmen ....p.c.	30.0	28.2	21.3	15.2	24.5
Clerical ....p.c.	10.5	14.7	21.0	20.8	17.3
Commercial ....p.c.	4.2	7.1	8.5	9.3	7.5
Business owners ....p.c.	8.4	12.5	16.4	23.9	14.7
Professional ....p.c.	2.3	5.5	13.7	22.8	10.1

* Reproduced by permission of the author and the publisher.

The fathers of the high-testing children, like their mothers, had had about three years more schooling than the parents of the low-testing group (eleven years instead of eight). This is no doubt related to the fact that they were able to occupy better paying jobs. A classification of the occupations of fathers, indicating something of the length of training involved, shows for the children with high I.Q. 22.8 p.c. professional and 2.7 unskilled labour, with these proportions roughly reversed for the children of low I.Q.

The low-testing children much more frequently came from broken homes, 17.1 p.c. of them living with one parent only, as compared with 9.4 p.c. of the high-testing group. More, too, lived with others than their parents though the proportion is small in both cases.

It is tempting, if futile, to speculate what might have been the effect on I.Q.'s if the environmental factors we have mentioned in the lives of the two groups of children had been reversed. Supposing an exchange of circumstances had reduced the high scores by ten points and increased the low scores by like amount, they would of course still have represented two distinctly different I.Q. groups—above 120 and under 100.

In all of the characteristics thus far noted, as Table [5] shows, the children with I.Q.'s between 90 and 130 occupy an intermediate position. In fact there is a consistent gradation from the first to the fourth level— the higher the I.Q., the greater the size and value of the home, the fathers' earnings, the length of the fathers' and mothers' education, and the smaller the family [pp. 35–37].

The foregoing data do not of themselves demonstrate very much. In fact, they are only the starting point for reflective thinking and further research. In our opinion, these statistical averages merely reflect rather crudely the pervasive presence of general social and economic conditions that constitute a locus of what might be termed superior, above average, below average, and inferior factors of the reactional biography surrounding the developing children classified into these various groups. Of course, the figures reported above undoubtedly disguise quite a bit of overlap and exceptions which could be understood only through a specific study of the reactional history of each of the individual children lumped into the four groups. Indeed, it is remarkable that the averaging process yields as neat results as those presented in the table.

VI. CHILDREN WITH INFERIOR SOCIAL HISTORIES: THEIR MENTAL DEVELOPMENT IN ADOPTIVE HOMES

For both practical and theoretical purposes it is important to know what can be predicted of the psychological development of children whose true parents are behaviorally deficient. Popular psychology would, of course, very definitely assert that since intelligence is inherited, such children are not worth taking a chance on for adoption purposes.

According to the hypothesis of the reactional biography, since every individual begins at a zero point and builds up his behavior during his psychological history, children of "feeble-minded" parents are thus behaviorally equivalent to other children, providing they are biologically normal. It is interesting to examine the results of studies that have followed the intelligence development of children of inferior parents adopted into average or better homes.

Mean I.Q.'s reported in the major studies in the field are 107.4 for Burk's group of 214 children tested at 8 years; 110.0 for Leahy's group of 194 tested at 9 years, 3 months; 111.5 for Skodak's group of 154 tested at 4 years, 4 months; and 101.7 for the 175 children in Freeman's group who were placed under the age of 2 years.

Skeels and Harms [7] did a follow-up study of 107 children placed in adoptive homes in infancy or under 2 years of age. All were selected from those Iowa Soldiers' Orphans' Home children who showed inferior social histories. Those in Group I had mothers with I.Q.'s of 75 or less as determined by standard intelligence tests. Group II consisted of children whose putative fathers were classified in such inferior occupations as unskilled or slightly skilled laborers. Group III met both of the requirements of Group I and II; that is, their mothers tested 75 or below *and* their fathers were known to be occupationally not above slightly skilled laborers. All the children were of white non-Jewish parentage, were

---

[7] Skeels, H. M. & Harms, Irene. Children with inferior social histories; their mental development in adoptive homes. *J. genet. Psychol.*, 1948, **72**, 283–294. (Reproduced by permission of the authors and the publisher.)

committed to the orphanage when less than 6 months of age, and were adopted under 2 years of age.

GROUP I: DEVELOPMENT OF CHILDREN WHOSE MOTHERS HAVE LOW I.Q.'S. Of the 107 children in this group, about 80 per cent were illegitimate. Their mothers' I.Q.'s ranged from 75 down to 32. All had been adopted prior to 6 months of age into homes selected in general for their satisfactory adjustment in the community. The foster parents were described as stable, intelligent, and dependable, and their occupational level was higher than that of the children's true parents but not so high as that usually found when the foster children are not specifically selected because of inferior social histories.

The average age of children at time of examination was almost 5½ years. The mean I.Q. was 105.5. Only 4 children in the entire group classified below the dull normal group with I.Q.'s of less than 80. In contrast to these four, 15 fell into the superior group with I.Q.'s above 120! When the subjects were grouped according to the occupational level of the foster home, there was a 4-point difference in favor of the occupationally superior homes. The average I.Q. of 32 children in the three upper levels was 108.6, while that of 54 children in the four lowest levels was 104.2. These differences are suggestive.

GROUP II: DEVELOPMENT OF CHILDREN WHOSE FATHERS HAVE LOW OCCUPATIONAL STATUS. Statistically, studies have shown a certain relationship between the I.Q. of children living with their own parents and the occupational level of their fathers. There has been general agreement in finding a progression upward from the unskilled-labor group to professional groups. However one interprets these results, the present study tested 111 children whose true fathers were classified as unskilled or slightly skilled laborers that were dependent upon odd jobs or casual farm work. Intelligence-test scores that were available for 75 of the true mothers of the children tested ranged from 40 to 110, with a mean I.Q. of 77.8.

The foster homes of the children in this group were somewhat superior to the homes of the subjects of Group I and markedly superior to the homes of their true parents. Their mean age at placement was 5 months, at examination time, 5 years, 1.5 months. The average I.Q. for the whole group of 111 children was 110.3.

Here only 2 children tested below 80 in contrast to 28 children with I.Q.'s above 120.

GROUP III: DEVELOPMENT OF CHILDREN WHOSE MOTHERS ARE RE-
TARDED AND WHOSE FATHERS HAVE LOW OCCUPATIONAL STATUS. Of the 31 children who met the above criteria and were tested, all were offspring of mothers whose I.Q.'s ranged between 40 and 75, with a mean of 62.6, and of fathers all but 7 of whom were in the lowest occupational classification. Their mean age at placement was 4 months, 13 days, and mean age at test was 5 years, 3.4 months. The foster home was much superior to the true home in regard to the education of the foster parents and their occupational level. The average I.Q. for this group of 31 children was 104.0. Again, it was found that 10 children placed in homes of the upper three occupational levels had an average I.Q. of 110.1, while 20 children in homes in the four lowest brackets earned an average I.Q. of 102.5.

CONCLUSIONS. Skeels and Harms draw the following conclusions:

1. Children of mothers with low intelligence or from fathers with low occupational status or from a combination of both, placed in adoptive homes in infancy, attain a mental level which equals or exceeds that of the population as a whole.

2. The frequency with which cases showing mental retardation appear is no greater than might be expected from a random sampling of the population as a whole, and the frequency with which cases having superior intelligence appear is somewhat greater than might be expected from a random sampling [p. 294].

VII. HOW ABOUT THE JUKES AND KALLIKAKS?
N. H. Pronko

Around the turn of the century the study of the "genealogy of degeneracy" was a popular pastime. Lengthy family pedigrees were accumulated which purportedly demonstrated the hereditary transmission of feeble-mindedness, alcoholism, criminality, laziness, prostitution, debauchery, and various other socially unacceptable conduct. In more recent years these investigations have been largely discredited, although they reappear from time to time to support hereditary doctrines. Since this type of study has been offered as recently as 1948 in support of the inheritance of behavior, we shall devote a little space to an evaluation of the two best-known pedigrees, the Kallikaks and the Jukes.

The Kallikak investigation, published in 1912, traced the genealogy of two lines, one "good" and one "bad," both originating with one Martin Kallikak, a Revolutionary War soldier of alleged respectable parentage and position. The "bad strain" resulted from an unconventional alliance with a presumably feeble-minded bar-maid (feeble-minded, presumably, because she was a barmaid), the progeny consisting of paupers, criminals, prostitutes, drunkards, the feeble-minded, and so forth. On the other hand, the "good strain" was composed of good and useful citizens. Goddard, who directed this study, was convinced that all of these social ills were inherited. The following quotation from Deutsch [8] on the Kallikak study needs no comment.

In the most famous of these studies, *The Kallikak Family*, the author tells us that field workers engaged in tracking down the descendants of the Revolutionary soldier and the servant girl were permitted to ascertain feeblemindedness in a person by merely "looking at" him or her. Evidence of feeblemindedness (and other defective and degenerate traits) was largly based on hearsay; in many cases it was deemed sufficient proof of mental defect if a person, deceasd two or more generations, perhaps, was reported to have been "a wild, immoral fellow," or a "plodding, dull and drinking fellow." And how, in the first instance, the author was able to ascertain that a "nameless girl" living in Revolutionary times, a poor servant maid unknown but for her genealogically convenient *affaire d'amour*, was feebleminded, is not revealed [p. 365].

Another famous study, that of the Jukes, was published in 1877. Belief in psychoheredity was very much in vogue at this time. Darwin's *Origin of Species* had appeared a few years earlier (1859), and popularizers of his theories, including his cousin, Francis Galton, had been applying "natural selection" concepts to be-havior. Galton, for example, in 1865 began publishing pedigrees of genius to support the theory of inheritance of behavior. Dugdale, however, who traced the Jukes through five generations, stressed the importance of environment in the destiny of this family. A total of 709 individuals was studied, 540 of them related by blood

---

8 DEUTSCH, A. *The mentally ill in America*. New York: Doubleday, 1938. Pp. 530. (Reproduced by permission of the author and the publisher.)

to the Jukes. Of this number, only *one* case of definite feeble-mindedness (idiocy) was found by Dugdale. Others interpreted the Dugdale study as indicating that intemperance, crime, pauperism, licentiousness, feeble-mindedness, mental disorders and diseases, in short, all social ills, were biologically inherited. Although the Juke family has a history of socioeconomic deprivation, there is nothing particularly startling in the frequency of diseases, injuries, or behavioral pathology in the 540 individuals of Juke blood or the 169 related by marriage or cohabitation, as Table [6], from Dugdale,[9] [p. 30] indicates. In fact, it would be surprising if frequencies this high were not found in a sample of comparable size in any family tree.

Table 6

Showing the Frequencies of Various Diseases, Injuries, Behavior Pathology, and Feeble-mindedness of 540 Individuals of Juke Blood and 169 Persons Related to the Jukes by Marriage or Cohabitation (X Blood)

Diseases, Injuries, and So Forth	Number of Cases		
	Juke Blood	X Blood	Total
Blind	10	1	11
Deaf and dumb	..	1	1
Insane	1	..	1
Idiotic	1	..	1
Tubercular consumption	1	1	2
Syphilis	29	13	42
Constitutional syphilis	22	3	25
Epilepsy	..	1	1
Deformed	1	..	1
Total	65	20	85
Total number receiving relief	33	15	48

VIII. A CASE OF AN "IDIOT-SAVANT"

Illustrative of individuals whose personality equipment shows extremes of behavioral effectiveness as well as ineffectiveness is the so-called "idiot-savant." Many such individuals have been studied and reported in the literature. It has been commonly supposed that every feeble-minded person shows no superior behavioral char-

---

[9] DUGDALE, R. L. *The Jukes.* New York: Putnam, 1877. Pp. 121. (Reproduced by permission of the publisher.)

acteristic or characteristics. This supposition is not supported by the study of the feeble-minded. The idiot-savant is characterized as a feeble-minded individual whose general behavioral equipment is inadequate, but who shows some distinct superiorities in some behavioral traits. Cases have been reported in which calculating abilities have been outstanding, although usually with some distinct process limitations. Cases of behavioral superiority in music, drawing and painting, mechanical skills, sewing, and memorizing behavior have also been reported.

The following case description is abstracted from a careful study and a detailed analysis made by Scheerer, Rothmann, and Goldstein.[10] The boy, who is identified by the name of L., was found to have an I.Q. of 50 at 11 years of age. When tested again at 15 years of age he was found to have approximately the same I.Q. level as measured by standard intelligence tests. His family history showed no evidence of mental deficiency. L.'s father was a businessman and his mother a school teacher. Grandparents on both sides were of average intelligence.

In 1937 an 11 year old boy, L., was presented by his mother to the writers for neuropsychiatric and psychological consultation. The complaints about L. summed up to this; he could never follow the regular school curriculum, like a normal child, or learn by instruction. His general information was alarmingly sub-standard; he had made progress in only a few school subjects, and even in these, his achievements were very limited. His motivational and behavior peculiarities had been an early concern of his parents. He had never shown interest in his social surroundings or in normal childhood activities. On the other hand, he had always excelled in certain performances.

Medical examination showed him to be healthy and physically well-developed with no signs of neurological disturbances and with a normal EEG (electroencephalogram) record. Follow-up examinations from his 11th to his 16th year, including laboratory tests, showed no physical abnormalities. The following description of L. is based on a great number of observations and examinations made during the years 1937 to 1943.

The first impression on meeting L. is that of an erratic and hyperkinetic child, driven by an urge to keep in constant motion. He seems

10 SCHEERER, M., ROTHMANN, E. & GOLDSTEIN, K. A case of "idiot-savant," an experimental study of personality organization. *Psychol. Monogr.*, 1945, **58**, 1–63. (Reproduced by permission of the author and the American Psychological Association.)

also to be governed by an ever recurring impulse to move all four fingers of each hand rapidly in a definite beat, rubbing them against the thumbs (in a snapping-like motion without the snaps). Alternating with extreme inattentiveness, self-preoccupation, and restlessness, he displays a friendly poise and stereotyped politeness, as when responding to or addressing people. Most of the time L. appears motorically or otherwise self-absorbed and socially aloof. However, he shows one unique interest in his human surrounding—an amazing phenomenon exhibited in the first minutes of the examination. Spontaneously, the boy asks each of us, "When is your birthday?" Given the date, he answers in a fraction of a minute. "Dr. G.'s birthday was on Saturday last year and Dr. S.'s birthday was on Wednesday." A glance at the calendar proves him correct. We call others to the scene, and with amazing swiftness, L. gives correctly the day of the week of every person's birthday. Moreover, he can tell at once exactly which day of the week a person's birthday was last year or 5 years ago, and on what day it will fall in 1945, etc. More closely examined, L. proves capable of telling the day of the week for any given date between about 1880 and 1950. Conversely, he can also give the date for any given weekday in any year of that period, e.g., the date of the first Saturday in May, 1950, or of the last Monday in January, 1943, etc. As much as we could determine he makes no mistakes in his calendar answers. Though L. unquestionably takes delight in the recognition of his feat, he never seems aware of its extraordinary character in the same sense as a normal person (e.g., the reader of this, if he could master such a task). On the other hand, it is known that, since his 7th year, he had developed a persistent interest in the birthdays of everyone he meets. For some time he had been surprising people he met only once before by volunteering their birthdays "on sight." This, of course, happened to the writers on many occasions. In conjunction with this specific memory he almost inevitably will know the day and date of his first visit to a place and usually the names and birthdays of all people he met there. He never fails to look for the date when he sees a newspaper, which otherwise does not interest him in the least.

This specialized interest and retention of L. is coupled with an impressive skill in rapidly manipulating and retaining numbers. His span for immediate recall is 7 digits forward and 6 backwards. He can also add up correctly the total of ten to twelve 2-place numbers just as quickly as one can call them out. In other respects his arithmetic achievements appear on the surface to be normal for a child of his age. Except for an unusual speed in those calculations which he can execute, he does not show any superiority. On the contrary, he makes errors in multiplying, adding, or subtracting larger numbers although he has received instruction in arithmetic. Here, as in other subjects, appears an inherent difficulty in learning by following instructions and explanations in a systematic way.

This kind of memory organization is indicated by L.'s performance in spelling, for which he shows an affinity similar to that for counting. He correctly spells many words forwards and backwards, orally or in writing. He will usually ask how a word is spelled when he hears it for the first time, and will never forget it. A word not taught to him this way he will spell out phonetically without hesitation. In contrast, he never inquires into the meaning of a word, so that he knows the spelling of many more words than he knows the pertinent meanings.

L.'s rigid trend towards developing skills and knowledge only on his own limited terms of play-like function and sheer manipulative interest reappears in his musical ability. He shows a surprising musical capacity and sensitivity together with equally surprising gaps. He has absolute pitch, likes to play the piano for hours without being taught. Although he has learned to read simple scores, he plays only by ear, e.g., such melodies as the "Moonlight Sonata" or "Three Blind Mice," and later, at 14, more difficult compositions, e.g., the "Largo" from Dvorak. Mostly, however, he will play monotonous sequences of his own fancy. He will rarely reproduce a tune he knows and then only on insistent demand. He loves the opera "Othello" to the degree of obsession, and can sing the "Credo," "Si ciel" and the "Adagio Pathetique" from beginning to end. He sings the accompaniment or the Italian words as they sound to him. Without knowing the language he reproduces it purely phonetically. His interest in music includes a preference for the operas of Verdi, for Beethoven, Schubert, and Tschaikowsky, all of whom he likes to hear on records. He prefers a victrola concert to music from the radio in which he never showed interest. He is able to recognize and place a heard composition, to identify its name, and to complete a melody, if he hears a part of it. At 12 he was taken to a competent musician who played a piano piece unknown to him. Asked to repeat it, L. did so, according to the musician, amazingly well . . . the melody correct, the accompaniment adequate. In contrast, L. never has profited from any systematic musical training. He has always refused to learn piano pieces by reading the scores, and would not pay any attention to them. He would never practice a composition nor readily repeat his musical performance on demand, and would not correct his mistakes when told to do so. It is not even certain whether he did grasp the errors which were pointed out to him. If he heard the same composition several times, he would improve his playing of it, but he never seemed to improve through practice. Occasionally he sat at the piano and played what appeared to be short compositions, but it was never possible to make him repeat them so that they could be fixated. Yet words and names related to music he retained almost indefinitely . . . [pp. 1–3].

L.'s case is instructive and shows among others things, how relative the term "idiot" really is. As a matter of fact, this term is so inapplicable to L. that the apparently contradictory label "idiot-savant" seems to suit better. He is truly lacking in certain specific behaviors, but, at the same time, he is exceedingly overdeveloped in certain other specific reactions—far above most persons.

9

ATTENTION

I. INTRODUCTION
John Bucklew, Jr.

Attending is not a distinct kind of response, in the sense that feeling or other responses are, but rather is the beginning part of every psychological response, or adjustment, that the organism makes. It is the organism's preliminary contact with some stimulus. For this reason, experiments on attending, although they may be concerned with a variety of actions—perception, feeling, attitudes, habits—will be found to emphasize the variables which operate in the initial phases of the total response.

The stimulus to which a person attends will be the one which he perceives and to which he carries out some final adjustment, such as approaching, avoiding, or speaking to or about something. Therefore, since attending is in a genuine sense a determiner of what will follow, its study becomes of some importance to the psychologist. The lover of visual arts, standing before a new painting, illustrates admirably the successive attention and perception phases of the responses he is making to the various qualities of the stimulus object. The complex aesthetic object before him requires more than a single glance for its proper appreciation, and so our aesthete must gain his comprehension of it through a series of responses to its parts and their relations.

What governs this continual shift of attention from one stimulus to the next? At first consideration, it may seem to be a purely random and chaotic affair, but it can be demonstrated that there are classes of factors which govern it. For a given person one stimulus object, or a group of objects, may possess a greater "attention value" than others. These various factors may be conveniently classified into (1) factors of the stimulus object (such as size or brightness), (2) factors of the person's history or reactional biography (attitudes, knowledge), (3) behavior in progress at the moment (momentary interests or needs), and (4) physiological conditions of the organism (fatigue, hunger).

As one might expect, the psychology of attention has been extensively applied in advertising and selling, for businessmen are concerned with what will attract attention to their merchandise and are usually willing to pay a great deal in order to accomplish this with maximum efficiency. The following reading is meant to serve as an introduction to the topic of attention by presenting some ways in which the term has been used and some classic experiments in this area. Subsequent sections show how stimulus factors, such as intensity of illumination and complexity of the stimulus, operate in directing or channeling the activity of people. But the organism and its conditions also play a determining role in the stimuli to which it responds. It will be demonstrated that a person's knowledge or information and his experiences sensitize him peculiarly to react to certain stimuli rather than others. Even his interests and attitudes operate in a similar fashion.

II. CLASSIC STUDIES OF ATTENTION

It should be pointed out that the term "attention" is employed in a variety of ways in psychological literature. The referents for this term fall into three main categories:

1. Attending reaction systems refer to the initial phases of behavioral events which involve either a shift in activity from one stimulus object to another or from one phase of an object to another phase of the same object. These shifts in activity are fleeting acts which initiate new behavioral segments and have been described in the preceding article.

2. Attentional posture or attentional adjustment is another referent for the term. Still another term so employed is "set." Here the fleeting shift in activity is not referred to, but a complete adjustment or behavioral segment in preparation for a subsequent adjustment is the referent. A soldier responding to the command "Attention!" would illustrate the type of behavior referred to in this use of the term. The performance of the postural adjustment

reaction is a final act in itself, even though it is preparatory to the performance of some later action. Notice that this attentional posture involves an attentional or contacting reaction system. If the soldier fails to get into contact with the command, he is precluded from perceiving it and executing it. This preparatory set may condition subsequent genuine attentional acts, as is shown in the Postman and Jenkins study discussed elsewhere in this chapter. Subjects "set" to perform one type of action contact the stimulus differently than do subjects "set" to perform other types of responses.

3. The third use of the term refers to a continuing series of behaviors in which the person is *preoccupied* with some task, such as reading a book or solving a set of arithmetic problems. An equivalent term for this "sustained attention" is concentration. It does not denote a unit of action or a phase of a single behavioral segment (attending reaction system) but is a nontechnical term encompassing perhaps thousands of discrete responses performed in the completion of some task. It, too, of course, involves attentional acts—each of the responses involved in the series is initiated by a contacting reaction system—and it may also involve set or preparatory attention adjustments.

Writers have not always carefully defined the term "attention" as they employed it, hence an extensive literature subsumed under this heading includes various combinations of the three general uses of the term described above. Clearly, attentional acts, i.e., the initial phases of behavioral responses, are not easily isolated for investigation because of their subtlety and brevity. Therefore, most studies have been concerned with the other sorts of attention described. Although nearly all behavioral segments are initiated by attending reactions, most studies have emphasized the later phases, perceptual, and final adjustments, since these aspects of the segment of behavior are more amenable to investigation. This has been true of the studies reported in other articles in this chapter as well as in the summaries of classic studies which follow.

One early investigation attempted to discover the rapidity with which a series of visual responses to a picture was performed. This was an indirect endeavor to get at contacting reaction systems. A picture was placed in front of the subject, and he was asked to fixate a particular point in the picture and press a key whenever he shifted to some other part of the picture. The methods of investigation were obviously quite crude, and the shifting reaction systems were in themselves not isolated. That is, shifting from the initial fixation point involved not only attending but perceptual reaction systems as well, and pressing the key required a shift in attention from the picture to the key. Further, new attentional and other reaction systems could occur without shifting to a new portion of the picture; one can perform a series of implicit (daydreaming) reactions, for example, under conditions such as the above.

Perhaps the investigator can best observe visual attending reaction systems in reading situations, particularly with the aid of cinemagraphic recording devices. The eye movements from one fixation point in the reading to another are for the most part genuine attending reaction systems. The comparatively new eye-camera techniques utilized by applied psychologists in the study of advertising, for example, also isolate contacting reaction systems. The fixation periods between shifts to new word groups in reading or new portions of a picture are not necessarily limited to single behavioral segments, however. A series of attending, perceiving, and various final adjustments may occur during a fixation.

Some of the classic studies of attending reactions utilized ambiguous figures, such as those drawn in reversible perspective. These objects, of simple design, are usually conducive to two, though occasionally more, sorts of reactions. They may be described as objects which, because of their construction, force attentional shifts from one of their phases to another and then back again. The familiar cubes and staircases are illustrative of these objects.

Such forced attention shifts with simple types of stimulus objects were noted by the aurist Urbantschitsch (1875) when he employed the watch test for hearing. He discovered that when the watch was held at a distance, the subject did not constantly hear it but periodically got into contact with it and then lost contact. Similar results were later obtained with various faint stimuli, and the term "fluctuation of attention" was applied to these shifts in activity.

"Set," or attentional posture reactions, were reported in early studies of reaction time. Exner, a Vienna physiologist investigating reaction time (1873), noted that there was a preparatory response before the RT (reaction time) stimulus was presented. This was studied in more detail by Lange (1888) who found that trained subjects could perform different sorts of preparatory adjustments and that their reaction times varied with those adjustments. It was discovered in these early studies that the preparatory reactions led to responses to time intervals. Unless the delay following a "ready" signal was varied, or the stimulus for the RT response was occasionally omitted, subjects came to perform the key-pressing response in anticipation of the RT stimulus.

The reader may have noted that the term "postural attention" is not too satisfactory in that some of the preparatory adjustments involve other than postural reactions. The Postman and Jenkins experiment, for example, is concerned not with postural adjustments but with preparatory orientations or attitudes toward the learning material that was to be presented. However, for want of a better term, we have used "attentional posture" to refer to these preparatory reactions in this chapter, since the behavioral configurations are similar when the preliminary responses are characterized by postural adjustments and when other features are more prominent.

Concentration or sustained attention has become a field of interest, particularly since the classic study by Morgan [1] on work under conditions of distraction and nondistraction. Morgan was interested in the techniques utilized by subjects in avoiding various sorts of potential distracters. Subjects were required to perform a task something like typewriting with an instrument containing 10 numbered keys. The apparatus was so devised that the pressure of the subject's fingers upon the keys could be recorded. A pneumograph about the chest furnished a breathing record.

The apparatus exposed a letter which the subject translated into a number according to a code and then struck the key containing that number. When the key was struck, another letter was immediately exposed, and so on.

The subject was allowed to work under quiet conditions for a time, then bells, buzzers, and phonograph records began to sound from all parts of the room. The noises continued for 10 minutes and a 10-minute quiet work period followed.

Morgan found that, since the subjects had had little preliminary training in this task, progressive improvement was made throughout the experiment. When the noises commenced, there

---

[1] MORGAN, J. J. B. The overcoming of distraction and other resistances. *Arch. Psychol.*, 1916, 35.

was some slowing down in work; they were functioning as distracting stimuli, and the subjects shifted to them instead of responding consistently to their task. However, within a few minutes the subjects regained their former speed and went on to further improvement. The distracters failed to function as stimuli after a brief time, and the subjects continued reactional preoccupation with their assigned task. The noises continued to operate as setting factors in this study in that during the noise-work conditions the subjects struck the keys with greater force, and breathing records and observations revealed that the subjects utilized the technique of talking to themselves while performing the task to avoid interacting with the distracters.

It was also noted that, when the noises ceased, there was often a momentary slump in work output, i.e., the change from noise to quiet also functioned as a distracting stimulus. Later studies have analyzed in more detail the behavior of individuals in distracting and nondistracting situations (see for example the experiment by Freeman in this chapter).

The articles in this chapter deal with the various referents for attention described above, or with combinations of them. They illustrate the need for detailed analysis of behavioral events if understanding is to be achieved, and, incidentally, point to the constant operational check the investigator must maintain upon his use of *terms* and the *referents* for which they stand.

III. THE EFFECT OF ILLUMINATION
UPON ATTENTION [2]

The most obvious visual element is the actual amount of illumination, whether it be provided by an electric sign, an illuminated poster board, or simply by a number of lamps in front of one's place of business. The general increase of attention with intensity of illumination needs little demonstration. It is interesting, however, to note a few instances in which an effort has been made to measure the relation between intensity and attention. Experiments were conducted with different degrees of illumination in a store window, and an observer was posted to count the pro-

[2] BURTT, H. E. *Psychology of advertising.* Boston: Houghton Mifflin, 1938. Pp. 473. (Reproduced by permission of the author and the publisher.)

portion of the people passing the store who stopped to look into the window. The results are summarized briefly in the accompanying table. The first column gives the amount of illumination in foot candles, and the second column, the corresponding percentages of the passers-by who

Table 7

Percentage of Pedestrians Stopping to View Window Display

Foot Candles	Per Cent
15	10
30	12
50	15
65	17
85	19
100	21

actually stopped to view the window. The added illumination produced an obvious increase in the attention value of the window display, although the two factors are not in direct proportion. Doubling the illumination, for instance, from fifteen to thirty foot candles merely increased the percentage of those stopping from 10 to 12. Attention lagged behind intensity, just as it has been found in other experiments to lag behind. The writer knows of a church that increased the attendance at its evening service about 50 per cent by the simple expedient of putting a few bright lights in front of the church building. Persons out walking on a pleasant evening with no particular destination would be attracted by the lights and come into the service. Figures similar to the above are not available regarding the effectiveness of illuminated outdoor displays, but there is every reason to suspect that they are quite valuable from the standpoint of commanding attention [pp. 179–180].

At any rate, the simple experiment described above does illustrate the point previously made that such aspects of the stimulus object as intensity do have a determining effect on an individual's response. In attempting to force an individual to "pay attention" to a particular stimulus object or situation, one of the variables that may be manipulated is the intensity of the visual (or auditory or olfactory) stimulus. Where there is keen competition for people's attention, as in the myriad signs of Times Square, New York, such other variables as color, novelty, and movement must also be introduced.

IV. A STUDY OF SOME ORGANISMIC FACTORS
INFLUENCING ATTENTION

The ability of the individual to perceive particular properties of stimulus objects is dependent upon a number of factors of the psychological field. Among these factors is the amount of time that the stimuli are exposed to the observer. If circumstances are such that the exposure is not sufficiently long, the subject may not be able to enter into appropriate psychological contact with the object. This does not mean, of course, that exposure time is the only factor of importance in determining whether the subject will enter into appropriate psychological relationship with the stimulus objects. Among other factors is the complexity of the stimulus object or objects.

Saltzman and Garner [3] used concentric circles as stimulus objects. In one experiment, the exposure time of the flashes on the screen was kept at ½ second. From two to ten circles were randomly presented. The subject was instructed to observe carefully and report the number of circles on each flash exposure. One, two, or three concentric circles could be perceived without error on each exposure. Four circles could be perceived correctly on about 90 per cent of the exposures. Five or more circles could be perceived correctly on less than 50 per cent of the exposures. Thus, effective contacting and perceiving reaction systems could be made to these particular stimulus objects in ½-second exposures only if no more than four circles were present. For the more complex stimuli, the ½-second exposure was not a sufficient time. But the efficiency of contacting reaction systems is not to be regarded as static. As a matter of fact, experimental factors were found to be as important here as in other classes of behavior. It was shown that, after some practice, stimuli as complex as *seven* circles could be perceived correctly more than 50 per cent of the time by the same subjects. A further factor determining the effectiveness of contacting reaction systems is the amount of knowledge which the subject had beforehand. When subjects were informed that stimuli with a range of from *two* to *ten* circles would be exposed, they averaged approximately 80 per cent or better correct on stimuli as complex

[3] SALTZMAN, I. J. & GARNER, W. R. Reaction time as a measure of span of attention. *J. Psychol.*, 1948, **25**, 227–241.

as ten circles. For the same amount of practice, subjects who did not know that the range was from two to ten circles perceived 80 per cent or better correct only on stimuli of five or less circles. In another portion of that study, Saltzman and Garner attempted to determine the minimum time for effective contacting and perceiving reaction systems by varying the time of exposure rather than the amount of material as above. As the complexity of the stimulus objects increased from two to ten, the amount of time necessary for efficient psychological interaction increased from approximately ½ second to 3½ seconds. Again, with practice, the time necessary for contact on the ten-circle stimulus reduced from 3½ seconds to slightly more than 2 seconds.

These findings lead the investigators to conclude that "attention span" is not to be regarded as an absolute quantity, characteristic of individuals, as has been held by some psychologists. The complexity of the stimulus which may be perceived on a single exposure varies for the individual with a number of factors. The variables that were shown to operate in the Saltzman and Garner experiment were the time of exposure, the complexity of the stimulus object, amount of information given the subject, and experience with the stimulus materials.

In chemistry, the student is taught that the characteristics of a chemical interaction, e.g., the speed with which it occurs, depend upon how finely the material is subdivided, the temperature under which that interaction occurs, presence or absence of catalytic agents, and so on. In psychology, the situation is no different except that it takes place on a different level. As with other behaviors, so with attention—what happens is a function of a multiplicity of conditions or variables in the field under observation. There is no easy listing of important factors. The investigator must be sensitive to their operation and determination in each instance.

V. A STUDY OF FIRST IMPRESSIONS
N. H. Pronko

Making a good first impression has long been considered one of the social graces. Psychological study of the topic poses the twin questions of what about a person attracts attention and what influences favorable judgment. Jacobson's [4] study of the first impressions of college students of one another reveals some of the attentional factors operating when one person observes another. The study was performed on 401 women students in a College Problems class for freshmen at Ohio University. The girls met in groups of 23, and their participation was enlisted by asking them if they would like to come up to the front of the class individually, speak their names, and stand for a minute while the others jotted down impressions of them. Although the study was performed early in the semester, some of the students were already acquainted with one another, so each observer was asked to record on the card her degree of acquaintanceship with the person she was observing.

The experimenter classified the impressions into five general categories and tabulated the positive, neutral, or negative judgments falling in each. The following table shows these categories, along with some typical comments falling in each. Table 9 shows the frequency of responses in each of the four categories broken down for degree of acquaintanceship.

Table 8

Classifications of Impressions, with Typical Responses

I. Physical characteristics
   A. Physique

1. Hair	"Pretty blonde hair"
2. Eyes	"Large eyes"
3. Eyebrows	"Eyebrows could be thinned"
4. Mouth	"Not very attractive mouth"
5. Nose	"Cute nose"
6. Teeth	"White teeth"
7. Complexion	"Too pale"
8. Dimples	"Beautiful dimples"
9. Figure	"Good figure"
10. Height	"Too tall for a girl"
11. Weight	"Should lose some weight"
12. Posture	"Good posture"
13. Carriage	"Carries herself nicely"
14. General Characteristics	"Very attractive face"
15. Masculinity-femininity	"Boyish in appearance"

   B. 16. Health   "Unhealthy looking"

[4] Adapted from JACOBSON, W. F. First impressions of classmates. *J. appl. Psychol.*, 1945, 29, 142–155.

Table 8 *(Continued)*

Classifications of Impressions, with Typical Responses

C. 17. Vitality	"Looks worn out"
D. 18. Voice	"Nice voice"

II. Intelligence
19. Abstract	"Looks brilliant"
20. Practical	"Looks efficient"

III. Clothing
22. Harmony of parts of costume	"Should not wear heels with ankle sox"
23. Harmony of colors	"Too many different colors"
24. Suitability of clothes to person	"Wears becoming clothes"
25. Suitability to occasion	"Suitable school clothes"
26. Manifestations of taste in dress	"Good taste in dress"
27. Fit of dress	"Skirt doesn't fit properly"
28. Remarks about clothing	"Pretty sweater"
29. Principles of art involved	"Bow too large for its position"

IV. Grooming
30. General remarks	"Dresses neatly"
31. Make-up	"Needs more make-up"
32. Hair dress	"Hair could be fixed differently"
33. Shoes	"Shoes could be cleaned"
34. Nails	"Too dark a shade of nail polish"
35. Cleanliness	"She looks clean"
36. Laundering	"Belt is a little soiled"

V. Psychological characteristics
21. Manifestations of emotions	"Afraid to smile in public"
37. Ascendant-submissive	"Dominant at times"
38. Expansion-reclusion	"Quiet"
39. Persistence-vacillation	"A bit flighty"
40. Extroversion-introversion	"Acts as if she would be nice after you know her but seems to have a wall you would have to break through first"
41. Self-objectification–self-deception	"Imagine she would be sincere"
42. Self-assurance–self-distrust	"Seems rather sure of herself"
43. Gregarious-solitary	"Very sociable or friendly"
44. Altruism–self-seeking	"Very kind to others"
45. Social intelligence	"Not always tactful"
46. Directed toward values	"Seems serious about college"
47. Radicalism-conservatism	"Very conservative type"
48. Observers' approval or disapproval	"Don't think I'd like her"
49. General responses	"A great deal of charm"

Table 9

Percentage Distribution of Responses (116 Observers)

Category	Don't Know Her	Know Her Slightly	Know Her Well	A Friend	All Groups
Physical	24.0	24.2	27.0	24.8	24.2
Intelligence	1.1	0.8	0.5	0.9	1.1
Clothing	15.8	14.8	12.2	13.3	15.4
Grooming	30.3	27.2	22.7	22.6	29.3
Psychological	28.8	33.0	37.7	38.5	30.2

Another human being is a very complex source of stimulation for an observer. Consequently, the factors which tend to attract attention are numerous and varied. Some of this complexity is revealed in Table 8. The nature of the stimuli for the first, third, and fourth categories is fairly apparent, but it is less so for the second and fifth. A moment's reflection, however, should convince us that the majority of stimuli for these must be the *behavioral patterns* (the walk, postures, voice qualities, facial expressions) which the students displayed before the class. Some of the comments listed, such as "afraid to smile in public," "quiet," would seem to substantiate this, although, in most instances, the remarks are too general to permit us to isolate the stimulus.

The frequency of responses given in Table 9 would appear to indicate that attention is more apt to be attracted to the behavior of another person rather than to his physical features. This seems particularly striking when we realize that the activity of the subjects in the experimental situation of this study was reduced to a minimum. In a free and unrestrained social setting, it would probably be even more true. The artificial conditions of the study probably placed a maximum emphasis on the physical, clothing, and grooming categories. The progressive increase in the psychological category with degree of acquaintanceship suggests that the behavioral adjustments of other people finally dominate as the most attention-compelling stimuli. This agrees with everyday experience.

A demonstration in support of this point has been frequently made by the author. After checking the roll or even lecturing for some time, he will turn to the blackboard and turn up his coat collar quickly, then turn around and ask the students to report the color and style of the instructor's necktie. Very few have observed it. Yet a rating sheet, given the students each semester asking them to evaluate the instructor, shows the keenness with which they observe his gestural, voice, and other personality features. It is doubtful if the physical characteristics (outside of disfigurements, unusual size, shape, and so on) have the same attention-compelling characteristics as the behavior of individuals. Certainly, with greater acquaintance or experience, behavioral characteristics of individuals seemed to dominate over nonbehavioral features in getting attention.

VI. THE DISTRACTING EFFECT OF NEARBY CARTOONS ON THE ATTENTION HOLDING POWER OF ADVERTISEMENTS [5]

John J. McNamara and Joseph Tiffin
Purdue University

"Sustained attention," or the performance of a series of responses to a complex object such as a magazine advertisement, is influenced by various features of the behavioral setting, like the presence of cartoons. This is shown in the following experiment.

In a recent series of experiments using the Purdue Eye Camera it has been possible to evaluate objectively the effect of cartoons adjacent to advertisements upon the attention holding power of these advertisements. The Purdue Eye Camera makes it possible to photograph the time spent upon each advertisement (or specific part of the advertisement) by a reader leafing through a magazine. The camera is so constructed that the magazine is placed unopened on an easel before the reader. The reader voluntarily opens the magazine and leafs through the pages at whatever rate he wishes, stopping for as long, or short, a time on each item of interest as he desires. The camera is driven by an electric motor which is activated by a silent switch so that it can be started and stopped without awareness on the part of the reader. By means of this arrangement, only eye movements occurring on the material being studied need be photographed. The reader is told that an investigation is being made of what interests him in the magazine. While he

[5] McNamara, J. J. & Tiffin, J. The distracting effect of nearby cartoons on the attention holding power of advertisements. *J. appl. Psychol.*, 1941, **25**, 524–527. (Reproduced by permission of the authors and the publisher.)

realizes that it is some sort of experimental situation, he is not actually aware at the time that his eye movements are being recorded.

In the present series of experiments, of which this report covers only one part, various groups of men and women readers from an industrial city were asked to leaf through a recent issue of the *Saturday Evening Post.* This magazine was obtained two days prior to newsstand release. The readers, therefore, had not had an opportunity to see the magazine prior to the experiment. The readers used in the study were divided into four groups. One group leafed through a standard issue of the magazine exactly as it appeared later on the newsstands. The other three groups leafed through issues which had been "doctored" as indicated below:

Group 1. Magazine unaltered.

Group 2. Magazine altered by blocking out cartoons near certain advertisements with printed material similar to the copy appearing around the cartoon.

Group 3. Magazine altered by interchanging certain advertisements and cartoons from left to right page (or vice versa).

Group 4. Magazine altered by blocking out cartoons near certain advertisements and changing advertisements from left to right page (or vice versa).

The reversal of left and right hand pages was not essential in studying the effect of cartoons, but was necessary for certain other parts of the investigation which are to be published at a later date.

One hundred and twenty readers were used in the experiment, but since each reader was allowed to see a given advertisement in only one of the four situations mentioned above, no single group contained more than thirty-five readers.

The result of the measurements are shown in Table [10]. This table reveals that of the ten situations studied, nine show a definitely greater average time spent by the reader upon the advertisement when the adjacent cartoon had been eliminated than when the cartoon was present as it appeared in the normal issue of the magazine. The only exception to this finding is the ninth item on the table, which shows a slight and statistically insignificant reversal. The averages show that for the five advertisements studied in ten positions, the average time spent with the nearby cartoon present was 2.94 seconds, whereas when the cartoon had been eliminated, this average was raised to 4.54 seconds. This difference of 1.60 seconds, or 54%, is 4.4 times its standard error and hence is significant from a statistical viewpoint.

Table 10 *

Mean Time in Seconds Spent on Five Advertisements in Ten Positions When Each Appeared with and without a Cartoon on the Same Spread

Advertisements Appearing in a Recent Issue of the *Saturday Evening Post*	Effect of Cartoons	
	With Cartoon	Without Cartoon
	Mean	Mean
Eastman Kodak on left page (1 page advertisement)	2.64	5.99
Eastman Kodak on right page (1 page advertisement)	3.69	6.39
Pyroil on left page (2 column advertisement)	1.77	3.24
Pyroil on right page (2 column advertisement)	2.81	2.94
Remington Rand on left page (2 column advertisement)	1.78	2.29
Remington Rand on right page (2 column advertisement)	2.64	4.60
Del Monte on left page (1 column advertisement)	1.58	2.00
Del Monte on right page (1 column advertisement)	3.20	5.39
Capital Stock on left page (1 page advertisement)	4.91	4.63
Capital Stock on right page (1 page advertisement)	3.69	6.70
Average	2.94	4.54

Difference = 1.60
S.D.$_{diff.}$ = .36
C.R. = 4.4

* Reproduced by permission of the American Psychological Association.

It should be emphasized that this study deals only with the effect of cartoons upon nearby advertisements when all other factors are held constant. It is likely—indeed, perhaps certain, when one considers the reader preference for cartoons—that a scattering of cartoons throughout the advertising section of a magazine increases the reader "traffic" through this section. This increase in traffic probably results in a net gain for the advertisements considered as a group. But when the traffic is held constant (as in this experiment) those advertisements which happen to be on a spread which does *not* contain a cartoon seem to be in the preferred positions [pp. 524–527].

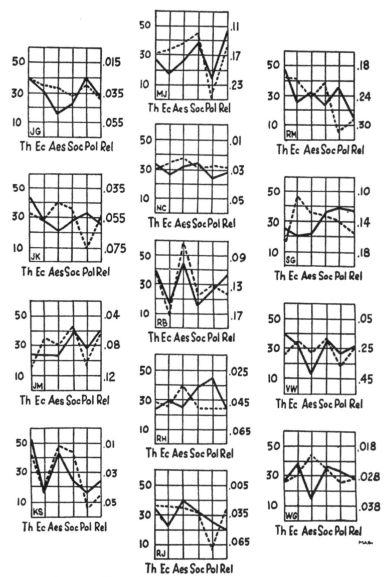

FIG. 24   Value profiles and time-of-recognition profiles of the subjects. The values tested by the Allport-Vernon Study are indicated along the abscissa. Value scores are plotted against the left-hand ordinate. Average recognition

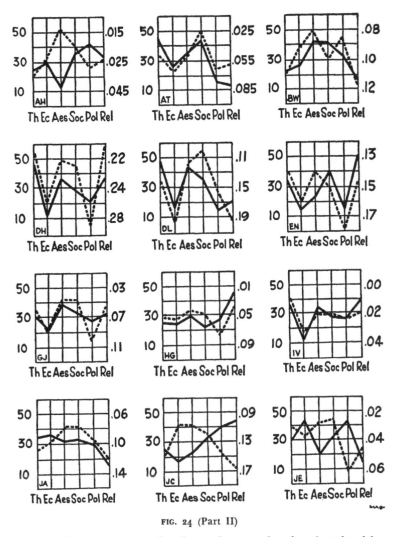

FIG. 24 (Part II)

times for the words representing these values are plotted against the right-hand ordinate. Solid lines represent value scores, dotted lines represent times of recognition. (Postman, L., Bruner, J. S., & McGinnies, E., Personal values as selective factors in perception.)

VII. CONDITIONS OF THE REACTIONAL BIOGRAPHY ARE IMPORTANT IN ATTENTION

A recent study by Postman, Bruner, and McGinnies [6] demonstrates that, in addition to conditions on the part of the stimulus object such as movement, repetition, change, suddenness, contrast, or intensity, other features of the behavioral field are important in determining the speed and ease with which an organism attends to and perceives an object. These are conditions of the reactional biography. The attitudes, interests, feelings, likes, and dislikes which go to make up the personality structure play a part in attending and perceiving events.

PROCEDURE.   Twenty-five college students served as subjects in this study. They were shown thirty-six words, one at a time, in a tachistoscope. The words represented the six values of the All-port-Vernon Study of Values Scale (a test sampling the individual's attitudes toward a variety of topics—theoretical, economic, aesthetic, social, political, and religious values or attitudes). These stimulus words are shown in the following list.

Stimulus Words Representing the Six Spranger Value Categories

Theoretical	Economic	Aesthetic	Social	Political	Religious
theory	income	beauty	loving	govern	prayer
verify	useful	artist	kindly	famous	sacred
science	wealthy	poetry	devoted	compete	worship
logical	finance	elegant	helpful	citizen	blessed
research	economic	literary	friendly	politics	religion
analysis	commerce	graceful	sociable	dominate	reverent

Each word was exposed in the tachistoscope three times for 0.01 second. If the subject did not attend to and correctly perceive the word, exposures were repeated at longer intervals. The subject's performance on this test of attending and perceiving was compared with his "values" or "attitudes" as sampled by the Allport-Vernon Study of Values. This scale was administered either several weeks in advance of or after the experiment.

RESULTS.   Figure 24 shows "time of recognition profiles" for each subject. The solid lines are the value or attitude scores obtained on the Allport-Vernon scale. The dotted lines are the aver-

---

[6] POSTMANN, L., BRUNER, J. S. & McGINNIES, E. Personal values as selective factors in perception. *J. abnorm. soc. Psychol.*, 1948, **43**, 142–154.

age recognition times for the six words representing each value. Note the marked tendency for the "high-value words," those representing dominant interests or attitudes for the individual, to be recognized at the shorter time exposures. Considering the sample as a whole, time of recognition varies with the value of the words, indicating that the conditions of the reactional biography which give these words their stimulus values are important features of attending and perceiving events. These results are statistically as well as behaviorally significant.

VIII. SET OR "PREPARATORY ATTENTION" IN LEARNING

Set or "preparatory attention," in this experiment by Postman and Jenkins,[7] refers to the preliminary adjustment of the individual to some sort of learning task. The experimenters hypothesized that the subject's performance would be optimal if the test employed for the retention of learning was the one expected by the subject but would be less satisfactory if the type of retention test was other than the one expected. "Attention" here refers to the orientation of the subject to the learning tasks as influenced by the instructions given him. As such, it indicates a definite adjustment of the subject to a complex behavioral situation rather than the split-second shift of activity from one object to another in initiating a new segment of behavior which also bears the name "attention."

The learning material in the Postman and Jenkins study consisted of twenty-five two-syllable adjectives which the experimenter read to a group of subjects. The list was read through a total of five times, with a 6-second interval between successive readings.

Prior to this learning phase of the study, different instructions were given to three groups of subjects. One group of subjects was instructed that they would be tested for learning by the *anticipative* method. They would be expected to attempt to anticipate and write down the word following the one read by the experimenter.

Free-recall instructions were given to a second group; they

---

[7] POSTMAN, L. & JENKINS, W. O. An experimental analysis of set in rote learning: the interaction of learning instruction and retention performance. *J. exp. Psychol.*, 1948, 38, 683–689.

were told that they would be given a sheet of paper on which to write down all the words that they could remember.

The third group received *recognition* instructions. They were told that after the words were read, a long list of words would be handed them and they would attempt to pick out of this list the words that had been read during the learning phase.

Following the learning series, either tests for retention were given as in the instructions, or the subjects were told that the test would be different from the one originally announced, and new instructions were given. Thus, subjects who had been instructed for *anticipation,* were tested by anticipative, free-recall, or recognition methods; subjects instructed for *free recall* were tested by free-recall, anticipative, or recognition procedures; and subjects instructed for *recognition* were tested by recognition, anticipative, or free-recall techniques. If the instructions given with regard to the type of retention test to be employed elicited different sorts of preparatory adjustments, if subjects responded differently with the word stimuli as a result of those instructions, retention-test performances should be highest when such tests were given according to the initial instructions.

The results, in terms of the average number of items correctly retained, appear in Table 11. An analysis reveals that the relationship of the learning instructions to testing procedure is quite

Table 11

Average Number of Items Retained under the Different Experimental Conditions. (Number of Cases on Which Means Are Based Appear in Parentheses.)

Test Procedure	Learning Instruction		
	Anticipation	Free Recall	Recognition
Anticipation	9.90 (40)	7.96 (25)	8.25 (20)
Free recall	15.00 (21)	13.60 (25)	11.17 (24)
Recognition	18.58 (12)	19.26 (23)	21.20 (25)

significant. With the *anticipative tests,* both free-recall and recognition instructions lead to poorer performance than do instructions to anticipate. With the *free-recall tests,* subjects instructed for recognition did not do so well as those instructed for recall. With *recognition tests,* subjects given both anticipative and recall instructions performed less satisfactorily than subjects instructed for recognition. The results of this experiment show that set, or the preparation of the subjects to attend to certain aspects of the word stimuli in the learning situation, definitely conditioned their later retention-test performances.

IX. "DISTRACTING STIMULI" AND EXPENDITURE OF ENERGY

"Distracting stimuli" are objects such as lights, sounds, movements, or persons which function to attract the attention of an individual from some other activity. These elicit a shift in activity from one object to another, and thus "distracters" are basically attentional stimuli. To avoid responding to potential distracters, particularly if they are intense, and to maintain preoccupation with the task at hand, increased effort on the part of the individual may be required, as Freeman [8] found in the experiment summarized here.

Freeman's subjects were two adults. They were required to perform tasks under conditions of quiet and of noise of approximately 50 decibels. The experiment was carried on for 12 consecutive days. Work periods were of 20 minutes' duration, divided equally between noisy and quiet conditions. These periods were preceded by 40 minutes of rest and took place in the morning when the subjects had been without food for 12 hours. This was done so that the subjects would be in a "basal" physiological condition, since consumption of oxygen was used as one index of the expenditure of energy. Consumption of oxygen was measured during the work periods and the last 10 minutes of the rest period. Action potentials (electrical activity of the muscles) were photographically recorded by means of a crystal oscilloscope and were employed as a second index of metabolic rate. These recordings were taken from the four limbs.

Noisy and quiet work conditions were alternated in a random fashion to avoid anticipation by the subjects. Addition problems

[8] FREEMAN, G. L. Changes in tension pattern and total energy expenditure during adaptation to "distracting" stimuli. *Amer. J. Psychol.,* 1939, **52**, 354-360.

printed on cards were shown to the subjects while they lay in a semiprone position. The subjects solved the problems and recorded their answers on a writing board. Freeman found that work output was only temporarily reduced upon the introduction of noises. Initially, the noises functioned to some extent as "distracting stimuli," but eventually the subjects were able to maintain preoccupation with the addition problems about as well during the noisy periods as the quiet. Concentration upon the addition tasks was not achieved without effort, however. Especially during the first few days, there was a considerable increase in expenditure of energy, as indicated by the amount of oxygen consumed during the noisy periods. The energy level gradually returned to about that established for work under quiet conditions.

Action-potential records were consistent with consumption of oxygen. They revealed that, under the early noise-work conditions, the subjects were more active than under quiet-work conditions, but that, on succeeding days, activity gradually reduced to near the quiet-work level. Under quiet-work conditions, the greatest electrical activity was found in the right arms of the subjects. Under early noise-work conditions, the other limbs showed striking increases in muscular activity, but under later noise-work conditions this activity had returned to about the quiet-work level. Activity was high in the right arm, of course, because this arm was used in writing answers. These findings indicate that the subjects' efforts at compensating for the noises in the early phases of the noise-work conditions involved increased tension and random-movement kinds of activity.

This study may be described as an investigation of sustained attention or reactional preoccupation with a given task under conditions of noise and quiet. In summary, it was found that when noises first were introduced, they functioned to elicit attention reactions; however, they did not continue to function in this way. The two subjects came to ignore or avoid them, but initially this avoidance was obtained at the expense of increased effort. Eventually, the subjects became adjusted to these new behavioral conditions and maintained their work output without marked increases in expenditure of energy. Without increased effort, they eventually learned not to attend to the noises, i.e., not to shift their activity intermittently to such stimulus situations. Again, the effect of the person's experience or history on attention is demonstrated.

SUMMARY. This chapter has dealt with a genuine behavioral fact, namely, attention. People working in a boiler factory learn to ignore surrounding noises. Others can sleep in an automobile running at high speed with motor roaring, horns blowing, and so on, but cannot sleep under similar conditions in their bedrooms. Students of birds, architecture, dress design, painting, or carpentry become highly sensitized to those stimuli with which they have had much contact in the past. Such experiences determine that individuals will react to certain stimuli and not to others. Other homely examples, such as the person sitting in his living room reading a paper but being almost literally forced to look out the window at every car in anticipation of his dinner guest, define the kind of behavioral fact we have analyzed here. The same person, when he is not expecting anyone, can pursue his reading of the paper without noticing the passing cars.

It is this initial phase of every reaction that we have scrutinized in this chapter—the head turnings, the postural and other shifts that bring the organism and stimulus object into such a psychological relationship that other subsequent adjustments are facilitated. We have found that factors on the side of the stimulus (intensity, size, movement, and so on) as well as those on the organism's side (previous experience, knowledge, attitudes, and set) are important variables in directing or selecting what stimuli will act on a particular individual.

10

PERCEPTION

I. THE NATURE OF "PERCEPTION"
N. H. Pronko

The kinds of behavior isolated in this chapter under the title of perception include the *recognition* of automobiles, airplanes, whistles, 25-cent pieces, pesos, or shillings, our homes and friends, and the odors, tastes, and feels of objects with which we have been in contact before. Since Aristotle, psychologists have acknowledged that in perceptual behavior objects *mean* something. For example, sounds are *identified* as the whistle of a steamboat or train, the putt-putt of a motorboat, the sounds of horses hooves, and so on.

How stimulus objects come to have meaning older systems of psychology explained in the following manner. First, it was said that there are *sensations* or elementary sounds, sights, or smells out of which *perceptions* are "created." In other words, the train whistle which we hear is at first a meaningless sound which is worked upon by a brain or mind or some equally mysterious synthesizing agent somewhere inside the person. Eventually, it emerges as an interpreted sensation or a perception. This process is said to occur anew each time one hears the sound.

An alternative theory considers that stimulus objects have no function prior to situations that bring organisms into contact with them. It is out of the chain of reactions involving organisms and stimulus objects that "perceptions" gradually emerge. At first, the infant does not perceive milk bottles, mama, papa, the kitten, streetcars, tugboats, and so forth. It does nothing with respect to these objects, and they do nothing to the infant. However, as it accumulates a historical series of contacts with such objects, they function in certain ways for the child, and vice versa. For example, the kitten is not simply an object but is perceived as something that scratches you if you pull its tail. Mama and papa are discriminated from other people and reacted to in specific ways. Eventually, whistles are not simply noises but are identified as the whistle of the five-fifteen or that of the boy next door.

To us, the significance of the alternative explanation suggested above is the attention which it calls to the developmental aspects of perceptual behavior. In our opinion, it is false to fact to treat perception as if it were something occurring at an instant of time. Rather, what is demanded is a framework that does not do violence to the connectedness or interrelatedness of the total sequence of specific reactions involved. We seem to be forced to expand our investigation to include the very first contact between the infant and a particular stimulus object, their subsequent interactions constituting a figure with other related perceptual interactions serving as background. The accompanying picture is intended to illustrate a few links in a multitudinous series of interactions involving an infant and a book. The first perceptual interaction is relatively simple as compared with the last one shown in which picture and word-perceiving reactions have been elaborated. However, the last reaction cannot be cut off from all those preceding it and studied in isolation. Of course, perceptual development continues beyond the last incident shown (Fig. 25).

The readings in this chapter bring out this essential point about perception. Whether during a short experimental session or over a larger life span of the organism, we see in a striking fashion how utterly important the interconnected series of events is in leading to the evolution of perceptual responses.

II. A CRITICAL REVIEW OF THE LITERATURE ON ABSOLUTE PITCH

D. M. Neu
Pennsylvania State College

Pitch discrimination and, more specifically, absolute pitch, have been a source of controversy and speculation for a great many years,

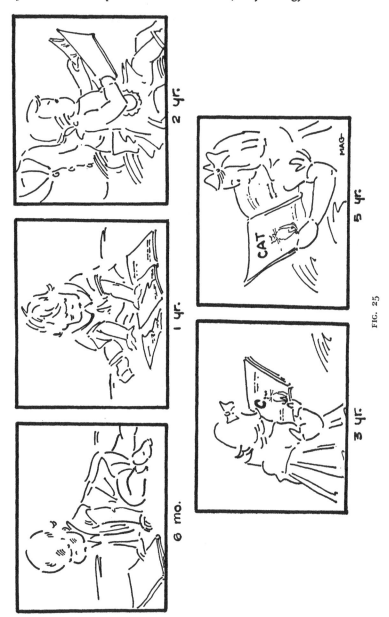

FIG. 25

beginning with Stumpf's discussion of Mozart's sense of pitch [10].[1] In general, the term "absolute pitch" is used to refer to an individual's naming correctly a particular tone that is sung or played on an instrument without comparing it to any other heard tone. The explanations of absolute pitch have been varied and many. Their inadequacy creates our present problem. More so than other "abilities," musical talent, and especially absolute pitch, have been traditionally explained as an inborn quality or faculty with which relatively few persons have been endowed.

In view of the fact that the inborn-quality explanation has been so generally accepted as an explanation of accurate pitch discrimination, one might hesitate to offer any other explanation if it were not a fact that no real evidence has been presented to prove the existence of such a quality. At best, it is a word. Moreover, if all the work concerning pitch discrimination is surveyed with an eye on the behavioral event known as "pitch discrimination," the evidence points away from any faculty or quality residing in the individual. Rather, the findings show that the discrimination of pitch (whether only relatively or very accurately) depends upon an evolution that has taken place during the individual's psychological history.

The performance of absolute pitch is defined by most writers as designating a heard tone correctly from memory alone without any other aid. In the opinion of the present writer, absolute pitch might be better defined as the discrimination and identification (by naming) of tones, without the aid of other tones, to such a degree that there are few errors. Of course, this is only a matter of degree from a comparison of a tone with a second tone presented directly to one.

RESULTS OF EXPERIMENTAL INVESTIGATION OF ABSOLUTE PITCH. Some main points in the results of experiments that Petran [7]

---

[1] The numbers in brackets refer to the numbered items in the bibliography on pp. 235–236.

FIG. 25 Development of perceptual behavior. This series of "snapshots" is intended to suggest that perceptual behavior originates during the history of the organism. Although the same object, a book, may be used in the 4½ year life span shown here, perceptions are not the same throughout. At 6 months the book may be simply discriminated from the background; at 1 year as something to be torn; at 2 years, pictures; at 3 years, letters, and at 5 years as definite words.

reviewed up to 1932 were that white notes on the piano are more often correctly judged than black, that notes in the middle range are judged more accurately than those in the extremes, and that there is a tendency to judge high notes higher than they actually are. Recently, Riker [9] showed experimentally that subjects with musical experience were able to judge pitch better in the middle range. All these results show greater accuracy with notes that are most frequently experienced. In other words, notes that are played and heard more often are the ones that are discriminated more sharply. Thus, absolute pitch shows a relationship to frequency of experience with certain tones.

As a matter of fact, investigators have been forced to consider experience. Stumpf [10] found that a bass player was better in judging tones in the lower ranges while a violinist was superior in judging or discriminating tones in the upper range.

Bartholomew [2] found that proficiency of subjects increased with the number of ear-training and harmony courses they had. Boggs [3], experimenting on herself, improved her judgment by paying special attention to overtones; and Kohler [4] did the same thing by concentrating on what he calls "body-tones."

The results of Mull's experiment [6] show that ability to judge notes correctly can be greatly improved by training. Mull states that in making judgment of absolute pitch, a higher degree of attention to the notes is more effective. She concluded that the importance of attention is indicated by (1) the immediateness and permanence of the learning, (2) the individual variability from day to day, (3) the fact that a stimulus which is not attended to has no noticeable effect, and (4) the fact that a good hearing of the note is necessary before judgment can be made. In the same connection, Riemann [8] said that some musicians have absolute pitch because of the frequent tuning of their instruments. Mull [6] and Wyatt [12] place special emphasis on systematic practice and the right kind of training in order to achieve improvement in pitch discrimination. Experimenting with college students, they found that a certain amount of pitch naming was acquired by musical as well as unmusical subjects. Wyatt showed that pitch discrimination of initially "pitch-deficient" adults was significantly improved after training.

Bachem [1] tells of a blind person without musical training who discovered his absolute pitch accidentally during a conversation with a possessor of absolute pitch, and he was able immediately to identify tones correctly after he knew how to denote them. Bachem admits that the large percentage and high degree of absolute pitch in congenitally blind persons show that inheritance is not the only factor. Of his 103 cases, 11 were blind since birth, and in none of these cases were there any relatives who had absolute pitch. Bachem also admits that there is an influence of forced attention to sound by the blind.

It is true, of course, that a musical environment may help the development of pitch discrimination because of the added opportunity to attend to tones. There is a decidedly higher percentage of absolute pitch in musical groups, particularly professional musicians. Bachem states, "Especially is this true of those with early musical training." He goes on to say, "It seems that attention to musical tones in early youth plays a predominant role in the development of absolute pitch" [1, p. 439].

Besides the statements made by these investigators, the results of many other experiments throw much doubt on the assumption that absolute pitch is an absolute inborn quality. Meyer [5] and Heyfelder attempted to train themselves, and their results show a high degree of correct judgments. After 2 weeks of practice, Kohler [4] could make 112 correct judgments out of 220, while Mull's data [6] show that practice increases the percentage of correct judgments from 40 per cent to 82 per cent!

In an experiment comparing subjects who said they had pitch-judging ability with those who disclaimed it, Riker [9] concluded that ability to judge pitch was not confined to specially trained or talented subjects. He also concluded that there were various degrees of accuracy in judging pitch and that it was ". . . a function of day to day experience with music [19, p. 346]."

ABSOLUTE PITCH IN CHILDREN. Probably the most significant and thorough experiment to show what effect age and practice have upon pitch discrimination was conducted by Wolner and Pyle [11]. Music teachers in three elementary schools selected pupils showing the greatest deficiency of pitch discrimination. From this group the seven poorest were selected. No pupil selected could distinguish the thirty-vibration differences on the forks. On the piano, in general, they could not distinguish differences of the octave, fifth, third, whole tone, or semitone. None of them could sing, although they had been in music classes from the first grade and were at the time of the experiment in the fifth, sixth, and seventh grades. There were three boys and four girls.

Each pupil received individual instruction and tests for 20 minutes each morning, 5 days a week. The whole number of hours spent in training was, on the average, 16 for each pupil, extended over a period of 81 days.

The definition and meaning of pitch, or "high" and "low," as distinguished from intensity, duration, and timbre, were strongly and repeatedly emphasized, particularly in the early days of training. The pupils were led to see the necessity of thinking of tones as one would think of a problem. Interest, attention, and concentration were worked for in the method of teaching.

Results showed that all seven pupils learned to discriminate perfectly the intervals of octaves, fifths, whole tones, and semitones in the range from A, sixteen tones below middle C, through A, thirty-four tones above middle C, a tonal range of four octaves! There was great variability in the time required to reach a given degree of efficiency, and in the response to methods and changes of methods. With forks, four of the pupils became perfect in distinguishing all the pitch differences from the largest, thirty vibrations, down to the smallest difference, one half vibration. Of the other three pupils, one learned to distinguish perfectly down to two vibrations' difference, another down to three vibrations' difference, and the third down to five vibrations' difference. The standard of perfection was 10 out of 10 trials correct.

Each pupil also improved noticeably in ability to sing. At the conclusion of the experiment, one pupil sang the words and music of several songs, with no trace of pitch deficiency, and also sang major and minor scales, chromatics, intervals, and tones picked at random. Another sang scales and intervals and the music of a song without words. Two pupils sang scales and intervals. The other three pupils sang, not perfectly, but with tremendous improvement over their initial efforts.

CONCLUSIONS. The statements made by the writers we have quoted and the results of the many experiments we have discussed certainly show the need for an adequate explanation of absolute pitch. The results show that:

1. Absolute pitch and lesser degrees of pitch discrimination can be acquired by individuals. Thus, it proves false the notion

that absolute pitch is some rare power over which we have no control.

2. Behavior that closely entails pitch discrimination, such as musical experience and musical training, allows a much better opportunity to develop keener pitch discrimination.

3. Pitch discrimination can be acquired readily in early age, which may be an indication that the younger the child, the easier it is to acquire new reactions.

4. The development of keener attention to stimuli makes for a keener development of pitch discrimination. Obvious examples of this are congenitally blind persons and child prodigies.

5. The subtlety of behavioral development is brought out by those individuals who have built up keen pitch discrimination and suddenly realize that they are able to perform such behavior.

From the above discussion, it is apparent that absolute pitch as well as other degrees of pitch discrimination can be accounted for as behavior developed within the lifetime of the individual. This means that the discrimination is due to the way in which the individual builds up reactions to sounds, and more specifically to the thoroughness with which he attends to tones (stimuli). Accordingly, the individual's reactional biography, built up from past experience, is the important factor in determining what sort of tonal discriminations he will make. It follows then that absolute pitch is nothing more than a fine degree of accuracy in pitch discrimination.

BIBLIOGRAPHY

1. BACHEM, A. Genesis of absolute pitch. *J. acoust. Soc. Amer.*, 1939–1940, 11, 434–439.

2. BARTHOLOMEW, W. A study of absolute pitch ability. Master's thesis, George Washington Univ., 1925, Pp. 123.

3. BOGGS, LUCINDA P. Studies in absolute pitch. *Amer. J. Psychol.*, 1907, 18, 194–205.

4. KOHLER, W. Akustische untersuchungen III. *Z. Psychol.*, 1915, 72, 159–177.

5. MEYER, M. Is the memory of absolute pitch capable of development by training? *Psychol. Rev.*, 1899, 6, 514–516.

6. MULL, HELEN K. Acquisition of absolute pitch. *Amer. J. Psychol.*, 1925, 36, 469–493.

7. Petran, L. A. Experimental study of pitch recognition. *Psychol. Monogr.*, 1932, 42, No. 6.
8. Riemann, L. Das absolute cehor. *Neue Musik-Zeitung*, 1908, 29, 515–516.
9. Riker, B. L. The ability to judge pitch. *J. exp. Psychol.*, 1946, 36, 331–346.
10. Stumpf, C. *Tonsychologie.* Leipzig: Hirzel, 1883.
11. Wolner, M. & Pyle, W. H. An experiment in individual training of pitch-deficient children. *J. educ. Psychol.*, 1933, 24, 602–608.
12. Wyatt, Ruth F. Improvability of pitch discrimination. *Psychol. Monogr.*, 1945, 58, 1–58.

III. A FIELD OBSERVATION OF PERCEPTUAL DEVELOPMENT

Suppose a person had been born blind and were suddenly made to see. How and what would he perceive in view of his total lack of previous visual experience? This has been an intriguing question down through the ages, but the answer has never been clear cut because the blind who recover their sight have had some degree of visual experience (no matter how vague) prior to restoration of their vision.

This is true in the case of George Campbell [2] who, at the age of 18, had a surgical operation which permitted him to see somewhere nearly adequately for the first time in his life. How perceptual reactions became built up is told in Mr. Campbell's own words, although we leave to the reader the task of translating the everyday language into technical, scientifically acceptable terminology.

I entered a new world.

The room was full of objects completely new and strange to me. I did not recognize what anything was, or what it was for, as I had practically no visual experience. Most people do not realize how much of their "seeing" is actually brainwork, reasoning and past experience. [3]

---

[2] Reprinted from *This Week* magazine. Copyright 1941 by the United Newspapers Magazine Corporation. (Reproduced by permission of the author and the publisher.)

[3] To us, "brainwork, reasoning and past experience" can only be popular psychology's equivalent for reactional biography.

The doctor took me to a window and said, "George, do you see that hedge across the street?"

"No, sir."

I had no idea what it was among those strange forms.

"Where," I asked in confusion, "is the far curb of the street?"

This might help me. I had often crossed the street and knew it more or less by footstep touch. He explained carefully which one of those forms the curb was—and suddenly I understood. Yes, I could "see" it now! I was so thrilled I could hardly speak.

I could hardly take my glasses off to give my aching, new-born eyes a rest. I was fascinated by the details and colors of household objects such as ash trays, chairs, vases, carpets, and the friendly radio that I had known largely by touch.

I didn't know which color was which. Before my operation I could tell fireman's red if it was placed a few inches from my eyes, or perhaps bright blue, but any blends or gradations were beyond me. I asked Mother what the other color in the sky was. She explained the small white spots were clouds. After a day or two I went to a fruit store and asked what the color of each fruit was. I bought yellow bananas, green limes, red-and-yellow apples, lemons, oranges, and other fruits. I studied their subtle colors as I ate them. Why, there were thousands of shades of green alone!

My reactions to colors were different from the average person's. Dark green was like loyalty and tradition; light green was like touching a baby's skin. Light blue, to me, suggested something clean and fresh, like a cold drink on a hot summer day. Purple was like the cold, clammy feeling you get just before it rains. Pink was like eating delicious candy. Scarlet was like the burning sensation I had in my finger tips when I touched something hot.

That evening I went to a movie. I do not remember what the picture was, or its plot. All was confusion to me—there were so many things portrayed I did not recognize, and I could only look at the screen for a few seconds at a time. When I did look, I tried to learn what *caused* certain noises. Sounds that were not made by visible people or objects, such as an outer door shutting, added to my bewilderment. After a while, my eyes gave out. I had to leave.

When I walked out of the theater it was dark. I looked up. There were the stars! To my surprise, no one was looking at them except me.

REDISCOVERED OLD FRIENDS. When I returned to high school, a few days later, I was in a predicament. An old friend would rush up to congratulate me. I would shake his hand, but until I heard his voice, I wasn't at all sure I knew him. During these first days I would often leave off conversation with boy friends in the halls to stare at pretty girls going by. *What* had I been missing? At first I had faulty judgment of distance. When I'd reach for an ash tray, my hand would go beyond it. So I learned to measure distance by trial and error, like a baby. My glasses were focused at two distances, for reading and for far off seeing. I had to learn to use them effectively. As I said, most people do not realize how much of their "seeing" is actually brainwork, reasoning and past experience.

It was a job for me at first to go up and down stairs. But I had too much fun in my new world to bother about stumbling occasionally.

IV. THE DEVELOPMENT OF VISUAL PERCEPTION IN MAN AND CHIMPANZEE [4]
Austin H. Riesen

Yerkes Laboratories of Primate Biology, Orange Park, Fla., and Yale University

The study of innate visual organization in man is not open to direct observation during early infancy, since a young baby is too helpless to respond differentially to visual excitation. A first attack on this problem has been made by investigating the visual responsiveness of persons born blind and later made able to see by cataract removal. To evaluate the apparent contradictions between these clinical reports and experimental findings with lower mammals and birds, chimpanzees were reared in darkness until sufficiently mature for the testing of visual responsiveness. The results, which corroborate and extend data reported for man by Senden, may require changes in current theories of learning and perception.

Two chimpanzees were reared in darkness to the age of 16 months. The animals were then brought periodically into the light for a regular repeated series of observations. By the time of the first observations the animals had developed postural and locomotor skills roughly comparable to normally reared chimpanzees of the same age or approximating in

---

[4] RIESEN, AUSTIN H. The development of visual perception in man and chimpanzee. *Science,* 1947, 106, 107–108. (Reproduced by permission of the author and the publisher.)

a general way those of a two-year-old human child. At this time the total light experience, received in half a dozen brief (45 second) episodes daily, as required by the routine care of the animals, was approximately 40 hours. At 21 months of age the female was brought permanently into normal indoor illumination. At the present writing the animals are 26 months of age. A full account of their behavior will appear in future publications.

The first tests of visual reactions with both subjects demonstrated the presence of good pupillary responses to changes in light intensity, pronounced startle reactions to sudden increases of illumination, and a turning of the eyes and head toward sources of light. In the darkness there was pursuit of a moving light with both eye and head movements. The eyes, however, did not fixate steadily on a light. During all tests episodes of a resilient "spontaneous" nystagmus occurred, the quick phase usually toward, and the slow phase away from, the light source. With the subject sitting stationary at the center of a rotating drum marked in alternating black and white stripes, tests for optokinetic responses were made. Characteristic pursuit eye movements with quick jerks in the opposite direction were obtained.

Aside from the reflexes just described, and the pursuit of a moving light, the two animals were, in effect, blind. The acquisition of visually mediated responses proceeded very gradually, with no evidence of any sudden increased responsiveness such as might be expected if, for example, the failure to respond was at first due to a general lack of attention of visual stimulation. No fixation of any object, still or moving, could be elicited in any of the early tests. For a long time there was no eye blink when an object was brought rapidly toward the eyes. An object brought slowly toward the face produced no response until contact was made, when the animal reacted with a quick jerk in the typical startle pattern. With the female this was observed for the last time on the 30th day after she was moved into the daylight room. Her first blink to a threatened blow in the face occurred on the 5th day, but occurred consistently only after 48 days, at which time she had been in the light for a total of 570 hours, was 22½ months old, and had for a month received some pushing around daily in short play periods with a younger but visually sophisticated chimpanzee.

Many repetitions of experience with objects presented visually were necessary before any recognition of such objects appeared in either subject. The feeding bottle, for example, was thoroughly familiar tactually and kinesthetically. If the bottle or nipple touched the hand, arm, or face, either animal promptly seized the nipple in its mouth. First signs of *visual* recognition occurred in the female when she protruded her lips toward the bottle on the 33rd meal, or the 11th day, following her shift into the daylight room. The first reaching for the bottle with the hand (done before 12 months of age by normally reared animals) appeared on the 48th meal, or 16th day in the light. With the male, whose visual experience was limited to mealtime, many more feedings were required before these responses appeared. The first reaching responses of both animals were grossly inaccurate.

A training procedure employing electric shock showed that the learning of avoidance responses was also an extremely slow and gradual process.

These results can best be interpreted in conjunction with the data of Senden. Lacunae in each set of findings, clinical and experimental, are in many respects filled by the other.

In the first place, there is no question that the chimpanzee subjects were well motivated. Sufficient hunger to produce whimpering, and shock severe enough to bring vocal protests, did not alter the fact of failure to "see." The similar slowness of learning of the human patients therefore can not be accounted for merely by a defect of motivation. The emotional disturbances would seem to have been the result of slow learning, just as Senden concluded, rather than its cause; that is to say, the patient lost some of his enthusiasm when he found how difficult it was to make effective use of the new and at first interesting sensations.

Secondly, the verbal assistance given the human patients makes it clear that the difficulty is not simply a failure to attend to visual sensations. With attention successfully directed to a newly-introduced stimulation, as attested to by the patient's partial success in describing it, learning to identify remained a tediously slow process, with the notable exception of color naming. Since color names were learned easily, it cannot be said that "visual attention" was absent.

The prompt visual learning so characteristic of the normal adult primate is thus not an innate capacity, independent of visual experience, but requires a long apprenticeship in the use of the eyes. At lower phylogenetic levels the period of apprenticeship is much shorter. The chick makes effective use of vision immediately upon hatching and shows further improvement of efficiency with the practice afforded by a dozen pecks. Rats reared in darkness, when first exposed to light, show no clear utilization of vision but learn to jump in response to visual cues within 15 minutes, and after an hour or two may be indistinguishable from the normally reared animal. The chimpanzees of the present study received 50 hours of exposure before the first visually mediated learning was evident; and man, to judge by some of Senden's cases, may require an even longer exposure.

The comparative data conform to the generally recognized principle that organisms whose potential adaptations to the environment are most complex, i.e., those that show the greatest intelligence at maturity, also require the longest period of development. This has generally been regarded as a period of maturation. The clinical and experimental data discussed here, however, show that this long period is also essential for the organization of perceptual processes through learning [pp. 107–108].

V. IS THERE AN IMAGE ON THE RETINA?
N. H. Pronko

It has been a conventional piece of "knowledge" of long standing that the eye is like a camera. Even the unschooled man in the street naïvely believes that the things that he sees are somehow focused on the back of his eye and that this "image," is somehow "transmitted" to the back of the brain, and so on.

In exploring this interpretation seriously, we should first note that "seeing," which is an almost universal characteristic of living things to some degree or other, is made unnecessarily complex by such a theory. The very first step here has obscured the matter rather than explained it. This difficulty alone should have been sufficient to overthrow such a theory, but tradition dies hard.

However, we continue to uncover more difficulties in pushing the problem further, for the reader will note that, once seeing is alleged to begin with a retinal image, how could the process be carried through the optic pathway without dogmatically attributing some imaginary characteristic to the visual pathways? Such scientific enterprise is arbitrary, indeed.

But, should we overlook the above difficulties, there are still others to plague us. How, in the first place, could the nerves project the retinal image onto the occipital lobes? No one has ever demonstrated the feasibility of such a versatility of neural functioning. But, if one were to forgive all of the foregoing scientific sins, and simply assume that *somehow* the image has got there on the brain, the problem still remains of explaining how *the organism* sees that image. Could it be that the eyes turn inward on the brain to see what the organism actually sees in front of it? Here is an obvious *reductio ad absurdum.* We started with an actual fact in which an organism sees something, but our interpretation has got us off the track, as it were, and failed to bring us back to the original event.

Nevertheless, we continue the examination of the long-lived explanation of how organisms see. Overlooking the preceding, you must still explain how the two cerebral hemispheres which are said to have the image on them could give a unified single view of the thing seen, inasmuch as they are separate structures. As such, they should show a crack or blank down the middle of the thing seen, but they don't. Should you attempt to show that perhaps these two portions of the brain are connected through the corpus callosum, the thick band of fibers that unites various portions of the two brain hemispheres, Ranson,[5] the anatomist, would refute such a claim. According to this investigator, apparently no one has established the presence of such connecting fibers, for he states that there are "few, if any" [p. 288] neurons interconnecting the specific visual areas of the two hemispheres.

How there could ever be an "image" on the retina to begin the whole series of the purely hypothetical acts should receive consideration, too. In the living organism, the retina is a transparent structure and so cannot reflect an image. Only in the dead organism does the retina become opaque enough to satisfy this condition. Furthermore, the retina does not permit a three-dimensional "representation" of the thing, since it is a two-dimensional surface. Then, the stray or scattered light of the eye also interferes sufficiently to invalidate the sharp focus of the image required by the traditional theory. Finally, no one has observed an image on the retina of a living person.

The belief in "the image" as described above has been borrowed from perfectly sound laboratory observations and descriptions that physicists have given us of their work on lenses. But, although such interpretations fit their own data, that is no reason for borrowing them to impose as a ready-made explanation of behavioral data. Let interpretation of light and lens functioning be limited to the subject matter from which they were derived. Then study visual reactions and interpret them in their own right.

---

[5] Ranson, S. W. *The anatomy of the nervous system.* Philadelphia: Saunders, 1942. Pp. 507.

Pioneering work at the Dartmouth Eye Institute shows that "visual space" and "physical space" do not have the one-to-one geometrical correspondence traditionally attributed to them. The following quotation from Luneberg [6] will give an indication of how the present work on vision departs from what might be called the eye-as-a-camera theory.

Actually, a visual sensation is the response of a living organism to physical stimuli. Thus, we can scarcely hope to find the explanation of visual sensations and their sensed qualities in the complicated chain of physical events by which the organism is stimulated. We must take account of other factors which are given by the organism itself and not by the stimuli. These are psychological factors determined by the purposes, expectations, and the experimental background of the observer.

By adopting this point of view we have to consider the following possibility. Objects can be identical in certain aspects of physical form and localization but are seen as objects which differ in these aspects. Vice versa, two sensations can be identical in all their qualities though related to different physical objects. That this is true even in the realm of binocular vision is clearly shown by some experiments carried out at the Dartmouth Eye Institute. A set of rooms with curved walls has been constructed; the walls are provided with curved window patterns. Every one of these distorted rooms gives the appearance of the same rectangular room, i.e., the same sensation is related to an infinite set of physically different rooms. In a second experiment, perspective patterns are drawn upon a vertical board. The apparent localization of the board changes strikingly if the pattern is varied though physically the board is not moved. An infinite set of apparently different localizations thus can be related to the same physical localization. We stress the point that in both demonstrations the observation is binocular.

We conclude from the above experiment that it would be futile to attempt to express the relation of visual and physical space in the form of a necessary one-to-one correspondence. The qualities of visual sensations are *not* uniquely determined by the physical stimuli [p. 3].

This selection was included to show how nonoperational techniques, as used in the past, have led to bafflement rather than clarification of such behavioral phenomena as seeing. While the

---

6 LUNEBERG, R. K. *Mathematical analysis of binocular vision.* Princeton: Princeton Univ. Press, 1947. Pp. 104. (Reproduced by permission of the author and the publisher.)

problems in this area are not by any means considered as solved at the present time, such operational pioneerings as that of Luneberg may give hints of more fruitful approaches to come.

VI. EXPERIMENTAL STUDIES OF ILLUSIONS [7]
N. H. Pronko

As an individual gains more experience, he becomes more sophisticated in his perceptions as in other reactions. The illusions have been utilized for the purpose of shedding light on the manner in which perceptions operate. One of these is the vertical-horizontal illusion in which a vertical line and a horizontal line of the same length are arranged in such a manner that the horizontal line "looks" shorter. Another is the Muller-Lyer illusion. Here, two lines of equal length are seen as unequal owing to the arrangement of arrows on the ends. Apparently, humans do not readily isolate portions of their surrounding world and react to those pieces as such. Rather, they react globally to the total situation.

Even infrahuman animals perceive the world in this fashion. In an experiment performed on chickens by Winslow,[8] two lines of very apparent different length were presented in a discrimination apparatus. The long and short lines were alternated from the right and left positions in a chance order. The chickens were rewarded with food if they approached the shorter line and punished with shock if they approached the longer one. After a few hundred trials, they were able to discriminate the lines with an accuracy of 80 to 90 per cent. The two lines were then drawn so that the difference between them was reduced, and training was continued. Other changes were introduced in order to prevent disturbance upon the later introduction of arrows. Eventually, two lines of equal length but with different arrangement of arrows, as shown in the accompanying figure, were presented to the chickens. Results showed that they continued to discriminate the line that to us appears shorter.

---

[7] WALTERS, SISTER ANNETTE. A genetic study of geometrical-optical illusions. *Genet. Psychol. Monogr.*, 1942, 25, 101–155.

[8] WINSLOW, C. N. Visual illusions in the chick. *Arch. Psychol.*, N.Y., 1933, No. 153, 1–80.

The following experiment was designed to answer the question as to what happens on this point developmentally with respect to humans. Is there a progressive decrease in the extent of this illusion as the person grows older?

Figures used were the Muller-Lyer illusion and the vertical-horizontal illusion. Both figures were drawn in black on white cardboard and so arranged that a knob in back permitted the experimenter to adjust the lines in the figure. A large screen hid all parts of apparatus except the illusions themselves.

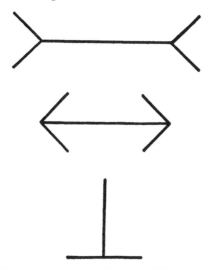

FIG. 26   The Muller-Lyer and vertical-horizontal illusions. Which lines appear to be longer?

A scale on the back of the cards permitted the experimenter to measure the amount of error, in millimeters, which the subject made in estimating the length of the lines to be equal.

Individuals of different ages ranging from 5 to 19 were used as subjects. Over 100 subjects were used at each of these age groups, except the 18-to-19-year group which had 93 subjects. Both sexes were included in the study.

Table 12 gives results for all age groups.

The average Muller-Lyer illusion scores decrease from ages 6 to 11, then increase from 11 to 14, and decrease again from then on. The mean vertical-horizontal illusion scores decrease con-

Table 12

Amount of Illusion in the Muller-Lyer and Vertical-Horizontal Figures
for Different Age Groups

Age Group	N	Muller-Lyer Illusion Mean Error (Millimeters)	Vertical-Horizontal Illusion
5[6]–6[5]	110	29.10	32.96
6[6]	106	26.62	32.34
7[6]	124	24.93	33.18
8[6]	101	23.91	33.20
9[6]	137	23.49	32.12
10[6]	162	23.76	23.45
11[6]	166	24.34	28.54
12[6]	139	23.36	28.27
13[6]	122	24.84	26.94
14[6]	108	26.71	24.96
15[6]	104	25.51	23.77
16[6]	111	23.61	24.63
17[6]	110	24.26	23.99
18[6]	93	24.59	25.36

sistently during early years and increase slightly in the last age bracket. Both sets of averages reveal a trend in the direction of a decrease in amount of illusion with increasing age, or the benefit of experience on perceptual reactions.

VII. THE EFFECT OF PROLONGED INVERSION OF THE VISUAL FIELD IN THE RHESUS MONKEY
J. W. Bowles, Jr.

Information regarding the developmental features of visual perceiving has been provided by Foley [9] in his study of prolonged inversion of the visual field, using a rhesus monkey as the subject. The effects of such inversion have interested psychologists for many years, particularly since the classic studies by Stratton

[9] FOLEY, J. P. JR. An experimental investigation of the effect of prolonged inversion of the visual field in the rhesus monkey (Macaca mulatta). *J. genet. Psychol.*, 1940, 56, 21–51.

(1896–1897) in which he served as his own subject. Foley has done pioneer work in this type of study with an infrahuman animal as the subject. It offers several possibilities for further studies. For example, as Foley points out:

> Visual inversion could be begun at birth, and could, with proper facilities, be continued indefinitely. Stimulational factors in the reactional biography of the subject could be far more rigidly controlled than in the human experiment [p. 33].

Instead of performing an experiment of the magnitude suggested above, Foley worked with an adult animal and over a compact time period. His subject was an adult female rhesus monkey approximately 9 years old. She had served in several previous experiments and was docile and tractable. The gross structure and function of the eye of the rhesus monkey are very similar to those of the human, hence the results of this experiment are of especial significance for comparative psychology.

The optical system used to achieve inversion was a pair of inverting unit-magnification telescopic spectacles. The lenses were mounted in aluminum tubes 20 millimeters in diameter. The tubes were fitted into brass bushings of an aluminum mask conforming to the animal's face. A leather headgear kept the mask in place and prevented any light from reaching the eyes except via the lenses. As a control, the animal was first accustomed to the mask, headgear, and tubes without the lenses. The tubes were of the same length and diameter as those containing the lenses and were constructed to give a visual field identical in size with that obtaining under conditions of inversion. The tubes were, of necessity, 75 millimeters in length, and the entire apparatus weighed 130 grams.

The lens system, which, unlike that employed by Stratton, was binocular, distorted the visual field 180 degrees in both vertical and horizontal dimensions. Further, near objects appeared distant and vice versa.

In initiating the experiment, a restraining apparatus was necessary to keep the animal from dislodging the mask. This kept the animal in as near normal a sitting position as possible. When the subject became accustomed to this apparatus, a series of training trials was instituted until the animal had learned to reach for food in the one of a group of eight food boxes that was lighted. It was hoped that this would later permit observation of the perceived location of stimulus objects in the visual field.

Following this training period, in which the animal wore the apparatus *without* the reversing lenses, the lenses were put in place and worn continually for 7 days (168 hours). The subject was at first restrained in the special chair except for exercise and observation periods. As the monkey became adapted and the risk of displacing the lenses decreased, the restraints were loosened.

1. FIRST DAY.   A marked tonic immobility was the immediate effect of putting on the lenses. The animal became purely passive in a bent-over posture. Every few minutes she raised her head, seemed to be looking around, and became again inactive.

The subject, during the periods of immobility, tended to grasp something with hands or feet. If nothing else was available, one foot was grasped with the other. If food was placed between the lips during these periods, no chewing or swallowing was elicited. After about 2½ hours, she ate some bits of an orange if they were placed in her mouth, but she would not transfer them from her hand to her mouth.

Eyes were closed a large part of the time, and, when she was forced to exercise by the examiner, eyes were probably closed while walking. Also, when placed on a high stool, she stepped off without hesitation and had to be caught, suggestive of eye closure.

2. SECOND DAY.   The subject was still immobile most of the time. Food was, however, transferred from hand to mouth. About noon of the second day, incoordination of arm and leg movements was observed, suggesting that the subject's eyes were open, and that the new visual conditions were an interference. Walking was incoordinated. After an unsatisfactory attempt, she refused to walk and squatted on the floor.

In the evening when bread was held before her, she reached out for it. When she failed to grasp it she became quite upset and tried to remove the lenses. When raisins were offered, she reached to the opposite side. This happened on twelve consecutive trials. She also underreached, failing to reach far enough. The same results were obtained with another food object; however, she began to compensate for her errors. After reaching and missing she, first in a random fashion and later more accurately, moved her hand until she reached the object. Thus, by the second day, visual adjustments were beginning to show modification.

3. THIRD DAY. The subject continued to show tonic immobility, with frequent twitchings of the entire musculature. Incoordination of movement was present during exercise, with forward walking inhibited. Bimanual coordination was definitely interfered with. In general, the subject showed improvement in making corrections for errors in reaching.

4. FOURTH DAY. Immobility persisted. Spatial localization errors still existed, but with less magnitude. In the afternoon, the animal was more active but still refused to walk forward.

5. FIFTH DAY. Little change was noted, but the subject was more active and attempted more often to move about the room.

6. SIXTH DAY. The subject was much more active. Seeing a cup of peanuts on the table, she climbed upon a chair and onto the table, climbing down again after peanuts that dropped on the floor. She engaged in much exploration but was easily upset. By evening of this day, few exploratory movements were required in reaching for an object. Forward walking on the hind legs was attempted for the first time, though balance was poor.

7. SEVENTH DAY. Spatial orientation was improved, coordination was good. She walked freely on the hind legs. She recognized her position in the laboratory and walked through various rooms, as well as climbing about the caging in a normal fashion. Objects were reached for with a small amount of trial and error, with no error on about 20 per cent of the trials.

8. EIGHTH DAY. The apparatus was removed at 2:00 P.M. on this day. Observations during the morning revealed that adjustment was virtually complete. Walking, climbing, reaching, and manipulating were essentially normal, indicating that visual perception was no longer disturbed to any extent. States of immobility occurred after periods of stress and strain but were of short duration and not intense.

9. POSTINVERSION PERIOD—FIRST DAY. Immediately after removal of the lenses the subject ran about the room. There was slight but definite incoordination, especially in climbing and jumping, but this did not persist. She did not walk erect but ran on all fours. After 5½ hours without the lenses there was still some interference in jumping. Jumping from the perch to the floor of the cage was inaccurate, clearly showing that the distance was misjudged. Visual responses built up during the 168 hours with the lenses were not immediately replaced with older seeing habits.

10. POSTINVERSION PERIOD—SECOND DAY. All behavior appeared normal except jumping downward, which remained inaccurate.

11. POSTINVERSION PERIOD—THIRD DAY. Readjustment was virtually complete, although the animal was hesitant in jumping down from chairs, stools, and the like.

In summary, in a period of 7 days during which inversion lenses were worn continually, this adult rhesus monkey showed essentially complete readjustment of visual responses. Minor and temporary difficulties were noted when the lenses were removed. Clearly, then, the developmental aspects of seeing are exceedingly important.

VIII. THE INFLUENCE OF TRAINING UPON PERCEPTUAL SKILL

Training in perceptual skills was found to be an important asset in the armed forces of World War Two. Accurate recognition of aircraft and ships under a variety of conditions was a valued skill for servicemen. Frequently, a plane would be visible for only an instant through cloud obstructions. A ship at night might be visible for only the instant of a flash of gunfire. It was important for "spotters" and men in combat action to identify the type of plane or ship and whether it was friendly or enemy. A good illustration of the influence of variables of the reactional biography upon perception is found in the training program planned by Renshaw [10] of Ohio State University.

Renshaw's procedure was to devise an apparatus that permitted high-speed exposures of pictures on a screen. Brief exposure was employed because it was felt that this would force the subject to see shapes coherently and unitarily. The perception required an active effort on the subject's part, sheer repetition of stimuli being useless in improving such perceptions. The results of this experiment fell in line with those secured from children and nonmilitary subjects. In general, there was a remarkable increase in the speed of perception.

---

[10] RENSHAW, S. The visual perception and reproduction of forms by tachistoscopic methods. *J. Psychol.*, 1945, 20, 217–232. (Reproduced by permission of the publisher.)

A sample of the early results with pre-flight cadets at the North Carolina Preflight School at the end of the third and tenth weeks of training is given in Table [13]. It should be borne in mind that by Session 15 about 15 planes had been introduced, each in six positions, and at Session 50 about 42 types of aircraft had to be identified. Digits "counting"—that is, the immediate estimation of numerousness—of planes or ships and short-stroke sketching, as well as projections of planes and ships in various positions were shown.

Table 13

Group Tachistoscopic Training—Navy Preflight Cadets

Per Cent of Planes * and Ships Correctly Identified	$N = 323$ Cumulative Per Cent Cadets (Session 15)	$N = 272$ Cumulative Per Cent Cadets (Session 50)
100	2.5	12.5
90	30.3	74.7
80	66.6	94.6
70	88.9	99.3
62.5	. . .	100.0
60	96.6	. . . .
50	98.8	. . . .
22.5	100.0	. . . .

* Forty slides were shown at ⅟₂₅ second in Session 15; 40 at ⅟₇₅ second in Session 50. The pretest averages of the two battalions before training showed no significant differences. Many of the views of planes used in the tests were not seen previously in the training sessions.

Ninety-five per cent of the 272 cadets correctly identified 80 per cent or more of the planes at ⅟₇₅ second exposures. One-fourth of all cadets correctly identified 90 per cent or better. Only 1 per cent failed to get approximately three out of four correct identifications.

Untrained American and British pilots given a similar test on operational air craft succeeded, at ⅟₂₅ second exposures, in one correct out of three [pp. 228–229].

Renshaw's work has further demonstrated the effects of training upon perception of nonmilitary stimuli. The technique of tachistoscopic or rapid-stimulus exposure has been shown to have important effects on improved reading skills. College students have been found, after tachistoscopic training, to have more than doubled their reading rate on literary materials (*Reader's Digest*) without handicapping comprehension. On more difficult reading matter, gains as high as 125 per cent were found as a result of perception training.

Results of training on digit perception offer an interesting illustration of what effective practice can accomplish. Dr. Sale Finkelstein, noted as a "memorizing and calculating genius," was submitted to such a training program as were average college students. The following quotations summarize the findings.

Within the first 60 days Finkelstein made marked improvement in his speed of perceiving and reproducing numbers. For example, at first a 21-digit number required an exposure of 9.23 seconds. This time was reduced during training to 7.18, 5.46, 4.90, 4.43, 4.14, 3.92, 3.50, and finally to 3.17 seconds. Fifteen-digit numbers reduced from 2.54 seconds to 1.47 seconds. Seven-digit numbers remained throughout the experiment at 0.003 second exposure, the shortest exposure within the 2 per cent error limit afforded by the apparatus at that stage of development. Finkelstein worked with numbers from seven to 42 digits in length. No one had previously made comparable records of speed and accuracy in perceiving visual forms. At first he was quite skeptical of any possibility of improvement from tachistoscopic training. As the experiments progressed, the only question was one of limits. Knight, Banner, and Schwarzbek attempted to discover this limit. After more than 70 training sessions devoted to the reduction of exposure time to a minimum on numbers of one length it was concluded that performance was still improving; that no ceiling was in sight, and that the ultimate attainment of limit was contingent upon the discovery and use of the best possible method, the control of motivation, and, more important *still*, the development of the perceptual skill of field structuring by the active observer to the maximum possible level . . . [p. 218].

After even relatively limited digit skill is attained . . . the indices of comprehension and speed in silent reading will show marked gains. And we shall show that from digit training alone, given on the horizontal retinal meridians, the visual form fields of the eyes are significantly expanded *in both the horizontal and vertical* axes. Shortly after Finkelstein's training began to exhibit results we sought to discover how far we could extend the skills of average college students with tachistoscopic exposures of digits.

One student (K) required 17 seconds to reproduce a 15-place number on his first trials. After about 50 20-minute practice sessions he was able to reproduce digit patterns of this length in 2.1 seconds. This is by no means a limit. Further practice would unquestionably have reduced this time. Another student (W) reduced his exposure time from 20 seconds to 1.45 seconds. During the present academic year one student (P) did a 9-digit number in 0.003 seconds; another (S) did a 12-digit number in 0.750 seconds. . . . The importance of the fact that ordinary college students can be trained to perceive visual forms at a level of skill which, because of the low performance standards we accept as "normal," may be classed as "genius," is very great . . . [p. 219].

IX. THE PERCEPTION OF OBSTACLES BY THE BLIND [11]
Milton Cotzin

Southbury Training School

The skill of some blind people in avoiding obstacles in their paths has long been a subject of special interest and speculation. The early explanations, based for the most part upon casual observation or poorly controlled experiments, have been highly fanciful and have led far oftener to confusion than to enlightenment. At one extreme are those theories which postulate that this skill results from the heightened acuity of one or more of the other senses, but there is no agreement among the theories as to which sense or combination of senses are involved. At the other extreme are those theories which maintain that such detection of obstacles defies natural explanation. This has led to the introduction of such terms as "facial vision," "warning sense," and "distance sense," and even "telesthesia," "paroptic vision," and "sixth sense." The blind are themselves unable to understand the behavior involved.

Because of the contradictions arising from speculation and experimentation during the past two centuries, Supa, Cotzin, and Dallenbach in 1941 undertook a series of carefully controlled experiments in an attempt to establish the fundamental basis of the skill. Seven experiments were conducted. The first three, Experiments 1 to 3, which were practice, exploratory, and normative, were given under conditions normal to the blind. Besides placing blind-

---

[11] Based on experiments reported in the following article: SUPA, M., COTZIN, M., & DALLENBACH, K. M. "Facial vision"; the perception of obstacles by the blind. *Amer. J. Psychol.*, 1944, 57, 133–183.

folds over the eyes of the subject, the conditions of everyday life of the blind were practically unchanged. In the last four, Experiments 4 to 7, various controls were introduced that reduced or eliminated certain cues. Four subjects, two blind and two with normal vision, served throughout the study. The blind subjects perceived obstacles from a distance and did this to a marked degree in their daily lives. Neither, however, could explain the basis of his judgment. One blind subject thought that hearing helped, but the other was of the opinion that sounds hindered. The two sighted subjects were unable at the beginning of the study to detect the presence of obstacles when blindfolded, and they expressed grave doubts concerning the possibility of learning to do so, although both were willing to try.

A series of experiments in this study consisted of 25 successful trials, i.e., trials in which the subject made his report without coming into contact with the obstacle, or 50 consecutive failures, i.e., trials in which he collided with the obstacle. Failures interspersed among successes were repeated until the number of successes reached 25. In the first six experiments, the eyes of the subjects, blind and sighted alike, were covered with pads of cotton and a flexible leather blindfold. Thus all the subjects were "blind" and all had their facial areas reduced by like amounts. Except for *experience*, the blind subjects had no advantage over the sighted.

In Experiment 1, the subject walked toward the end wall of a large experimental hall from varying starting positions; the obstacle was stationary, but the subject's starting position was varied. In Experiment 2, the subject walked from a fixed position at the wall to a masonite screen which was placed down the hall at varying distances from that point; the position of the obstacle was varied but the subject's starting position was fixed. In Experiment 3, the subject, starting from varying positions, walked down the hall to the screen that was placed at varying distances from the starting point; the position of the obstacle and of the subject's starting point were both varied. Each of these three experiments was performed twice, once as Series A, with the subjects wearing shoes and walking on the hardwood floor; and a second time as Series B, with the subjects in stocking feet, walking on a carpet runner.

From these preliminary experiments, the following information was obtained:

1. The blind subjects perceived obstacles at a distance with a high degree of success, since they brought to the study the experience of a lifetime, as well as the "tricks of the trade." Neither was

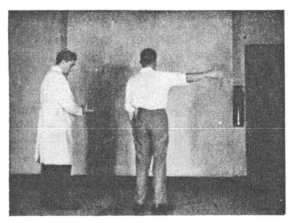

FIG. 27 Blindfolded subject signals with his raised right arm that he perceived the wall. (Figs. 27 through 38 from Supa, M., Cotzin, M., & Dallenback, K. M. "Facial vision"; the perception of obstacles by the blind.)

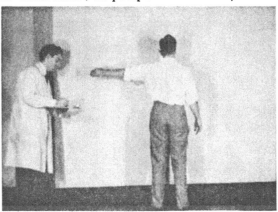

FIG. 28 Blindfolded subject signals with his raised left arm that he has approached the wall as near as possible without touching it.

able to explain his skill, but each favored one of the classic theories. One of them thought his judgment was based on hearing, the other that the perceptions were matters of facial pressure.

2. Neither of the sighted subjects, at the outset of the study, perceived obstacles at a distance while blindfolded. They soon

learned, however to do so. Under the highly favorable conditions of Series 1-A they rapidly acquired this skill. Their learning was so rapid that after their first successes, following an initial run of failures, they seldom collided with the obstacle.

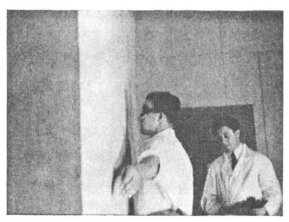

FIG. 29 Showing how closely blindfolded subject approaches the wall.

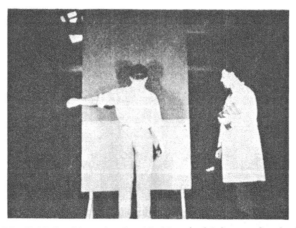

FIG. 30 Blindfolded subject signals with his raised left arm that he has approached the masonite wall as near as possible without touching it.

3. On the whole, the reports given by the subjects during and after the various series of experiments contributed little to the understanding of obstacle perception. Nevertheless, some insight into the problem was obtained from the subjects' observations. The blind subject who thought at the beginning of the study that

his "obstacle sense" was based entirely upon cutaneous pressures localized in the forehead, and that sounds played no role, was less certain of his claim at the conclusion of the preliminary experiment. In the experiment of Series 3-B, in which the intensity of the sounds of his footsteps was greatly reduced by stocking feet and a carpet runner, he found himself, as he reported, "listening for the obstacle." He further stated that the "pressure sensation did not feel anywhere near as strong as before." The other blind subject, who came to the study with the firm conviction that audition was the basis of the blind's perception of obstacles, completed the preliminary experiment with that belief undisturbed.

In the B Series of every experiment, in which the intensity of his footsteps was greatly reduced, he walked toward the obstacle with his head turned to one side; he claimed that he was turning his better ear toward the obstacle. The sighted subjects, who approached the problem naïvely and without prejudice or theoretical bias, offered little in the way of explanation. Their earlier explanations that they were perceiving "facial pressures" were soon relegated to their own imagination. The sighted subjects noted that during the experiment they had to shuffle their feet and make some noise so as to perceive the obstacle.

Besides furnishing norms with which later performances could be compared, the results of the preliminary experiments set the problems of the main experiments.

Experiment 4 attempted to test the variant of the "pressure theory," that the basis of the "obstacle sense" rests upon pressure sensations aroused by reflected air currents or air waves. If those sensations are the basis of the perception, the subject should collide with the obstacle when conditions were so set that "air waves" could not contact his skin. What does the subject do under such conditions? To answer that question, all of the exposed areas of his skin, the face, head, arms, and hands, were covered, and the procedure of Experiment 3 was repeated.

In this experiment, in which there was no possibility of stimulation by air waves but in which sound could be used as a stimulus, it was found that all subjects detected the presence of the obstacle. The blind subject who had previously adhered to a pressure theory finally admitted his dependency on sound. He said, "I do not get an impression of the screen until I hear some little sound. I find myself scraping my stockings on the carpet in an endeavor to make a little noise." The other subjects pointed out that when they could not hear well because of the reduction in sound due to the veil, they were uncertain about their perceptions. Behavior of both the sighted subjects indicated their dependence upon sound.

Experiment 5 was attempted to answer the question whether

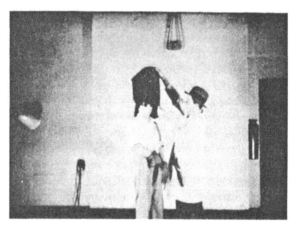

FIG. 31   A heavy felt veil, gloves, and a hat are worn by blindfolded subject to eliminate the possibility of pressure changes upon cutaneous areas.

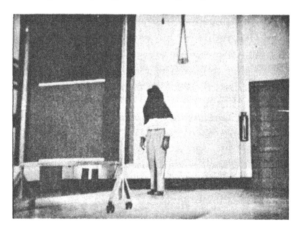

FIG. 32   Blindfolded subject still walks toward the wall with confidence. He perceived it on every trial.

echoing sounds are necessary for the perception of obstacles. To answer it, the subject's ears were stopped, leaving the normally exposed areas of the skin open and free for stimulation by air waves, air currents, sound waves, and so on. If, under those conditions, the subject failed to perceive the obstacle, the "pressure theory" would be disproved. The subject's ears were stopped by means of an ear defender, a series of beeswax-cotton shields over the concha and the pinna, layers of cotton batting, ear muffs, and elastic bands. Under such conditions all of the subjects were deaf to ordinary sound. The hearing loss was approximately 65 decibels. Except for the blindfold which had been used in the previous ex-

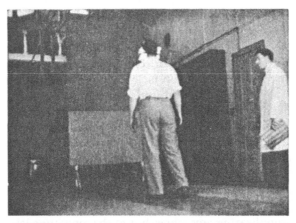

FIG. 33 Blindfolded subject approaching the wall with hearing eliminated.

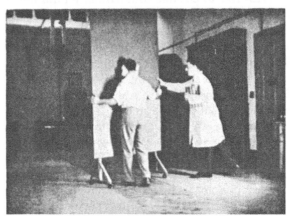

FIG. 34 Blindfolded subject, with hearing eliminated, runs into the wall.

periments, the subject's face was uncovered and open to tactual stimulation. The procedure and instructions were the same as in the control experiment, Experiment 3. Under such conditions, none of the subjects in either Series A or Series B was able to detect the obstacle but collided with the screen in 50 consecutive trials in each series. The posture of the subjects during the approach was very different from that in any preceding experiment. They walked with heads thrust forward, as if they were straining to hear, which they were, as their verbal reports proved. The result of this experiment indicated that sounds were necessary for the perception of obstacles.

Since it was possible that the loss of hearing in Experiment 5 could have been responsible for the subjects' failure to perceive the obstacle by means of cutaneous pressure, Experiment 6 was set up to determine whether pressure stimulation of the exposed areas of the skin by reflected "air" or sound waves was a sufficient condition for the perception of obstacles when hearing was left intact. In other words, could the subjects succeed in perceiving the obstacle when the face and other exposed areas were free and open to stimulation and when hearing was not eliminated nor adversely affected? This problem was met in Experiment 6 by means of a sound screen—a constant, continuously sounding tone of moderate intensity produced by means of an electrically driven tuning fork of 1,000 cycles conducted by long, pliant wires to a set of headphones worn by the subject. Such a sound screen prevented the subject from hearing any echoes but at the same time left his face and other areas free to possible stimulation, yet did not eliminate or affect adversely the subject's hearing except that the only sound heard was the tone.

With the substitution of the sound screen, the procedure and instructions were the same as in Experiment 5. Once again, it was found that all of the subjects ran into the masonite screen in every trial, i.e., for 50 consecutive trials. The behavior of the subjects was similar to that in Experiment 5. They walked slowly and more noisily than in any of the preceding experiments, and some of the subjects approached the obstacle with hands held apprehensively before them. The results of this experiment indicated that the subject's failure to perceive the obstacle in the preceding experiment was due not to a hypothetical deleterious effect of the loss of hearing upon tactual perception but to the absence of all the cues which were eliminated by the earplugs and pads, and which were submerged by the sound screen in this experiment. Once again, the conclusion that sounds are a necessary condition for the perception of obstacles seemed reaffirmed.

In Experiment 4, where the subject's exposed areas were

hidden, stimulation by an air medium had been eliminated. There still remained the possibility of perception being made by the cutaneous areas by means of reflected sound waves upon those areas. Experiment 7 eliminated the sound waves that might stimu-

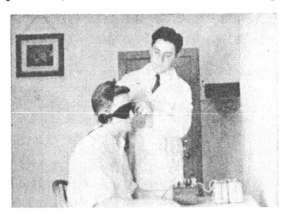

FIG. 35 The sound-screen, which makes hearing ineffective, is being placed on subject.

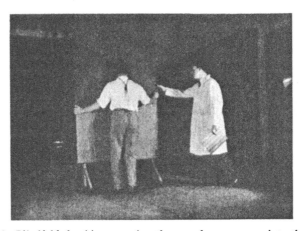

FIG. 36 Blindfolded subject, wearing the sound-screen, runs into the wall.

late the exposed areas of the skin but did not exclude sounds from the ears. The final experimental conditions were obtained by placing the subjects in a soundproof room and thereby removing their exposed cutaneous areas from any stimulational effects. The subject had to judge the experimenter's approach to an obstacle by means of the sounds transmitted electrically to headphones on his ears, so stimulation was limited to sounds. Seated comfortably in a soundproof room and wearing high-fidelity earphones, the subject listened to the sounds of the experimenter's footsteps during the latter's approach to the obstacle. The sounds of the experimenter's footsteps were carried to the subject by means of a microphone which was carried shoulder high by the experimenter and connected to the headphones of the subject through a power amplifier. In addition, the subject in the soundproof room held a transmitter which was connected to headphones worn by the experimenter so that they were able to communicate with one another as occasion demanded. The experimenter, starting at varying distances from the obstacle, walked to it at a rate which suited the subject. He stopped at the instruction of the subject or continued until he bumped the microphone against the wall.

Even under the unusual conditions of this experiment, all the subjects were able to perceive the obstacle. They permitted the experimenter to strike it with the microphone not much more frequently than they did in the control experiment, Experiment 3. In addition, all of the subjects reported that they were able to judge the experimenter's approach toward the wall by means of the transmitter sounds, and they stated furthermore that the sounds of these footsteps were different from those they heard when they themselves were doing the walking. They reported that they based their judgment upon changes in the sound of the experimenter's footsteps which occurred when he came near the wall.

The results obtained from the seven experiments led Supa, Cotzin, and Dallenbach to conclude that the pressure theory of the "obstacle sense," insofar as it applies to the face and other exposed areas of the skin, is untenable, and that sound stimuli are both necessary as well as adequate for the perception of obstacles.

The work of Griffin and Galambos, in 1941, on the sensory basis of obstacle avoidance by flying bats corroborates the findings of Supa, Cotzin, and Dallenbach insofar as both studies show the perception of obstacles to be responses to sound stimuli.

In 1947, Worchel and Dallenbach, using ten deaf-blind individuals, selected on the basis of their ability to get about alone, showed that these subjects did not detect and could not learn to detect obstacles at a distance. In addition, they proved that the pressure theory is untenable, and that auditory stimulation is both a necessary and a sufficient condition for the perception of obstacles by the blind. The auditory explanation sustained by the result of this study could be regarded as an accurate description of the facts.

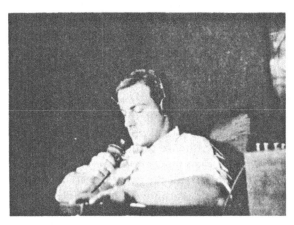

FIG. 37   The subject in the soundproof room judging the experimenter's approach to the wall. He tells the experimenter when to proceed and when to stop.

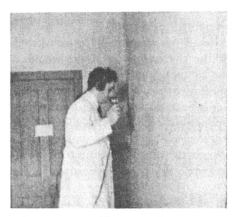

FIG. 38   The experimenter approaching the wall with the microphone. The subject is in the soundproof room with earphones. He listens to the sounds of the experimenter's footsteps and judges the approach to the wall.

Cotzin pursued the investigations further in an attempt to discover the range of audible frequencies in which the subject perceived obstacles and also to determine the specific aspects of sound which were the basis of the perception. He suspended a carriage from three horizontally spaced wires stretched tautly 9 feet from the floor, through the center and length of the experimental room. A loud-speaker and microphone were attached to this carriage which was moved smoothly and noiselessly along the wire track by means of a variable-speed, reversible, d-c motor and chalk-line belt. The subject was stationed in a soundproof room and could move this apparatus in a forward direction at varying speeds; the experimenter controlled the direction of its movement and its maximum speed. The sound stimuli used were (1) a thermal noise, and (2) pure tones of 125, 250, 500, 1,000, 2,000, 4,000, 8,000, and 10,000 cycles generated by an oscillator. These sounds carried by the loud-speaker were picked up by the microphone and transmitted to an amplifier, thence through an attenuator, to the subject's headphones in the soundproof room. A communication system between the subject and the experimenter consisted of a telephone microphone and earphones for talking and a bell and buzzer system for signaling.

After the sound carriage had been placed by the experimenter at a given distance from the obstacle, the subject moved it forward at a rate determined by himself and stopped it when he detected the presence of the obstacle. Once again, the subjects were two blind and two sighted individuals.

The first series of experiments concerned the detection of the wall with the thermal noise as the sound source. In these studies, all the subjects were successful in making correct judgments. Such performances were paralleled by reports of changes in the sound as it neared the obstacle. In order to determine that the change upon which the subjects' judgments were based was in the sound source, a series of experiments in which the carriage was moved toward the obstacle without the loud-speaker turned on was set up. Every subject failed consistently in each trial of the series.

The final series of experiments was conducted with "pure tones" as the sound stimuli. All of the observers, blind and seeing alike, failed to detect the wall when tones other than 10,000 cycles were used. With this tone, as with the thermal noise, the perception was based upon a rise in pitch as the sound source neared the obstacle.

Measurement by the continuous method of limits of the loudness of the thermal noise in terms of decibels above the intensity limen revealed no differences when the sound source was 0 feet or 6 feet from the obstacle. The rise in pitch, which is the stimulus for the perception of obstacles when footsteps or thermal noises are used as the sound, is explained by the fact that the incident and reflected sound waves of the complex tone set up a stationary wave pattern in which certain components are strengthened and others weakened. As the complex sound approached the obstacle, progressively higher frequencies were heard as louder, thereby giving the perception of an apparent rise in pitch. The explanation of the results with the 10,000-cycle tone is not easy. Differences in reflection and absorption of high and low frequencies by the obstacle may be the explanation. In any case, the results of Cotzin's study corroborated those obtained with bats by Griffin and Galambos, who found that bats avoid obstacles by sounds emitted by themselves which are in the range of the 50,000 cycles. On the basis of Cotzin's results, it is believed that the high audible frequencies are the important cues in the perception of obstacles by the blind. Such an interpretation is borne out by observation of the everyday activities of blind people who are skillful in perceiving obstacles and by the sighted subjects who learned to perceive obstacles in the above experiments. To help them in their perception of obstacles, these people resort to "artificial noises," such as jingling coins or keys in their pockets, snapping their fingers, slapping their thighs, whispering, hissing, whistling, and so on. Such sounds contain many more high than low frequencies.

The empirical methods employed by Supa, Cotzin, and Dallenbach solved the age-old problem of the perception of obstacles by the blind. Casual observation and occult explanation have given way to results based upon controlled experimentation. The factual knowledge that the blind perceive obstacles by means of auditory cues can now be utilized validly in teaching many blind people to become more independent in their everyday activities and in helping those newly blinded by accidents or wars to make a quicker and more satisfactory adjustment to life.

X. SOME DIFFICULTIES WITH "PRINTERS' ERRORS" [12]

The more experienced we become as readers, the faster and more "short-circuited" does the whole process become. Experimental work has shown that we do not "take in" every single letter of the text that we read. It is more like a hop, skip, and jump affair. We "grasp" at the whole configuration, be it word or phrase, and if the resemblance between it and that word or phrase as we earlier saw it is close enough, the perception is consummated. This tendency to read wholes must be counteracted by the proofreader. At his work, he must substitute more analytic perceptions for the rapid skimming of the general shapes of words which he practices in his reading off duty. The following selection indicates the difficulty that the early printers had in putting aside their daily reading habits while checking errors in printing. Because of its frequent occurrence in proofreading, this mode of perception is also referred to as the proofreader's illusion.

In spite of the utmost care, the King James version was from the outset bedeviled by printers' errors. The two impressions of the first edition were known respectively as "the Great Hee Bible" and "the Great She Bible" because the one rendered Ruth III.15 as "Hee went into the city," while the other read, "She went into the city," both forms still appearing in modern Bibles. Another error that has never been corrected was the substitution of "at" for "out" in Matthew XXIII.24, giving the oft-quoted mistranslation, "straining at a gnat." There was also much inconsistency in the spelling of Hebrew names, some of which has never been eliminated.

The errors were, in fact, so numerous that a revised edition was called for as early as 1615, to be followed by others every few years. In each new edition, however, new errors cropped up. That of 1631 was called the "Wicked Bible" because it gave the seventh commandment as "Thou shalt commit adultery." Cromwell was reputed to have paid out a thousand pounds in bribes to the 1638 revisers to induce them to change "we" to "ye" in Acts VI.3 so that the power of appointing officers

---

[12] BATES, E. S. *Biography of the Bible.* New York: Simon and Schuster, 1937. Pp. 183. Reprinted from *Biography of the Bible* by permission of Simon and Schuster, Publishers. Copyright, 1937, by Ernest Sutherland Bates.)

should seem to have belonged to the people instead of to the Apostles. An elaborate edition put out by the University of Oxford in 1727 was nicknamed the "Vinegar Bible" because a headline to the parable of the vineyard in Luke XXII read "The Parable of the Vinegar" [Pp. 124–125].

11

IMPLICIT OR "THINKING" BEHAVIORS

I. WHAT IS "THINKING"?

N. H. Pronko

To the man in the street, "thinking" appears as a wraithlike process and is usually attributed to the workings of the "mind." Steeped as he is in mentalistic thinking, this subtle action baffles description in any other terms. Fig. 39(A) shows what might be termed a "one-variable theory" of "thinking." The comic-strip feature is intended to convey the etherealness with which "thinking" is enshrouded. The person who is relatively inactive and lying on a couch and recalls or "thinks of something" readily convinces himself that the "thinking" must have come from inside, so subtle is this class of action. The layman can conceive of "thinking" in no other manner than as something out of the blue that wells up inside him.

People do "think"; that is an obvious fact. Yet to arrive at the description discussed above does not help much in any attempt at understanding this type of psychological activity. On the contrary, it appears to have led us into greater mystification than that with which we started. Obviously, for scientific purposes, this is not a satisfactory state of affairs. For that reason, we shall back up and try another type of explanation.

Within an objective framework, "thinking" gets a more precise formulation than the "one-variable theory" of the man in the street. First, we note that the striking feature of behavior so designated is that the organism interacts with an absent stimulus object. One can certainly recall last month's concert or last year's family reunion, and one can also be embarrassed again "merely

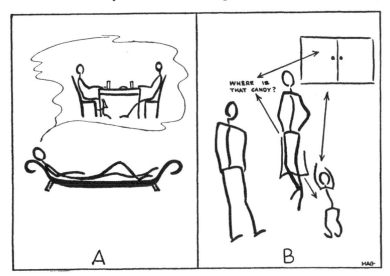

FIG. 39 (A) The popular or mentalistic theory of "thinking." Here "thinking" is thought of as occurring "somewhere" inside the organism for no apparent reason—a kind of spontaneous action unrelated to anything else. This might be considered as a "one variable" theory of thinking. An objective view would look for other variables such as substitute stimuli in the person's own behavior or setting factors. (B) An objective theory of thinking behavior. Here the action of the infant responding to the absent stimulus object is related to the mother's word "candy" which serves as a substitute stimulus for the actual candy. Thus, the child's action is not thought of as "welling up" inside him but as an occurrence involving a substitute stimulus as well as the absent stimulus object. The thinking behavior in A would be handled similarly.

thinking" of his most embarrassing moment. Similarly, humiliating, frightening, or grief-inducing experiences can occur again long after the original situations that called out such reactions.

To take a rather simple case: A child of 2 years has been given a bag of candy by a doting relative. Both in his past history as well as in the present situation, the "noise," "candy," has been repeatedly used on such occasions. Eventually, the mother hides the candy bag in the kitchen cupboard in the child's presence. The next day someone inadvertently uses the word "candy." Immediately, the child gets disturbed and makes reaching movements toward the cupboard in which the candy was hidden. During all this time, the candy has been out of sight and the child has reacted to it out of sight. The question is, how can he do that?

Obviously, the same infant could not have behaved in this

fashion on the day of his birth. However, by being handed sweets that were simultaneously called "candy" a number of times during his 2 years of existence, eventually the word "candy" alone elicited much the same sort of behavior as did the bag of sweets. In other words, by responding to the objects "candy" as the word is spoken, in time, the word alone is adequate to elicit such activity. When this stage has been reached, we may say that the word functions as a substitute stimulus, i.e., it substitutes or "pinch-hits" for the candy bag. The principle at which we arrive with our analysis is that reactions to absent objects originate in the same fashion as do all other reactions, namely, out of direct response to those stimulus objects. The added feature here is that, instead of the absent object, some other stimulus object functions as the other variable related to the individual's action. How it can perform such a function may be understood only in terms of its inseparable association with the absent object in a series of past behavioral events. Note that for a French-speaking child the noise, *bonbons,* would have to be used to elicit a reaction to candy out of sight, and that this would not function as a substitute stimulus for an American child.

An aged woman has just buried her husband. She has returned home from the funeral but is still "grief stricken." She weeps and will not be comforted. The striking feature about her behavior is that the dead husband is not there before her now. This, again, is a response to an absent stimulus object. How it originated can be easily traced out of the series of preceding events, for we can observe the widow's violent grief responses as she looks upon her husband for the last time. The group departs from the cemetery and the widow is now at home, yet her sorrow is as great as it was at the funeral. Reactions to absent stimulus objects are not always subtle (inapparent). As for substitute stimuli in this case, need we look any further than the dead husband's watch, pipe, clothes, books, and many other things that were so intimately connected with him and which "pinch-hit" so effectively for him now?

In the case of the afore-mentioned child, the substitute stimulus was by no means a subtle or inapparent affair. In fact, we can operationally predict that presence or absence of the word "candy" results in presence or absence of the "implicit response" (i.e., to the absent stimulus object). The case of the widow also shows that, despite the absence of the dead husband, her action is just as complete to the last detail (sobbing, moaning, crying) as when the corpse was before her. Thus, the action of the organism can be the same *in absentia* of the stimulus object as in its actual presence.

There are instances, however, in which the action of the substitute stimulus is of such a delicate sort that it is apprehended with difficulty if at all. It is these "thinking" acts that frustrate the layman. The following incident illustrates the point.

Mr. Jones is walking in a particular section of town when he catches himself humming the Scottish tune, "Loch Lomond" whose lines go, "I'll tak' the high road and you'll tak' the low road," and so on. Curious to know what "made him think" of that particular song, he begins to look for substitute stimuli. Taking special notice of his whereabouts, Jones observes that he has just passed the intersection of High Street and Maxwell Lane and immediately recalls the phrase from another Scottish song which runs, "Maxwelton's braes are bonnie" and in the next instant the portion of the song mentioned above. He is satisfied that the street names acted upon him as subtle substitute stimuli to elicit action explainable in no other fashion. Apparently, the organism participates in psychological reactions in which the stimulus variable is not always discernible (even to him) at first inspection.

An intricate type of implicit response follows when the substitute stimulus is quite obvious but the action of the organism is inapparent. (This term is not to be misinterpreted to mean "psychic" or "mental," but is used very much as the term "inapparent" might be used when applied to neural "action" or catalytic "action." These latter are also far removed from the kind of action illustrated in a landslide, explosion, or falling objects. One does not see nerves jump or even move; yet they "act" but in an inapparent way.) Here, the organism performs acts that are remnants of former acts. The recall of some past experience belongs here. In this case, a stimulus which substitutes for the absent one nevertheless elicits some degree of the organismic response that was formerly performed to that absent object.

There is one further step in the possible complexity of the variables involved in implicit behavior. The organism's own action can serve as a substitute stimulus. Because his action was connected with a certain stimulus on a former occasion, the action occurring at a given time to a stimulus can evoke the action that *was* performed to the absent stimulus. This is, by definition, an implicit response. An example of an individual whose dizzy or nauseated condition "reminds" him of some similar past situation is to the point.

Similarly, the person who daydreams performs a series of implicit reactions that serve as substitute stimuli in a kind of chain reaction. These latter are the most complex because the stimulus *and* response variables are both so delicate in their operation that only cooperation of the subject or other intimate study of each individual will reveal their details. However, regardless of their intricacy, implicit actions can be traced out of grosser and more direct forms of action through a series of stages in the manner suggested above. In any case, we are dealing with vestigial or remnant action.

EXPERIMENTAL STUDY OF IMPLICIT ACTION. Experimental studies of implicit behavior support the interpretation developed above. For a good many years, it has been known that when human subjects engage in "mental arithmetic," silent reading, and other of the more subtle activities, there is some degree of involvement of muscle action, very often so incipient that the subject himself is unable to detect it.

Some of the older work seems to show a degree of localization of such muscular activity; thus, if subjects worked arithmetic problems without paper and pencil, the musculature of the speech organs showed incipient action. On the other hand, if subjects *"visualized"* certain scenes, eye muscles would show involvement while *movements* that were "thought about" such as "thinking about" running a race resulted in definite tensions in leg muscles. The subject might not be able to detect these tensions because they were too vestigial, nevertheless they were recorded.

Among the more recent work along these lines is a study by Shaw [1] who studied the distribution of incipient muscle action during a variety of psychological performances.

Shaw's technique consisted of attaching electrodes to various portions of his human subjects and, by means of an oscillograph and amplifier, photographing the action potentials occurring in the muscles. With this procedure, he capitalized on the known

---

[1] SHAW, WILLIAM A. The distribution of muscular action potentials during imaging. *Psychol. Rec.*, 1938, **2**, 195–216. (Reproduced by permission of the author and the publisher.)

fact that when living tissues are functional, one phase of their functioning involves electrical activity. The greater the amount of muscle (or nervous) activity, the greater the changes in the accompanying action potentials. Much should be made of the point that the two phenomena are merely concomitant and that one is not "cause" and the other "effect," because the latter explanation is often given in the popular journals. In summary, then, Shaw used changes in the action potentials as an index of subtle muscle activity.

The next question is: Did a study of such action-potential changes make any psychological sense? In order to answer this question, Shaw required his subjects to "imagine" themselves engaged in a number of different acts. There was a considerable amount of deflection occurring in all four limbs when they imagined squeezing a hand dynamometer with the right hand *while in a state of rest*. The important point to note is that this implicit action is not localized. It involves the whole organism, although there is a focus of activity in the right arm. Shaw concludes that "during the imaging of squeezing a hand dynamometer in the right hand the muscles of the right arm are more active than they are during rest" [p. 201].

Another part of the experiment required subjects to imagine typing the alphabet in which increase in action potentials of a statistically reliable sort occurred in both arms but not in the legs.

When subjects were asked to image themselves singing, there tended to be an increase in action potentials from the arms during the time they were so engaged. There was also a moderately strong tendency for an increase in action potentials during the time subjects engaged in imagining playing a wind instrument.

In conclusion, Shaw writes:

> There appears to be an increase in muscular action potentials from nearly all of the muscle groups tested during the imaging of the various tasks. There is no good evidence of localization to the muscle groups commonly thought to be involved in such performances. While such action potentials seem to be necessarily concomitant as shown by the report of the unsuccessful subjects and the control groups, they are not localized in any particular part of the body nor are they exclusively peculiar to imaging since other workers have shown that action po-

tentials accompany other implicit activities also. The distribution of these action potentials seems to indicate that during the revival of vestigial responses one can expect to be present any muscular activity that accompanied the original response [p. 215].

In our opinion, the most important result of Shaw's work is to "demystify" thinking. There is no basis for the "one-variable theory" of mentalistic, popular psychology to the effect that "thinking" is a spooky act occurring in some alleged "mind." On the contrary, operational instrumental techniques show that imaging and the like are also interactions involving an organism and absent, past stimuli. And, when one concentrates on the organism's side of the picture in such *events,* one finds incipient muscle movements that bear a certain relationship to his past action when he was actually confronted with those stimuli. The essential difference is that some other stimulus substitutes for the absent one, and that the organism's action is stepped down or reduced in degree, not in kind.

Granted that the action is subtle and inapparent, nevertheless that is no reason for relegating "thinking" to a class by itself, separate from other kinds of stimulus-response units. All sciences have certain data that are simple and others that are complex and inapparent; neural action, catalytic action, electrical activity, and gases that have no odor, visibility, or taste but only weight are examples from different sciences. However, these are not relegated to the supernatural realm. For example, no biologist is mystified by nerve action, yet nerves do not act in a visible way. Only the application of instrumental techniques gives any index of when and how much activity goes on in them, but such study yields results in the way of scientific knowledge. So, for "thinking" and the rest, when studied operationally and naturalistically, they yield results in the way of sound knowledge. Actually, despite bad theory, where one knows another's responses and the connection between the latter and their stimuli as well as the interconnection between stimuli, one can "predict" and "control" the other's implicit responses. This has happened down through the ages between parents and children, husband and wife, and between lovers. Intimate acquaintance with all the variables involved has meant a knowledge of kind, as well as time, of occurrence of implicit or "thinking" actions.

II. HOW SUBSTITUTE STIMULI FUNCTION

N. H. Pronko

Razran [2] has conducted an interesting study which, according to him, was designed to study "thinking in different languages." If the expression is to be taken literally, we would prefer the interpretation that what Razran did was to study "thinking *with* (or by means of) different languages."

Before noting the details of his experimental procedure, it is important to consider Razran's reactional biography, since it was he that served as subject in this experiment. He was born in Russia, came to the United States at the age of 19, began the study of German and French at the age of 9, Polish at the age of 16, English at 19, and Spanish at the age of 22. It was his native language, Russian, and the five acquired later that were selected for use in the experiment. The word "saliva" from each of these six languages was the specific word employed. As controls, the same word from an unfamiliar language (Gaelic), a nonsense syllable, and no extra stimulus were also employed.

In order to have a quantitative index of the degree of familiarity of each of the six languages employed, Razran made tests of speed of association, speed of reading, and extent of vocabulary in each. The number of words uttered in each language in a 3-minute period with eyes closed constituted the first test. Tests of speed of reading were made by a comparison of the number of pages per hour read in *La comtesse de Charny*, a novel by Alexandre Dumas. Copies of this novel in the six different languages employed were obtained from the New York Public Library, divided into six equal but random groupings of chapters, and one grouping in each language was read for five hours. The number of unfamiliar words in the material read was counted; these constituted an index of vocabulary range.

EXPERIMENTAL PROCEDURE.   Nine 1-inch cards were used. On seven of the cards was printed the word for "saliva"—one printed in each of the six languages the subject knew and one in the unfamiliar Gaelic. One card was blank and one contained a nonsense

---

[2] RAZRAN, G. H. S. Salivating and thinking in different languages. *J. Psychol.*, 1936, 1, 145–151. (Quotation reproduced by permission of the publisher.)

syllable. The cards were shuffled by an assistant and placed in a box. Razran's mouth was dried of accumulated saliva by means of a dental-cotton roll. The assistant then drew a card from the box, at which moment Razran inserted a previously weighed but dry cotton roll under his tongue and continuously reacted to the word exposed (with eyes closed) for 2 minutes. At the end of that interval, a new stimulus card and new cotton roll were given to the subject, and the same procedure was repeated until all nine cards had been exposed. After each trial, the cotton roll was weighed in order to determine how much saliva had been secreted to that card. After each series of nine cards, there was a seven-minute pause. Four series constituted an experimental session, and there were nine such sessions so that each card was presented thirty-six times. Averages were then computed of the amount of salivary secretion to each stimulus card. The results and relationships with familiarity of the language used are shown in Table 14.

Table 14

Average Milligrams of Saliva Secreted to Stimulus Word (Saliva) in Different Languages with Corresponding Speeds of Association and Reading and Vocabulary in These Languages for the Subject Employed

Language	Average Salivation (Milligrams)	Speed of Association (Words in 3 Minutes)	Speed of Reading (Pages per Hour)	Vocabulary Range (Unfamiliar Words in 50 Pages)
Russian	812.4	81	43	1
English	594.6	131	52	3
German	417.1	54	27	27
French	307.2	33	23	41
Spanish	302.1	21	18	68
Polish	286.4	20	16	76
Gaelic (unfamiliar language) ..	207.4			
Nonsense syllable (QER SUH) ..	194.6			
No extra stimulus (control)	216.2			

The reader will note that most secretion occurs to the Russian word, even though English superseded that language in the subject's later life. Perhaps this result indicates that the earliest years of the reactional biography are the most important. When objects have no stimulus function, they may acquire values which will have priority over later acquisitions. As to the other languages used as stimuli, we quote Razran.

Thinking in either of the writer's wonted speaking languages (Russian and English) elicited more saliva than thinking in the best of his reading languages (German), which in turn caused greater secretion than thinking in any of three less mastered reading languages. Finally, thinking in languages even with which the writer's familiarity was rather limited (French, Spanish, and Polish) still produced reliable increments in salivations, but keeping in consciousness a word meaning *saliva* in a totally unknown language had no effect upon the salivary secretions [pp. 147–151].

We differ from Razran's interpretation of his experiment in one important respect. As the language of the preceding sentence as well as of the title of his paper implies, there are alleged to be two activities going on—salivating *and* thinking. In our view, the salivating *was* the thinking, although, of course, there were probably other components in the organism's response in addition to salivary secretion. But dealing with the salivary aspect of the reaction, we consider this as a remnant reaction of a salivary response performed by the subject to a wide variety of stimulus objects in his past. These stimulus objects included also the word "saliva," which was connected with the act of salivating through its use as a label for that act. The difference between former reactions, in which directly present stimulus objects elicited such action, and the experiment here discussed is that, in the latter situation, those objects were absent and were substituted for by the words for *saliva* in the various languages employed.

The way in which the substitute stimuli worked here is also instructive. The most striking feature of the salivary secretion is the variability in amount of secretion. However, this variability is not chaotic but shows definite relations to the psychological history of the subject. Stated generally, we might say that priority and/or frequency of their occurrence in the past determine how effectively they operate as substitute stimuli. On a strictly dictionary basis, all these seven words are equivalent. Not so from a psychological viewpoint. Here their specific connection with a certain individual's behavior counts. How many times and how effectively were they related to interactions in which the subject actually secreted saliva to stimulus object? That this occurred with the Russian and English words in accordance with some such relationship is indicated by the heavy flow of saliva (812.4 and 594.6 milligrams, respectively) when these words were used as substitute stimuli. On the other hand, the Spanish and Polish words have less connection with the subject's past history and function much less effectively, the former yielding a salivary flow of 302.1 milligrams and the latter 286.4 milligrams. Note that the unfamiliar Gaelic word gives 207.4 milligrams and the nonsense syllables (QER SUH), 194.6. Since the blank card elicits 216.2 milligrams, we may consider this last as a continuous or basal (i.e., physiological) flow and, therefore, state that because these last three stimuli were not connected with the subject's past reactions, they did not elicit vestigial salivary secretions during the experiment. As to the rest, they present a gradient of salivary secretions. Thus, the Russian, English, German, French, Spanish, and Polish words are arranged in the order of their efficacy as substitute stimuli. Put another way, the salivary secretions of the psychological reactions involved are vestigial in a descending order of their listing. Salivary secretions to the Russian word are least remnant, whereas they are mere remnants to the infrequently used Spanish and Polish words as substitute stimuli. How they relate to details of Razran's reactional biography may be teased out from the data given in the other columns.

In conclusion, Razran's results show that implicit or "thinking" interactions may be studied in detail as to their specific configuration, the variables or substitute stimuli which elicit them, and the relationship of these substitute stimuli to the organism's prior contacts with other stimuli. In essence, these acts need no longer be interpreted as "psychic" or "mental" happenings but may be handled as concrete if subtle behaviors—remnants of former acts and all subject to empirical or operational manipulation and analysis.

III. AFTERIMAGE RESPONSES
N. H. Pronko

The field of afterimage responses has been neglected in recent years, partially, perhaps, because such studies depend primarily upon the subject's observing and reporting his own behavior (commonly called "introspection") and therefore have not been deemed suitable for "objective" psychology. However, afterimage reactions are definite forms of interaction of organisms and things and must be included in a classification of actions in which human animals engage.

Difficulties of description also have been a handicap to studies of this sort. Physiological variables have been of obvious importance, but just how they related to an organism performing an afterimage response has perplexed many psychologists. Notice, however, that this type of action fits the general form of all implicit behavior. In the afterimage response, the organism is out of contact with the original stimulus and therefore is interacting with it "by proxy." The physiological (retinal) features serve in this case as the substitute stimulus, in a behavioral field suitable for this sort of action; that is, a field which includes the necessary illumination, "projection" screen, and orientation of the subject toward afterimage action rather than preoccupation with some other sort of activity.

Morsh and Abbott,[3] of the University of British Columbia, report a series of studies of so-called "eidetic imagery" of school children, from which the succeeding selections are quoted. Eidetic imagery was, at one time, considered a distinct kind of implicit response, in which the subject would look at an object for a while. He then shut his eyes or looked upon a gray screen and still reacted as if the absent object were present, answering questions about its color and other characteristics. In other words, this was a vivid or rather complete response in absence of a stimulus object for which there was a substitute stimulus. The findings reported here show the nature of complex afterimage responses as well as suggesting the range of individual differences which obtains in implicit action. It also throws doubt on the validity of the eidetic image as a distinct type of imagery.

. . . some 411 subjects from a large city school were individually tested for visual imagery. They varied in age from 6 to 17 years and ranged in school achievement from the first through the eighth grade. These subjects were for the most part Canadian-born Orientals, approxi-

---

[3] MORSH, J. E. & ABBOTT, H. D. An investigation of after-images. *J. comp. Psychol.*, 1945, **38**, 47–63. (Reproduced by permission of the authors, the American Psychological Association and the Williams & Wilkins Company.)

mately 50 per cent (205) being of Japanese and 27 per cent (109) being of Chinese parentage. The rest (with the exception of two Negroes) were white children.

An attempt was made to duplicate the technique employed by investigators of eidetic imagery. The visual stimuli used were bold black and white drawings which measured approximately 6 by 8 inches, of interest to children and containing a number of definite details. The most successful stimulus picture is reproduced in Figure 40. The subjects stood about three feet from the pictures and regarded them for 40 seconds in good daylight. The stimulus was then removed and the subjects were required to fixate a neutral gray cardboard [pp. 54–55].

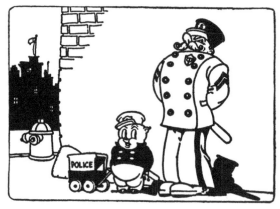

FIG. 40 The policeman picture in black and white. "If I could only be a policeman!" (Marsh, J. E., & Abbott, H. D., An investigation of after-images.)

On the basis of this and similar experiments, the investigators came to the following conclusions:

The after-image behavior of over 700 young subjects was studied using with some subjects the "blink" method with the dark-adapted eye and with others the fixation of pictures after the technique of Klüver. A grading scale was worked out in order to classify subjects according to their after-image performance. The present investigation revealed nothing to substantiate the claim that some special "eidetic" ability exists. After-image ability of a marked degree might be termed "eidetic" but it should not be implied that any sharp difference exists between so-called eidetikers and non-eidetikers. After-image abilities of a random group of subjects appear in a continuum. It is highly improbable that there is as Kobusch says a continuum of steps between the pure eidetic image and the pure memory image. The eidetic image is merely a vivid after-image, due probably to persistence of activity in the retina [?]. There seems, however, no real reason why the ambiguous and misleading "eidetic image" phraseology should be maintained. It is suggested that the term eidetic imagery be dropped from our already overburdened psychological terminology.

1. The incidence of varying grades of after-image ability on a scale of five steps was found to be: A (highest ability), 9.3 per cent; B, 9.8 per cent; C, 19.1 per cent; D, 31.7 per cent; E, 30.1 per cent.

2. Of 256 child subjects 69.6 per cent saw an after-image of a picture. The after-sensations were reported as: grays only, 8.6 per cent; all or in part complementary colors, 13.3 per cent; positive images only, 48 per cent.

3. Of 22 subjects who reported gray after-images, 18 were weak in color discrimination as shown by the Ishihara Test of Color Blindness.[4]

4. There appears to be a definite, positive relationship between age and ability to experience after-images.

5. Boys did not appear significantly different from girls in their after-image abilities.

6. From the present data after-image ability and intelligence appear to be associated though the correlation is not high.

7. Studies of the relationship between after-imagery and performance in spelling, English composition, and art revealed a statistically reliable relationship in the case of art achievement, an insignificant but strong trend for association in the case of spelling, while there was no more than chance relationship with English composition [pp. 62–63].

In other words, students who were proficient in art and spelling tended to be better imagers, although superiority in English composition showed only a chance relationship.

IV. EXAMPLES OF BORDERLINE IMPLICIT ACTION [5]
J. W. Bowles, Jr.

Conditioned response and implicit reactions to substitute stimuli have traditionally been confused. The conditioned stimulus has

---

[4] The fact that people who do not perceive colors well do not perform vivid implicit color reactions shows how the latter derive from the former.

[5] LEUBA, CLARENCE. Images as conditioned sensations. *J. exp. Psychol.*, 1940, **26**, 345–351. (Reproduced by permission of the author and the American Psychological Association.)

been called a cue or signal for the unconditioned stimulus, i.e., a substitute for it. For example, in the classic Pavlov experiment in which the dog learned to salivate to the buzzer as well as to the sight of food, the buzzer has been called a signal for the appearance of the food. The results of many investigations show, however, that the conditioned stimulus cannot be properly described as a substitute for the original. In the case of the above example, the salivary response to the buzzer is not identical with the response to food. In the case of conditioned motor reflexes, conditioned movements are much different from reflex responses to unconditioned stimuli such as electric shocks. The same is true for other conditioned responses. This means that the organism has built up a new, *direct* response to the conditioned stimulus and that the latter is not "pinch-hitting" for the original unconditioned stimulus.

Clear-cut implicit actions differ markedly from conditioned responses. A remembering event in which an individual, seeing the date marked on the calendar pad, goes to keep an engagement would be an example. The encircled date does "pinch-hit" for the original stimulus (the person with whom the engagement was made). Similarly, a person angered by a picture that reminds him of an enemy would be performing an implicit-feeling action.

Between conditioned and implicit actions, however, are borderline events that are partially conditioned reactions but show some implicit features also. The series of experiments reported by Leuba belong in this category (he refers to them as images as conditioned sensations); some are essentially conditioned responses; others, particularly those involving perceptual actions which are in themselves semi-implicit, might be classified as implicit, or conditioned, or both.

The plan of our experiments was briefly as follows: During deep hypnosis two stimuli, such as the ringing of a bell and a pin prick on the hand, were applied simultaneously to the subject for some half dozen pairings; before being awakened from the hypnosis, the subject was told that he would remember nothing that had happened during the hypnosis (post-hypnotic amnesia); a few minutes after being awakened, he was subjected to a succession of stimuli among which was one of the two stimuli originally applied, say the bell ringing; he was instructed to report at once if he experienced anything, visually, tactually, or in any other sense modality, besides the usual direct effects of those stimuli. Almost without exception, imagery (conditioned sensations) was immediately reported upon presentation of the conditioned stimulus. After the bell ringing, for instance, the subject reported itching and pain on his hand, though he had no recollection of being pricked there previously or having ever heard that bell. The conditioned pain-tactual sensations appeared automatically and immediately upon the bell ringing—much to the subject's surprise.

The conditioning was performed under deep hypnosis for two reasons. (1) The concentration of attention and absence of distraction during hypnosis should facilitate the conditioning process and should lessen the likelihood of conflicting imagery which might nullify whatever conditioning had occurred. (2) A subject upon awakening from deep hypnosis has usually forgotten what happened during the trance. This forgetting can be made dependable by a suggestion of amnesia. Complete post-hypnotic amnesia—spontaneous and/or induced—was present in all our subjects and was an essential prerequisite for discovering whether imagery could be associated with a stimulus without the consciously remembered associations postulated by the classic laws of association.

These experiments, carried out as opportunity afforded during the past ten years, were performed on several subjects by several experimenters. The subjects were all college students; most of them students in General Psychology at the time of the experiment. The hypnosis was ostensibly entirely for some therapeutic or other practical non-experimental purpose, such as a class demonstration. As far as we could tell, the subjects were always completely unaware of the nature of the experiment.

The experimenters were either the writer, or one of his students with sufficient theoretical and practical background in hypnosis to be entrusted with the conduct of a hypnosis demonstration before a class in General Psychology. The method of inducing hypnosis was the standard one of concentrating upon some monotonous repetitive or continuous stimulus, such as the ticking of a clock or a point of light, while suggestions of relaxation, peace, and sleep were given. Most of the subjects had been hypnotized several times before the experiment was conducted and had repeatedly shown the signs of deep hypnosis such as anesthesias, hallucinations, and post-hypnotic amnesia. Most of the experiments were conducted either in the writer's office or in a departmental partially sound-proof room.

The following protocols describe all the experimental sessions with all the subjects. The first two experiments were of a preliminary, exploratory nature.

SUBJECT P. W., EXPERIMENTER C. L. 1929. E pricked S's hand several times with a sharp object while ringing a small bell. Post-hynotic amnesia suggested. After waking S up and exchanging a few words with him, E rang the bell. S moved one hand toward the other that had been pricked and said he had just felt something there.

SUBJECT C. B., EXPERIMENTER V. R. 1936. After S had been hypnotized, he was asked to look at the image of a Chinese pagoda thrown on a screen and to listen to a victrola record. After he had been awakened, the victrola record was played again and he was asked to draw something—anything that came to mind. He reproduced the Chinese pagoda in some detail. When asked what made him draw the pagoda, he said he did not know. He did not remember having seen one for a couple of months. He did not remember having heard any music since he came into the room.

SUBJECT D. G., EXPERIMENTERS A. M. AND C. L. 1936. After deep hypnosis had been produced, one experimenter struck a can sharply while S was tapped on the hand six or seven times with the flat side of a ruler. S jerked slightly, especially with his head, each time. Post-hypnotic amnesia was suggested and then S was awakened. After a brief conversation, S was told to report if he heard, saw, or felt any sensations while one of the E's performed various actions. E picked up various objects, stamped, banged the table, and hit various objects with the ruler including the can. The first two times the can was hit, S jerked back his head; but on no occasion did he report any experiences other than those caused directly by the stimuli actually used. (While hypnotizing S., A. M. had suggested to him that he would hear nothing, and pay attention to nothing, but A. M.'s voice. The fact that A. M. forgot to remove this sensory limitation before proceeding with the experiment may account for the failure of conditioning to occur to an auditory stimulus.)

SUBJECT D. G., EXPERIMENTERS A. M. AND C. L. 1936. After S had been hypnotized by A. M. he was poked gently in the side with a ruler and told to look at the object in front of him. The object was a nickel plated watch held about eight inches from S's eyes. He was given 3–5 seconds to look at it. The combined poking and looking were repeated about six times allowing 10–15 seconds between trials. The S was then told that he would remember nothing that had happened while he was under hypnosis; he was also given some post-hypnotic suggestions concerning a class demonstration, and was awakened in the usual manner. After he was awakened A. M. told him to lie on the cot and gave him a blank card to look at. The card was placed at about the same position where the watch had been held. S was told to report anything he experienced while A. M. performed various operations. S was reminded to look at the card closely. A. M. then walked about the room and hit various objects with the ruler. Then A. M. poked S in the ribs with the ruler in the same way as had been done previously during the hypnosis. S immediately said, "Hey, wait; what the dickens!" He reported that a ring had formed on the card as soon as he had been poked. When poked in the ribs a third time he reported that the ring appeared again and that it had a black dot in the center and was silvery. S was not able to report any other details concerning the image on the card. He was somewhat startled and puzzled at the phenomena. Later as he was walking about the room, he picked up the stop-watch box from the table and immediately exclaimed that the ring he had seen on the paper was a watch; that he was quite sure of it.

SUBJECT D. G., EXPERIMENTERS A. M. AND C. L. 1936. The S was hypnotized by A. M. and the same phenomena as usual were used to make sure that S was in a deep stage of hypnosis. While C. L. snapped a cricket, A. M. pricked S on the back of the hand with an algesiometer. The stimuli were paired five times with an interval of 10–15 seconds between pairings. After being awakened, S was told to report anything he experienced while the E's did various things. As soon as C. L. snapped the cricket S jerked his hand back from where it was lying on the chair arm and exclaimed that something had pricked him on the hand and rubbed the spot which A. M. had pricked, while S was under hypnosis. To no other stimulus that we tried, would he respond, but every time the cricket was snapped his hand jerked back and he reported feeling a pin prick.

SUBJECT D. G., EXPERIMENTERS A. M. AND C. L. 1936. A. M. again hypnotized the S and then told him to pay attention to C. L. The latter held a small bottle of creosote under S's nose and asked him to smell it every time it was placed in that position. In the meantime A. M. had taken a ruler and rubbed S on the right arm with it just as C. L. held the bottle of creosote under S's nose and told him to smell it. Rubbing on the arm followed by the smell of creosote was repeated five or six times and then the S was awakened and told to report anything he might experience. A. M. then proceeded to hit or rub various objects with the ruler even rubbing the S's leg without getting any response from S; but as soon as his arm was rubbed, he sniffed the air and said that something smelled funny and that an odor had just entered the room. When he was rubbed on the arm again he said the odor was stronger but that it did not last long. S asked A. M. if he could smell it and he said no. S seemed quite puzzled. Making it appear as accidental as possible, A. M. again rubbed S's arm and S again reported smelling some strong odor—"something like a tarred road"—"like creosote" he finally said. The smell appeared only when the right arm was rubbed, no other stimulus that A. M. tried was successful. S was very puzzled by the appearance of the odor and wanted to know what it was caused by. He said it appeared suddenly and was unmistakable but that he could not see why it appeared.

SUBJECT J. D., EXPERIMENTER C. L. 1938.　S was shown an E.S.P. card with a rectangle on it for about one minute while E tapped on a metal filing cabinet with a ruler. Shortly after being awakened S was given a blank white card and told to gaze at it fixedly and told to report if anything appeared on it. E jiggled his keys, and walked up and down the room, banged a book, cleared his throat, and tapped the file with a ruler. At this last stimulus S said: "There it is; I cannot tell exactly what, but it is some kind of a mathematical figure." When asked what color it was he replied that it had a "black outline." When shown a pack of E.S.P. cards, he picked the rectangle out as the figure he had seen. The figure appeared on the card each time C. L. tapped on the file, but disappeared quickly.

SUBJECT J. D., EXPERIMENTER C. L. 1938.　E pricked S about eight times with an algesiometer on the fleshy part of the right hand between the base of the thumb and index finger while tapping the top of a small can with a pencil. On awakening, S was requested to report whenever he saw, felt or otherwise experienced anything in connection with a series of stimuli. E stamped on the floor, rattled a brief case and so on finally tapping the can with a pencil. S at once scratched the previously stimulated area on his right hand with the left one and said that "it smarts and itches." He stopped scratching as soon as E stopped tapping the can and started to rub again as soon as the tapping was resumed.

SUBJECT V. F., EXPERIMENTERS D. B. AND C. L. 1936.　D. B. showed S a small pen and ink drawing of a fish while S moved his arm back and forth at the elbow nine or ten times. After he was awakened, S was asked to tell C. L. whenever he saw, tasted, heard, smelled, or otherwise, experienced anything as he made various movements. He was then told to move his right leg, then his left leg and then to move his right arm back and forth. At that point he reported that something came into his mind but he could not tell exactly what. When given a blank piece of cardboard to look at, he saw "a fish on it, about two or three inches long and ⅛ of an inch wide at the tail. It fades away when I stop moving my arm." The fish reappeared when the arm was moved back and forth. . . . From the protocols it is apparent that the conditioned sensations (images) were frequently accompanied by objective responses, such as a movement toward, and a scratching of, the itching hand; or a wrinkling up of the nose and sniffing movements as the creosote was imaginatively experienced. These movements were quick spontaneous responses following immediately upon the conditioned stimulus and substantiated the subject's introspective reports. Usually, the overt movements started before the subject reported the presence of imagery.

The subject was invariably surprised and puzzled by the conditioned sensations. They came suddenly out of nowhere and vanished equally suddenly. They were entirely involuntary and automatic. After the conditioned stimulus had been repeated a number of times, the subject usually consciously realized that the imagery always followed that particular stimulus. He still wondered why that peculiar connection existed.

The conditioned sensations were frequently so intense and vivid as to be mistaken for actual sensations; the subject thought that he was really smelling an odor or that he was really being pricked on the hand by some sharp object; but the images were also fleeting and difficult to examine. They appeared and disappeared with the conditioned stimulus and if that stimulus was continued they soon grew faint. The subject could rarely name the image correctly at once; the stop watch was a silver ring with a point in the center; the creosote was a powerful penetrating odor; the rectangle was just the outline of a figure; but the image was always referred to the correct stimulus from among a number of stimuli.

Hull reports the appearance of a phenomenon, similar to that described in this article, as an incidental observation in an experiment by Scott designed to discover what difference, if any, existed between the conditioning, under normal and trance conditions, of finger withdrawal by pairing buzzer and shock. "Several of these (totally amnesic) subjects . . . when stimulated by the buzzer alone, reported the feeling of having received an electric shock on the fingers. At least one of his subjects insisted that he had received a *bona fide* shock though the experimenter was positive, from testing the apparatus, that no shock could have been received."

The hypnotic state served the same purpose as the hunger drive, the soundproofing, and the exclusion of extraneous stimuli in general, in Pavlov's conditioned response experiments. It limited the subject's attention to the pertinent stimuli, and thereby enabled the experimenters to demonstrate a fundamental psychological principle whose functioning in everyday life is frequently obscured by the simultaneous presence of many stimuli and many responses.

Our experiments indicate that after an inadequate stimulus has been present a number of times, while an individual is experiencing certain sensations, it will by itself automatically, and without the intervention of any conscious processes, produce those sensations. An image can, therefore, be considered as a conditioned sensation [pp. 345-351].

V. THE STIMULUS-RESPONSE RELATIONSHIP IN DREAMS [6]

M. M. Makhdum

Makhdum, using the reports on dreams of several subjects, has analyzed relationships between stimulus conditions and the perceptual nature of dreaming. Under one heading, he places those dreams in which the "sensory content" of the dream directly represents the nature of the stimulus. The dream may be close to the waking reaction to the same stimulus condition, or it may be abnormally distorted in the dream. The first instance is illustrated by a dream in which the subject felt very thirsty and drank glass after glass of water without lessening his thirst. Upon awaking, he found himself to be actually very thirsty. In the second case, the subject dreamed of seeing three snakes standing on end. When he awoke, the three snakes were transformed into three vertical pieces of wood which formed the back of the chair next to the bed. The subject had been sleeping with eyes partially open but evidently in the dream state had responded abnormally to a visual stimulus object.

Under another heading, the author lists dreams in which the acting stimulus only plays a small part or is only referred to in some manner during the dream. In this case, the connection between the actual nature of the stimulus and the nature of the dream is more remote. The following dream is an illustration.

---

[6] MAKHDUM, M. M. On the stimulus-response relationship in dreams. *Indian J. Psychol.*, 1939, 14, 87-90. (Reproduced by permission of author and publisher.)

D dreams that he and a friend of his are in the upper story of a house. His friend has a pamphlet with him. They are going to read it. D asks his friend to see that the door of the room is fastened lest someone should intrude upon them. D goes on insisting on this, pointing to the door, till he wakes up. He finds that his servant is knocking at the door. To D it appeared that the knocks began after he had woke up. But the servant had been knocking for a fairly long time before D was aroused.

In this dream the door plays a major part but there is no one *knocking* at a door.

In another dream D finds that he has got up from sleep. He looks at the alarm clock and discovers that it is about to ring. He feels very anxious to close down the alarm before it has begun to ring to save inconvenience to his companions who are sleeping nearby. He thinks over it again and again till he wakes up. Then he hears the alarm ringing. On examining the clock he learns that it has been ringing during his sleep, since it has now almost run down. Before going to bed he had wound up the alarm to its full capacity [p. 90].

Down through the ages, dreaming has puzzled mankind. The preceding discussion as well as the following one should suggest the possibility of dealing with dreaming within a stimulus-response framework the same as with other behaviors.

VI. A CONCRETE CASE FOR WOODWORTH'S HYPOTHESIS ON THE CAUSE OF DREAMS [7]

Euri Belle Bolton

A. THE PROBLEM. Woodworth has proposed a hypothesis on the cause of dreams which he has never had time to follow through with experimental or other controlled observational studies. In regard to it, he says:

I also was led by my readings and records to a hypothesis on the cause of dreams that I have often wished I had published, as it has a certain resemblance, along with a difference to Freud's conceptions which were published a few years later. Ives Delage had pointed out

[7] BOLTON, EURI BELLE. A concrete case for Woodworth's hypothesis on the cause of dreams. *J. Psychol.*, 1943, 16, 273-284. (Reproduced by permission of the publisher.)

that we do not dream of matters that fully occupy us during the day, but of something else. I thought I could see that we dreamed about matters that had been opened up but interrupted or checked during the day. Any desire or interest aroused during the day, but prevented from reaching its goal, was likely to recur in dreams and be brought to some sort of conclusion that was satisfactory in the dream, while the activities which had probably taken much more time were conspicuous by their absence from the dream. But the wishes "fulfilled" in the dream, according to my idea, were of any sort—sometimes mere curiosity—and the suppression of them which had occurred during the day might be the result of external interruption as well as of moral censorship.

He gives the following concrete example to support the hypothesis stated above:

In one case I dreamed of getting a clear view of the name on a street car that I had tried vainly to make out during the preceding day. Here we have a relatively superficial interest, though a genuine interest, since my curiosity had been aroused to know whither a certain line of cars led; and it is quite probable on the face of it that this unsatisfied curiosity caused the reappearance of the street car in the dream.

This view regards the dream as largely uncontrolled, free, associative thinking similar to imaginative activities of waking life. It agrees with the Freudian concept of dreams only in recognizing the wish-filling function of some dreams.

Freud advanced the following assumptions to explain dreams: (a) strong forces of suppressed tendencies find expression through the dream; (b) the relaxed influence of the censor during sleep makes the dream possible; (c) dreams are a compromise resulting from the conflict between the repressed unconscious forces of the id and conscious force of the super-ego; (d) dreams represent "latent content" or "dream thoughts" which have to be interpreted through the free associations of the dreamer and when these fail to reveal any "latent content," the dream must be interpreted by fixed symbols which represent wishes or urges of a sexual nature; (e) the dream is a hallucinatory experience and its function is to insure the continuity of sleep, and (f) dreams are a regression to primitive mechanisms. In regard to the last hypothesis, he says, ". . . on account of the same process of regression, ideas are turned into visual pictures in the dream; the latent dream thoughts are, that is to say, dramatized and illustrated."

Freud's explanation of dreams would not account for the dreams of writers which have been similar to their creative activity of waking life. A number of writers have, however, given introspective evidence that their dreams have been fruitful sources of inspiration for creative productions which have been perfected during waking life. Downey has summarized such evidence from a number of writers including Stevenson, Coleridge, Masefield, and Edward Lucas White. Woodworth, on the other hand, explains the two processes as essentially the same, though the thinking activity of the dream is less controlled than the creative thinking of waking life. He says:

Dreams follow the definition of imagination or invention, in that materials recalled from different contexts are put together into combinations and rearrangements never before experienced. The combinations are often bizarre and incongruous.

B. DESCRIPTION OF THE DREAM AND A BRIEF ANALYSIS OF ITS CAUSES. On the morning of January 28, 1942, I was awakened just before the usual time for getting up by a very vivid dream. I was walking down a street of a city, no part of which I recognized, when I suddenly saw a young girl who had a fair complexion and blond hair walking toward me on the opposite side of the street. She was arguing with a Japanese soldier who was dressed in the uniform of his own country, and was trying to persuade him to give her a small closed box which he carried. He suddenly challenged her to race with him in climbing to the top of a telephone pole which stood on the same side of the street on which I was walking. The girl accepted the challenge, but after they had climbed for only a short time, she said something to the soldier and he handed the box to her. She climbed for a moment very rapidly, then threw the box back across the street, climbed down the pole, and outran the Japanese to get it. She refused to return it because she thought it contained important papers of the government of the United States. The Japanese soldier became very angry. Up to this point I had heard no words spoken, but the meaning seemed clear from their actions. I then heard the soldier say in English that she had deceived him and had not played fair. She replied that she would have attempted to climb to the top of the pole if there had been a nurse near to help her in case of an accident.

Just at that moment an American soldier in khaki uniform came up. His uniform looked like that of the Marines, but it could have been that of the regular Army. I do not remember the details very well except that he wore a helmet and carried a rifle. I did not hear what he said at first, but he seemed to be reproving the Japanese soldier for violating international law. Then using his rifle held in both hands as a baton he began singing. The first words I heard were: "We always fight in the open." Then I missed a good deal and heard the conclusion of the song:

> "Rah, rah; rah, rah; rah, rah; rah, rah;
> We'll get them yet; we'll get them yet;
> We'll get them at Singapore."

After the last line I waked suddenly.

The events of the preceding day and of those immediately before which seem to have been influential in causing the dream will be given briefly. The annual Institute of Human Relations was being held at the college. I was working under pressure in order to attend as many of the programs of the Institute as possible. When I went home to lunch Mrs. X, with whom I live, told me of the news broadcasts she had heard that morning. One was that it seemed as if Singapore would soon be lost, and another was that some Japanese soldiers had been discovered tapping wires to get military secrets from our government, but that the F.B.I. was not permitted to tap wires generally in order to discover saboteurs. She was somewhat concerned over Singapore and thought that our government was making a mistake in regard to wire tapping. I wanted very much to say that if we lost Singapore, we would win it back and that we could win the victory over the Axis nations without adopting any of the Nazi unethical methods, but because of a lack of time for a discussion of the problems, I stood several minutes without making the comment in spite of a very strong desire to do so.

The work of the afternoon and attendance at the evening lecture caused the above incident and the war news to be forgotten. I had read a few days before a newspaper story of the passage by Congress of the bill which permitted the organization of the WACS for service in the army, but the story stated that the officials of the Navy had refused to permit women to enter this division of military service because they feared that women could not live up to its high standards of integrity. I had been quite surprised at such a view about women and thought that because they are as intelligent as men, they could, with training, become as clever as men in discovering the military secrets of the enemy or in guarding our own. I had in one of my classes a student who was preparing to enter a school of nursing. I had a few days before the dream occurred shown her a letter from a school of nursing urging that more students enter this profession in order to meet the war demand for nurses. There was a war poster on the bulletin board by the door of one of the classrooms in which I was teaching on which there was a picture of an American soldier wearing the uniform of the regular Army; he wore a helmet and carried a rifle. I had a number of times noticed small boys commenting about a similar poster, urging young men to enlist in the Marines, which was for some time exhibited in front of the local post office.

The memories left behind by the above situations seem to have been organized into the pattern of a dream which was evidently the result of the checking of the strong desire to comment on the news broadcasts which were discussed by Mrs. X. This seems to be a concrete case which supports the theory of dreams which Woodworth has suggested.

The writer has a strong attitude of interest in the improvement of vocational and civic opportunities for women. Because of this attitude, the newspaper story referred to above aroused a desire to see some opposition to the view of the Navy officials in regard to women being permitted to serve in the Navy. The desire had been aroused each time a paper had been read after the first reading of the news story, but had reached no satisfactory solution at the time of the dream. The incongruous encounter of the girl with the Japanese soldier was evidently a visualization of the thought that women could meet the difficult situations of dealing with enemies and it was influenced by the memory of the broadcast about wire tapping. In his explanation of intelligence as a mechanism, Peterson says, ". . . the effects of stimuli persist for a time—often for long periods—and enable the organism to suspend action and respond with more organic completeness to the general consistency of the situation, both inner and outer." G. W. Allport has pointed out that attitudes have a directive effect on the thinking and activities of the individual during waking life. To the extent that dreams approach the coherence characteristic of the creative thinking of waking life, it would seem that they would also be influenced by persisting attitudes.

Dorcus and Shaffer, who accept Dunlap's theory that dreams may produce integrative results that vary from those of a very low degree of directed association to those which approach the coherence and connectedness of waking life, think that dreams must be interpreted not only in terms of the problems and everyday experiences of the one who dreams, but also in terms of his personality. These concepts of the behavior of the organism which explain dreams by the same principles of stimulus-response adjustments characteristic of waking life are more fruitful for scientific analysis of dreams than the Freudian hypothesis that they represent "latent thought content" of the unconscious which must be interpreted by means of universal symbols. The experimental studies of dreams in response to controlled external stimuli are not reviewed here. The incongruous dreams of this type are undoubtedly examples of incomplete or inaccurate perception due to the low level of integration at which associative thinking is taking place.

There are two important problems of the thinking activity involved in the type of dreams resulting from an incompleted activity which have not been studied experimentally. The first is why should an activity that has been aroused during the day but has not been carried through to a satisfactory conclusion recur again in dreams. The second is why does visualization in terms of dramatic action occur in dreams and why does such action have meaning to the individual without a verbal interpretation of those actions. There are, however, experimental results from studies of other problems which seem to have value in explaining these processes involved in dreams.

Lanier has recently shown that "mixed" judgments of affectivity in response to stimulus words are accompanied by higher galvanic skin responses than stimulus words that arouse unequivocal effects of pleasantness, unpleasantness, or indifference. A preliminary study also indicates that—"Those words which elicit a relatively high skin resistance change tend to be remembered better than other words." He says that the galvanic skin responses may be an index to a degree of organic tension as Landis and Hunt have suggested, and if this is true it indicates that the heightened level of tension accompanying the reaction to certain words increased their memory value. It is also possible that activities begun but left in an unsatisfactory state of incompletion arouse heightened organic tension and this gives them greater intensity value in directing the associative recall of dreams than those activities that have reached a satisfactory conclusion. Two of Lewin's students, Ovsiankina and Zeigarnik, have shown experimentally that if tasks are interrupted before completion, they tend to perseverate or create what Lewin calls "tension systems" which drive toward discharge through a resumption of the interrupted activities. Zeigarnik found that the interrupted activities are better remembered than similar activities that have been carried through to completion.

Hollingworth, who on the basis of his concept of redintegration in thinking activity gives a descriptive account of dreams, says that the tendency of incompleted activities to recur in dreams is due to their greater tendency to perseveration than that resulting from activities that are carried through to completion. His criticism of the Freudian concept of suppression is given in the following statement:

Such indications also suggest that the doctrine of suppression which is so emphatic a part of the Freudian account is for the most part superfluous. It is not the *suppressed* but the *unexpressed* that is likely to be involved in the dream. It is not uncommon for the "wish" involved to be one not yet clearly formulated, articulated or verbally or otherwise reported or identified. It is this lack which constitutes its incompleteness. . . . In the dreams of sleep, as in the day dreams of waking leisure, it is the established patterns of thought, the insistent tendencies, and specially the uncompleted or unfulfilled and hence perseverative processes that lie in the most active condition of readiness. It is these processes that are most readily excited by stimuli from the outside world; by stimuli originating within the organism, and by other neural patterns that have elements in common with them.[8]

The experimental results of the studies of Lanier and of Ovsiankina and Zeigarnik suggest that the perseverative nature of unfinished activities referred to by Hollingworth is due to the affective conflict resulting from the thought processes at the time experienced.

The second problem of visualization or imagery in dreams is explained by Freud as the return of the individual in sleep to a primitive mode of thinking. He says that the interpretation of the meaning of dreams without words is similar to all of the thinking of primitive man before he developed language. Hollingworth says that dreams are experienced in a state of drowsiness which is a condition of "dissociation" intermediate between deep sleep and the controlled thinking of the waking state. He accounts for imagery in dreams as due to the substitution or confusion of cues or symbols. Of this phenomenon, he says,

At one moment an object, person, or situation is represented by one symbol, perhaps words spoken; the next moment words lapse and images take their place; in turn, imagery is abandoned and perhaps some current sensory process, such as the noise of machinery, the beat of the engine through the timbers of a ship, become the symbol to which is attached the meaning.

He, like Woodworth, thinks that dream activities are similar to the imaginative activities of waking life and that poets and novelists

---

[8] We prefer to speak here in terms of reactions to absent stimulus objects via a substitute stimulus. How could a stimulus arise spontaneously from within? Within what?

who do descriptive writing when in a state of slight drowsiness or fatigue are likely to use more symbolization in the forms of metaphors and similes than when they write in a very alert state of thinking [pp. 273–280].

VII. IMPLICIT BEHAVIOR AND PROBLEM SOLVING [9]
Karl Duncker

Even though the following experiment might well be used to exemplify the influence of past behavior on perception, such as the factors usually discussed under "set," it best illustrates the judging of objects in relation to others and the testing of hypotheses found in problem-solving behavior.

Certainly, the uses to which objects will be put depends upon how these or similar objects have been employed in the past. Thus, the possibility of a particular object acquiring a variety of stimulus functions may be seriously hampered if that object has acquired a relatively fixed value for an individual. Duncker's experiments show this hampering or restricting effect. For instance, he finds that first using a pair of pliers for a conventional purpose of twisting nails seriously interferes with the possibility of using them in some novel situations.

This experiment also illustrates the role of implicit behavior in problem solving. Hypotheses may be tested as presolutions, and answers found without overt manipulation of objects. In this sort of "manipulation," the subject is responding implicitly to the objects before him as if they were interrelated in different ways. Notice that although some problem solving may be implicit, not all is of this sort. For example, trial-and-error problem solving is not.

How an object is "thought about" or implicitly reacted to is determined by many variables in the total situation. Among others, is the *fixedness* of the object. If an object is needed and sought for, it is not likely to be reacted to if it is *fixed*. For example, a chimp in need of a stick as a tool is not so likely to perceive a tree branch in this relationship as it would a detached branch leaning against a tree or lying on the ground. Of course, a human or chimp who

---

[9] DUNCKER, KARL. On problem solving (tr. LEES, LYNNE S.). *Psychol. Monogr.*, 1945, 58, No. 270. (Reproduced by permission of the American Psychological Association.)

had reacted in past situations by tearing off a branch from a tree
would be capable of such performance in subsequent situations.

On the tree it is a "branch," a part of the visual figural unit "tree,"
and this part character—more generally, this "fixedness"—is clearly
responsible for the fact that to a search for something like a stick, the
branch on the tree is less "within reach" than the branch on the
ground [p. 85].

An object may also fail to function in a needed way if it has
recently functioned in some other way. For instance, a stick that
has just been used as a ruler is less likely to come into use as a tool
for other very different purposes, e.g., a stick to hold a window
up or to use as a back-scratcher. Duncker refers to this condition
as "functional fixedness." It might be restated this way: An object is needed for a certain purpose, a certain function. What
effect will its previous usage in a totally different situation have
upon its role in a subsequent behavioral situation? Duncker would
not distinguish between objects or tools actually manipulated and
objects "thought about" or those reacted to implicitly or at a distance.

EXPERIMENTAL PROCEDURE.   Objects in daily use (boxes, pliers,
and so on) were selected for the experiment. The subjects used
these in their accustomed way first and were later required to select
them from a confused array of objects on a table but for a very
different usage.

Each problem was given in two settings; (1) without preutilization of the crucial object and (2) once after its utilization in a
certain fashion. Two groups of subjects were used. One half of
them were presented with the problems in the order (1) without
preutilization, (2) after preutilization, (3) without preutilization,
(4) after preutilization, and (5) without preutilization. The other
half of the subjects were presented with the problems in the opposite settings. In this way, the order of settings as well as the order
of the problems was made independent of individual differences
among the subjects.

THE PROBLEMS

The following is a short description of the five problems and of the
experimental technique.

THE "GIMLET PROBLEM."   Three cords are to be hung side by side from a wooden ledge ("for experiments on space perception"). On the table lie, among many other objects, two short screw-hooks and the crucial object; a gimlet. *Solution:* for hanging the third cord, the gimlet is used. In the setting a.p., the holes for the screws had yet to be bored; in w.p., the holes were already there. Thus, F_1 (Function 1): "gimlet"; F_2 (Function 2): "thing from which to hang a cord."

THE "BOX PROBLEM." On the door, at the height of the eyes, three small candles are to be put side by side ("for visual experiments"). On the table lie, among many other objects, a few tacks and the crucial objects: three little pasteboard boxes (about the size of an ordinary matchbox, differing somewhat in form and color and put in different places). *Solution:* with a tack apiece, the three boxes are fastened to the door, each to serve as platform for a candle. In the setting a.p., the three boxes were filled with experimental material: in one there were several thin little candles, tacks in another, and matches in the third. In w.p., the three boxes were empty. Thus, F_1: "container"; F_2 "platform" (on which to set things).

THE "PLIERS PROBLEM." A board (perhaps 8 inches broad) is to be made firm on two supports (as "flower stand or the like"). On the table lie, among other things, two iron joints (for fastening bars and the like on stands), a wooden bar perhaps 8 inches long (as the one "support") and the crucial object, the pliers. *Solution:* this pair of pliers is utilized as the second support of the board. In the setting a.p., the bar was nailed to the board and had to be freed with the help of the pliers; in w.p., it was only tied to the board. Thus, F_1: "pliers"; F_2: "support."

THE "WEIGHT PROBLEM." A pendulum, consisting of a cord and a weight, is to be hung from a nail ("for experiments on motion"). To this end, the nail must be driven into the wall. On the table lies, among other things, the crucial object: a weight. *Solution:* with this weight (as "hammer"), the nail is driven into the wall. In the setting a.p., the weight is given expressly as pendulum weight (with the string already tied to it); in w.p., a joint serves as pendulum weight. Thus, F_1: "pendulum weight"; F_2: "hammer."

THE "PAPERCLIP PROBLEM." A piece of white cardboard with four black squares fastened to it is to be hung on an eyelet screwed into the low ceiling ("for visual experiments"). On the table lie paperclips, among other things. *Solution:* a paperclip is unbent, one end is fastened to the eyelet and the other put through the cardboard. In the setting a.p., the four black squares must previously be attached to the cardboard with paperclips; in w.p., on the other hand, they must be glued to it. Thus, F_1: "something for affixing"; F_2: (unbent) "hook."

The differences among the five problems are to be discussed later. The general instruction for all the problems ran as follows: "You will receive several little technical tasks. For solution, certain objects are needed which you will find among the objects here on the table. Everything which lies on the table is completely at your disposal. You may use what you like in any fashion you wish. Please think aloud during the experiment, so that I may hear as many of your ideas as possible, including those which you take less seriously."

With each problem there lay on the table—aside from the objects already mentioned—all kinds of material, partly less suitable and partly completely unsuitable for the solution, such as paperclips, pieces of paper, string, pencils, tinfoil, old parts of apparatus, ash-trays, joints, pieces of wood, etc. Each problem had its own inventory. (No object was put at the subject's disposal which might be better suited to the solution than the object then crucial.) The objects lay in apparent confusion, but in definite places. The crucial object never occupied a prominent place.

The experiments were *evaluated* in two ways: (1) the solved and unsolved problems were counted. Of course, a problem was counted as "correctly" solved only when it was solved by use of the crucial object, which, as stated, was always the best and simplest of the possible solutions. A problem was broken off as unsolved if for two to three minutes the S produced no more proposals, and if at the same time his attitude had become so negative that no more sensible ideas seemed forthcoming. (2) The proposals preceding the solution and different from it, the "pre-solutions," were counted (but only with those experiments in which the correct solution was finally found, as otherwise measurements 1 and 2 would not have been independent of each other). As "pre-solutions" counted not only those actually carried out, but also proposals merely formulated, also such as the S rejected as unsuitable [*sic*]. If, however, an object was only "grazed," i.e., just touched or picked up quite briefly and silently laid aside again, the fact did not count as a pre-solution.

Of the two methods of evaluation just described, the first is naturally the more adequate and by far the more important, while the second is rather superficial and dependent on chance influences. We shall find, however, that both methods yield results which are essentially in agreement.

PRINCIPAL EXPERIMENTS AND PRINCIPAL RESULTS

The principal result of the experiments is immediately evident from Table [15].

Table 15

Problems	Number of Subjects	Number of Problems Solved	Number of Problems solved (Per Cent)	Average Number of Presolutions per Problem
w.p. { Gimlet	10	10	100	0.3
Box	7	7	100	1.3
Pliers	15	15	100	1.9
Weight	12	12	100	0.8
Paper clip ..	7	6	85.7	0.8
Arithmetic mean ..	..	..	97.1	1.0
a.p. { Gimlet	14	10	71.4	1.6
Box	7	3	42.9	2.3
Pliers	9	4	44.4	2.3
Weight	12	9	75.0	0.8
Paper clip ..	7	4	57.1	1.5
Arithmetic mean ..	..	..	58.2	1.7

We see that the results of the a.p. (after preutilization) experiments clearly deviate from those of the w.p. (without preutilization) experiments in the expected direction. This holds in both measurements, which are independent of each other, and not only for the average of all five problems, but also within each single problem. Only in the weight problem are the two averages of pre-solutions equal.

Therefore, we can say: *Under our experimental conditions, the object which is not fixed is almost twice as easily found as the object which is fixed.*

The quantitative results were supported and clarified through qualitative findings. When, at the close of an a.p. (after preutilization) experiment, the S was asked: "Why have you not used this object" (the crucial one), or, "Why have you used it only so late?", the answer was frequently: "But that is a tool," or "Such a use would not be suited to the material," or "I thought it was there simply for . . . (F_1)" [pp. 85–88].

From the above results, we may conclude that the way an object is "thought about," evaluated, judged, or manipulated with relation to other objects is a function of how that object has previously been utilized or related to objects. Such previous usage has a hampering effect on some novel usage demanded of the person. It is as if the person were stimulus bound—not capable of freeing himself from his accustomed response to that object. It is our opinion that the creative individual in any field is the one who can free himself from such hampering effects as were here demonstrated. He is the one who puts objects into new relationships and ascribes to them new functions.

12

FEELINGS

I. THE RESPONSE SIDE OF AFFECTIVE OR FEELING INTERACTIONS
N. H. Pronko

Feeling "blue," depressed, resentful, anxious, angry, afraid, being in love, jealous, and so on, are only a few of the rich variety of affective reactions in which humans are involved. Not only are they important as reactions proper to objects that "move" us, but they occur concurrently as phases of such interactions as fighting, working, playing, eating, dancing, skating, waiting, and the like. In fact, we doubt if they are ever totally absent in the behavioral repertoire of organisms.

Some of these affective acts are quite apparent. This would be true of a "grief-stricken" individual. The person trembling from fear or perspiring freely, breathing rapidly or weeping is quite obviously "doing something." The difference between these activities and those called "effective" in contrast to them is that the latter involve the organism "doing something" with respect to some object or person such as picking something up or writing on paper with a pencil or striking keys as on a piano or typewriter. In affective interactions, the action is concentrated within the organism, although the preposition "within" is not to be misunderstood as implying an alleged "mind." While the examples listed above include gross or crude affective action, there are many subtle affective responses that are not so readily open to inspection. Anxieties and tensions furnish ready illustrations.

Inquiry into further details about affective interactions shows one prominent feature, namely the widespread involvement of the organism. Sweat glands, tear glands, adrenal glands, stomach, intestines, heart and lungs, and many other organs in a diversity of patterns participate in these interactions. The everyday phrase, "He (the organism) was greatly moved," is richly descriptive of the essential features of the activity centered on the organism's side of the picture. Effective interactions, in contrast, would be those which might be described as *"organism moves something,"* i.e., performs some movement with respect to something.[1]

Since the action in affective behavior is rather difficult to observe, its understanding has not progressed so far as has understanding of overt reactions such as key pressing. As a matter of fact, mysticism has held tenaciously to this department of psychology, with the result that these reactions have been thought of as "states," "mental states," "states of mind," and so forth. The primary reason for this state of affairs has been a traditional "body-mind" type of theory. Then, too, it has been easier for the man in the street to think of "action" when someone "pushes" or "pulls" something, and subtler forms of activity have usually gone by some other name.

It is our contention that affective behavior may be treated as concretely as any of the most overt acts. Let us assume that a human animal is born as transparent as a jellyfish. Imagine at what a disadvantage such an organism would be! By using a number of provocative stimuli, one could observe many dramatic shifts in its activity. Now the spleen muscles clamp down and push out a tremendous amount of reserve blood into the circulatory system. Such changes in the distribution of the blood supply effect blushing and paling. Increased or decreased lung action is immediately observable as our transparent animal becomes excited or calm and relaxed again. Provoke him again, and you can comment literally, "Your blood pressure is rising, old man!" At still another time the heart rate (pulse) is sharply and suddenly increased. Tear secretion and sweat-gland action occur. Stomach and intestinal contractions are speeded up or inhibited.

Our hypothetical animal could not have a single affective secret from us. Everything would be aboveboard and immediately observable. But humans are not transparent, and therein lies the crux of the matter. Just because they are not is no reason why we should become mystical and introduce "minds" into the picture

---

[1] While there may be behavioral events not readily classifiable into either of the above categories, the two opposed classes here employed serve to bring affective action into sharp focus.

to confuse us further. These visceral acts need not be considered as bodily changes either "accompanying" or "causing" feelings. The gland, skin, and visceral activities *are* the psychological responses of the organism! That's all there is; there is no more. It is in this fashion, among others, that the organism responds to stimulus objects.

These activities have been built up during his reactional biography just as his walking, talking, skills, and so on, have been acquired. It so happens that walking, talking, and skill reactions are performed with more or less discrete or integrated but *movable* portions of an animal's hands, arms, legs, and head. In affective reactions, *nonmovable* organs predominate. While it is possible for the arms to be stretched and moved so as to embrace the beloved, the heart (and other visceral organs) cannot do so because they are stationary. Because of the fixed position of the visceral organs, only very limited action is possible. Consequently, when the sentry sees an enemy, he shoots the gun with his hands and arms. His heart, lungs, and other visceral organs cannot manipulate the gun. It is true that the organism reacts to the sight of the enemy soldier with the viscera, but only insofar as they are anchored within the visceral region. These reactions are in terms of accelerated or inhibited normal action of the specific structures involved and constitute affective behavior when they occur in psychological events. The manipulation of the gun constitutes the effective class of response.

One more point should be made regarding the diffuseness of the organismic action during affective behavior. The question might be put thus: How is it that the organism responds in the widespread, diffuse fashion observed in feeling events? Some light on the answer to this question comes from the diagram of the autonomic nervous system and its connection with the organs and systems that we have been discussing. The reader will note how heart, liver, stomach, adrenal glands, and so on, are interconnected by this network of nerves. When the uninitiated public speaker reacts to his audience in the affective way commonly called "stage fright," his sweat glands, heart, and salivary glands are active in certain ways. The first two systems show more rapid action, while the salivary glands show an inhibition of salivary secretion. For this reason, the speaker may pour himself a glass of water from the pitcher traditionally placed before him.

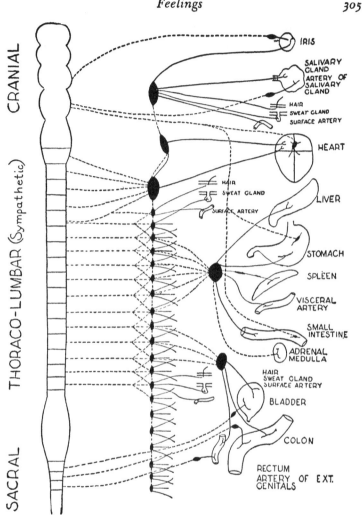

FIG. 41 Significance of the interconnection of the visceral organs. Since the variety of organs is intimately connected via the autonomic nervous system there is little wonder that they can all "fire off" in unison in the widespread action apparent in affective behavior. Thus, increased heart, lung, adrenal, tear, and skin gland action can occur simultaneously in a variety of patterns.

The important point concerns the reason for the involvement of these widespread organismic portions. Undoubtedly, it is because they are connected with each other that these organs participate in a particular coordinated activity. In a sense, it is correct to say that the heart is connected with the tear glands, with the surface arteries, with the spleen, and so on. The total action, involving as it does widely separated organs, is made possible as a result of the intricate connections between those parts. The specific coordination of visceral action occurring in the case of any particular individual can only be understood in terms of what configuration of action occurred in his early conditioning. Only in this way can we know why one person blushes while another shows cessation of stomach action, and so on. Finally, even though organisms are not transparent, affective interactions can be studied by such instrumental techniques as lie detection and fluoroscopic observations. Perhaps twentieth-century psychology will put an end to the "mental-states" treatment heretofore accorded affective interactions and will handle them as naturalistically and concretely as it has handled conditioned reflexes.[2]

One final point: Many workers have used the terms "feelings" and "emotions" synonymously. We have preferred to follow sound semantic principles and have used these two terms for rather different behaviors. The term "feelings" will be used to designate the behavior described above, while the term "emotion" will be used as a label for disrupted or disorganized behaviors as treated in the next chapter. Since some textbooks talk about "feeling responses" when the use of the word "emotions" would be more apt, this word of caution is necessary. However, the student need not be confused, because the usage here is clearly designated and consistent.

II. ADOPTING PATTERNS OF ANXIETY

Striking resemblances in the temperamental characteristics of members of the same family are most often attributed to heredity. Here Cameron [3] shows the subtle process by which the child builds

---

[2] With instrumental techniques, we do no more than the physiologist does when he applies such methods to the study of nervous action, heart activity, or bone conditions with the aid of galvanometer, oscilloscopes, or X-ray photography. All are alike inapparent.

[3] CAMERON, NORMAN. *The psychology of behavior disorders.* Boston: Houghton Mifflin, 1947. Pp. 622. (Reproduced by permission of the author and the publisher.)

up anxieties through unwitting "modeling" by parents. It is only by ignoring the operation of such conditions that one can appeal to "heredity."

Anxious adults make anxious parents and help to create an atmosphere of uneasiness in the home. The child, long before he is able to identify or understand what is upsetting him, tends to react to the prevailing insecurity with his own anxiety reactions. Thus, adults who are continually starting, exclaiming, ducking, cringing or crying, when danger seems to threaten them, are likely to have children who do the same. Indeed domestic animals also develop anxieties in the presence of anxious adults, so that an habitually apprehensive master is likely to have an apprehensive horse or dog. Likewise the anxious attitudes, gestures and inflections of an adult in relation to darkness, fire, animals, lightning, sex, high places, hospitals, sin and a hundred other topics, favor the acquisition of corresponding behavior in the child who is exposed to these reactions. This was brought out dramatically in the 1940 London air raids when it was found that adult anxiety reactions were more effective anxiety excitants in children than the terrific barrage of noise, fire and destruction [pp. 266–267].

III. STOMACH ACTION IN STRONG FEELINGS

In recent years, it has been shown that duodenal ulcers can be produced in laboratory and domestic animals by several means. One is continually to stimulate the production of acid secretion into the stomach by administering histamine. Another way is to stimulate continually the vagus nerve in dogs. Both of these methods utilize physiological techniques.

Although these artificial methods can produce ulcers, they are not factors ordinarily operating in humans in the production of ulcers. Previous experimental work on humans has shown that sometimes gastric function seems to increase as a result of certain feeling-arousing stimuli, and sometimes it seems to decrease. Studies of patients having stomach ulcers indicate that many of them have been subject to protracted emotional upsets involving conflict, anxiety, guilt, hostility, and resentment. These situations must be studied in a historical way involving organisms and stimulus objects and the manner in which they affect each other.

Wolf and Wolff [4] had the opportunity to study a 56-year-old man who, in early childhood, had suffered an accident which had occluded his esophagus. Since that time he had been forced to feed himself through a gastric fistula (artificial opening in the stomach). The opening had formed a collar of tissue around it essentially similar to that of the stomach cavity itself. Thus, it was possible to take samples of acidity directly from the stomach and to observe changes in the coloring of the gastric mucosa. The latter is an indication of change in blood flow. Also the observers occasionally took records of stomach contractions by means of the balloon-inflation technique.

The subject was in excellent health with no chronic stomach complaints. He was employed in the medical laboratory where the experiment was conducted and was described as shy, sensitive, proud, stubborn, and slightly suspicious. He was physically small, had little schooling, was married, and had one child. He was considered to be fun-loving but conscientious.

The subject's stomach was examined over a period of time, and the experimenter attempted each time to estimate his feeling and other reaction patterns in such terms as contentment, joy, gratitude, dejection, fear, guilt, anxiety, and the like. It was recognized that these were not clear-cut "states," but it seemed possible to recognize the dominant mood or feeling at any time. No attempt was made artificially to create emotion or feeling responses in the subject, but several incidents occurred in the laboratory and the man's home life which made it possible to observe stomach acidity, activity, and vascularity during several kinds of feeling interactions.

GASTRIC CONDITIONS DURING RELAXATION AND WELL-BEING. Stomach contractions were usually low in amplitude and rhythmic, with a frequency of about three per minute. Color value of mucosa was at point 50 on a stomach color scale calibrated by Munsell's method. Hydrochloric acid output per hour was around 3 to 5 cubic centimeters of 0.166 normal hydrochloric acid. A close correlation was noted between hyperemia and acid production.

GASTRIC CONDITION DURING FEAR AND SADNESS. The subject experienced fear one morning when an angry doctor came in look-

---

[4] WOLF, S. & WOLFF, H. G. Evidence on the genesis of peptic ulcer in man. *J. Amer. med. Ass.*, 1942, 120, 670–675.

ing for a record which had been misplaced (or possibly lost) by the subject, who was lying motionless and pale on the laboratory table during the episode. During this time the gastric mucosa also became pallid, and acid production fell. When the paper was found, the stomach promptly returned to normal. A similar expression of stomach function was also noted during sadness.

GASTRIC CONDITION DURING ANXIETY, HOSTILITY, AND RESENTMENT. Later, another incident occurred in the laboratory which enabled the experimenter to note changes during anxiety, hostility, and resentment. The subject had been working on an extra job after hours for one of the staff members. This doctor had complained that the man was slow and inefficient, and on this morning came to tell the subject that he would not need him any more. The patient responded quietly, but his stomach was quickly red and engorged with blood, and the stomach folds became thick and turgid. Acid production jumped up sharply, and vigorous stomach contractions started.

The experimenter reported such changes frequently during hostility and resentment. It was found that it was easy to create small hemorrhage points in the stomach wall during such conditions.

A slight stroking with dry gauze could result in small erosions and bleeding points. Sometimes stomach contractions themselves produced such bleeding points. Ordinarily, these points are quickly covered with mucus and heal within 1 day. But the experimenters were able to demonstrate that, if the protective functions of the mucus do not operate efficiently, then a small erosion in the stomach lining would enlarge into a lesion having the usual appearance of a stomach ulcer. This seemed to result from the continual action of gastric juice on the unprotected erosion point. When this was covered over with petrolatum, it soon disappeared completely.

The accompanying figures show the variation in color of the mucosa and of acid secretion for different feeling reactions of the subject. Especially noteworthy here is the correspondence between stomach conditions and types of feeling reactions, and in D, the prolonged hyperfunction of the stomach while the subject was enduring sustained anxiety.

The authors conclude:

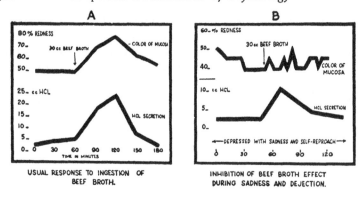

USUAL RESPONSE TO INGESTION OF
BEEF BROTH.

INHIBITION OF BEEF BROTH EFFECT
DURING SADNESS AND DEJECTION.

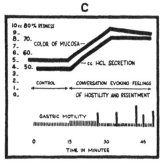
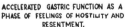
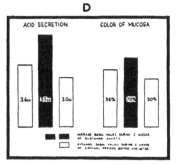

ACCELERATED GASTRIC FUNCTION AS A
PHASE OF FEELINGS OF HOSTILITY AND
RESENTMENT.

PROLONGED GASTRIC HYPERFUNCTION ACCOM-
PANYING SUSTAINED ANXIETY FOR TWO WEEKS.

FIG. 42 Showing gastric motility acid secretion and color of stomach mucosa as participating factors in affective reactions. B and C show that they are not the same in sadness and in hostile responses. (Wolf, S. & Wolff, H. G. Evidence on the genesis of peptic ulcer in man.)

The reason why our patient has not acquired peptic ulcer may be that the hyperemia and hypersecretion which we have observed in the presence of conflict have been relatively transitory. He is not the sort of person who harbors grudges or maintains emotional stress for prolonged periods. Usually he expressed his feelings either in words or in action, and his more serious conflicts were relatively short lived. Since the occurrence of gastric hyperfunction in certain emotional settings has been demonstrated, however, and since the destructive power of excess gastric secretion has been established, one may infer that these emotionally charged situations are involved directly in the genesis of peptic ulcer in man [p. 675].

IV. ASTHMA AS A REACTION TO
A LIFE SITUATION

N. H. Pronko

There is no doubt that living organisms, each with an individual biochemical make-up, show a differential sensitivity of their tissues to a variety of substances. Dust, ragweed, kapok, cottonseed, feathers, and timothy are six substances that commonly cause such allergic reactions. On the other hand, Sunday-supplement sections have publicized what they have called a "psychosomatic" basis for asthma. These somewhat spooky accounts are in terms of a "mind" affecting a "body." It is our purpose to throw light on the possibility of an asthmatic reaction performed to life situations involving frustration, insecurity, hatred, and other "emotional" circumstances but without reference to a "mind-body" framework.

Our discussion to this point implies that there are two kinds of phenomena, physiological and psychological, that may be labeled as "asthmatic" reactions. The first may be handled as a response of the respiratory tract of an organism, which may be understood completely in terms of the peculiar biochemical make-up of the tissues of that system and of the chemical make-up of the irritating substance. Modify or control one or the other of these two variables, and you modify or control the reaction. This discussion is based on the following article: [5]

However, not all cases of asthma fit such a description, for there are individuals with asthma in whom no specific sensitivity to such extrinsic factors as inhalants can be demonstrated. Others, in whom skin sensitivity exists, do not always have symptoms when the test substances are inhaled. On the other hand, symptoms may be present under circumstances in which there is no exposure to them. Considerable evidence has accumulated indicating that psychobiologic factors are of great importance in the production and propagation of symptoms of asthma [p. 380].

Obviously, these cases are not to be understood in the same way as those discussed above.

---

[5] TREUTING, THEODORE F. & RIPLEY, HERBERT S. Life situations, emotions and bronchial asthma. *J. nerv. ment. Dis.*, 1948, 108, 380–398. (Reproduced by permission of the authors and the publisher.)

Although as long ago as 1926 some investigators suspected a possible psychological basis for asthma, it was not until comparatively recently that McDermott and Cobb showed the presence of "emotional factors" in 37 out of a series of 50 unselected cases.

In the study reported here, Treuting and Ripley made a medical and psychological study of 51 patients, 28 of whom showed positive reactions to one or more of the six common allergy-inducing substances mentioned earlier. Subjects showed the characteristic wheezes, rattles, and "snoring" noises found in asthmatics. Of the 51 patients, only 2 showed asthmatic reactions when they were exposed to the substance to which their skin had reacted positively. In 30 cases, there was no such connection apparent, while in 19 cases, no information was available on this point. Study of a possible relationship between asthma and the season of the year showed seasonal variation in 5 cases, probable relation in 7, and unknown in 2 while the other 37 patients had asthma without relation to the season of the year.

With emotional reactions the opposite was true. In 36 cases symptoms occurred in certain situations and following certain emotional reactions on the part of the patient. The situations usually involved other members of the family or some aspect of the patient's work. In 12 cases there was no apparent correlation between the symptoms and emotional factors; and in one case, there was no available information, since the patient flatly refused to discuss her problem [p. 381].

ASTHMA AND IMMATURE PERSONALITY

Thirteen patients were studied thoroughly during an interview following injection of sodium amytal which was given to relax the individual for more careful personality study or in an attempt to abolish or relieve an attack of asthma. In general, these people showed an immature personality; they were moody (depressed), egocentric, anxious for prestige and praise, tense, insecure, unable to share with others, overdependent on others, unable to assume responsibility, quarrelsome, troubled with guilt feelings, sexually maladjusted, and so on.

One patient developed asthma in the Army at a time when he was just about to be sent overseas. Another patient had an attack at the time of his marriage after the war; he had not had asthma during the war. However, when he was about to be sent to a school for training in Military Government which would have meant overseas duty, he had such a severe outbreak of asthma that hospitalization and cancellation of orders were necessary. Still another patient showed an outburst of asthma when he was having trouble with his studies. As his problems were solved, his asthma improved, as did his marital situation. The histories of several patients showed relationships to outbursts of feelings of jealousy, as in the case of the birth of another child in the family of one patient. In another, such attacks occurred during the birthday celebrations for an older brother in the family and during the family's preoccupation with the latter's admission to college. One patient dated the beginning of her asthma to the occurrence of a fire which burned her house down. A male patient of 23 years suffered a first attack when his father died and it became necessary for him to give up his plans to prepare for the law. This patient wheezed when his father's death was discussed. Quarrels were also factors in precipitating asthmatic attacks.

An Analysis of Two Cases

The following two cases, given in greater detail and with an accompanying graphic representation, show a definite relationship between the patients' asthma and certain specific life situations of a different order than "tissue irritants."

A 24-year-old housewife complained of attacks of wheezing with dyspnea, which began when she was a child of two, but had only become troublesome in the previous two and a half years. She was the youngest of 5 children, of parents of Italian descent and Roman Catholic religion. She had always been extremely close to her mother, who was oversolicitous.

As a girl, she had always "loved night clubs and excitement." She began to go out often with young men when she was 17, and fell in love regularly. As soon as the courtship grew serious, however, she would find herself unable to decide to marry her suitor.

Two and a half years before she sought treatment, she became pregnant, while still unmarried, and had an abortion performed at two months. The incapacitating attacks of asthma began at that time. She benefited by the opportunity to talk these things over with a sympathetic listener, and her symptoms improved.

Two years later she was admitted to the hospital with asthma, a few weeks after her marriage. She had entered into matrimony after

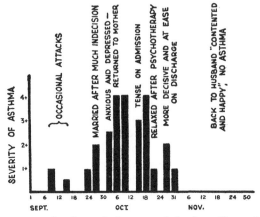

FIG. 43   Occurrence of asthma during a period of conflict and indecision, associated with mounting tension and anxiety. With resolution of the problem and attendant feelings of contentment, symptoms subsided. (Treuting, Theodore F., & Ripley, Herbert S., Life situations, emotions and bronchial asthma.)

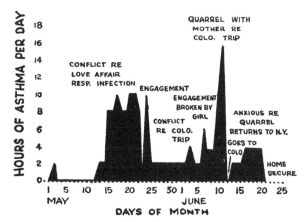

FIG. 44   Asthma associated with attempt to leave home and establish independence. Symptoms improved upon return to home and mother. (Treuting, Theodore F., & Ripley, Herbert S., Life situations, emotions and bronchial asthma.)

the usual amount of indecision, spent the week-end with her husband, and developed severe asthma. She returned to her mother and he, to his. When seen, she was depressed and anxious. She had found it especially hard to leave her mother, on whom she had been very dependent, and had difficulty getting accustomed to marriage and making plans for her own establishment. While in the hospital, she decided to return to her husband, and did so, feeling happy and content and without symptoms [Figure 43, pp. 383–384].

This woman illustrates the overdependence which was seen almost invariably, and the inability to establish independence and adult self-sufficiency. She further illustrates the characteristic indecisiveness and the difficulty of making a satisfactory sexual adjustment.

A 21-year-old hospital employee had had asthma since the age of two years. He was the only child of American-born parents of German-Czechoslovakian extraction. His father, now dead, was an alcoholic, violent when drunk, who paid little attention to his son at other times. His mother was a suspicious, complaining woman, who reminded her son constantly of his obligation to look after her, and also blamed him and his illness for the death of her husband.

The patient had one six-month period, three years earlier, during which he was entirely free from symptoms. He had been ill in bed with asthma, and had risen to investigate the sounds of commotion in the kitchen. There he discovered that his father had died very suddenly. He was shocked by this event, and his wheezing disappeared entirely. Because his asthma had left him, he enlisted in the Navy, but after being away from home for a few months, he began to worry about his mother, and about being away from her. His symptoms returned, and he was discharged.

About two years later, he made another abortive attempt to establish his independence. After much indecision, he decided to become engaged to the young woman with whom he had been going out, and also decided to travel to Colorado, perhaps to live. After a week, the girl broke the engagement, but he was still resolved to take the trip, at any event. He had a violent quarrel with his mother, on the eve of his departure, in which she charged him with deserting her, among other things. At this time his symptoms of asthma were of 4-plus intensity, and he left for Colorado in this setting. Once on the train, his asthma disappeared, but shortly after his arrival, he began to worry about his mother, developed more symptoms, and decided to return home. His asthma subsided as soon as he arrived there [Fig. 44].

More recently, after much conflict, he decided to continue his education at an out-of-town college. This time he seems to have established more independence, and has been away for one year with little difficulty.

Again, the great dependency of these individuals is illustrated. Making a decision seemed to help. The patient's immaturity and tendency to make decisions and plans which were not well thought out are also evident. Symptoms developed at an early age, and undoubtedly served to bring him some attention which he would not otherwise have received from his rejecting parents [pp. 383–384].

ASTHMA AND ALLERGY

Five patients who displayed a 2- to 4-plus sensitivity to various pollen extracts were exposed to the appropriate pollen, in a concentration of 50 to 100 grains per square centimeter, by inhalation during interviews. This was a quantity sufficient to produce symptoms. The pollen was circulated in the room by a fan and without the knowledge of the patient. Although in each case there had been a history, in the beginning, either of purely seasonal asthma, or of exacerbation of attacks during the pollen season, in no instance did asthma develop under these conditions. There were numerous instances, however, in which, during a routine interview, sometimes for so ordinary a purpose as taking a history, patients who entered the room breathing quietly began to wheeze when their life problems were first touched upon.

This same procedure has been carried out with nose reactors— patients with vasomotor rhinitis. In one case, who displayed a 3-plus skin sensitivity to ragweed pollen extract, exposure to the pollen resulted promptly in both objective and subjective evidence of increased nasal congestion and secretion. At the time of this experiment, the patient was depressed and worried, and felt hopeless about her situation, since all of her problems seemed to have assumed overwhelming proportions. When the experiment with the pollen was repeated subsequently, there was no response from her nasal mucous membranes. This time, some of her problems had been resolved and she felt more secure and hopeful about the future [p. 391].

SUMMARY

In the present series of unselected cases, it has been evident that the development of asthmatic attacks has been related to the patient's life situations and accompanying emotional reactions. Some of the patients have had positive skin reactions, some have not. In general, it has been felt that there was little, if any, correlation between the specific attacks of asthma, during the period of observation of these patients, and the reaction of the skin. Five patients who were skin-sensitive to pollen extracts were exposed to the pollen by inhalation during the interviews. Although in each case there was either a history, originally, of purely seasonal asthma, or of exacerbation of attacks during the pollen seasons, in no instance did asthma develop under these conditions; however, on numerous occasions during the course of an ordinary interview for the purpose of obtaining a history, patients who came in breathing quietly began to wheeze and developed the physical findings of the typical asthmatic attack [p. 394].

COMMENT. Traditionally, the cause for asthma has been sought exclusively in some substance which, when brought in contact with an organism's tissues, elicited exaggerated muscular or secretory activity of the portion concerned. Undoubtedly, asthma may occur on such a basis, in which case it may be understood as a physiological event. However, not all of the cases described above were of this sort. As a matter of fact, we may assert that in most cases such factors could be ruled out. While, perhaps, there were instances in which there may have been an initial history of a physiological asthma, this reaction, once available, came to be performed on a basis which is definitely psychological. In the latter case, the reaction called asthma is performed to a stimulus situation that is specific to each of the individuals concerned. A historical basis for the relationship of the organism and the particular stimulus object or situation involved becomes apparent. The "tissue-irritation" theory does not apply, for these are responses that illustrate the adjectives typical of behavioral events. Here we find demonstrated differentiation, integration, variability, modifiability, delayability, and inhibition. That is to say, the asthma that occurs is specific for each individual on a historical basis—a troublesome daughter, difficult domestic conditions, marital difficulties, and so forth. Not everyone, but the specific individual studied, reacts in this manner. Nor do all the stimuli that surround the person involved affect him this way. Furthermore, they are integrated into his other behavior. They do show variable features. They can be changed and even "cured" (i.e., modified or reacted to with a substitute response). They are also capable of various degrees of inhibition or delay, and, finally, they can be elicited without inserting pollen on sensitized nasal and other respiratory tissues.

In our opinion, the asthmatic reactions included under the

psychological order of events discussed here are accurately described as affective or feeling interactions. Whereas other individuals weep, get angry, blush, perspire, "skip a beat" or "catch their breath" when they are *affected,* the persons discussed here show a behavioral configuration that takes the particular pattern described and which *resembles* the kind of reaction that may occur on a purely physiological level. There is no need for "body-mind" dichotomies; merely a description of the variables involved and a specification of the historical or lack of historical features of such events suffices.

V. SUBSTITUTE STIMULI AND CRIME DETECTION
N. H. Pronko

Each of three volunteer students from an experimental psychology class is handed a plain sealed envelope prepared by the instructor but shuffled and distributed by another student. Two contain sets of instructions for going to separate rooms to read magazines found there. The third person has drawn directions for committing a "crime." No one in the class knows which student got which envelope.

Obviously, the student cannot be asked to perform acts that are immoral, unethical, or illegal. Yet, if the experiment is to be successful, we must get him to perform affective behavior *during* the crime. We must "get a rise" out of him in that situation.

Previous to the experiment, we secured a dead and smelly pigeon (found on the campus), a slightly decayed chicken head from a poultry house, ether, dissecting scissors, and a description of the shocking sexual customs of savages.

The third subject, whose identity is unknown to us, is to work with these materials. He must go to a certain office and, according to instructions which he found in his envelope, he must cut out the tongue from the chicken's head and apply a drop of ether to the "wound." Following that, he stands on a chair and puts his hand into a box located on a high shelf, pulling out the decaying bird and discarding it in the wastebasket. He next settles down in a chair and reads about harvest customs (pertaining to sexuality) of Melanesians. Most students react with some degree of affective response in the situation which we have contrived.

At a certain time, all three students come back to a specified place and await individual "cross examination," during which time they are held "incommunicado." They are successively put on the "witness stand" where each is connected with impressive-looking apparatus as he sits behind a brilliantly lighted one-way-vision screen permitting the "jury" to see him but not vice versa.

Each then submits to the following procedure. A pneumograph is attached around the chest. This is an elastic rubber tube with a coiled spring inside that permits contraction and expansion of the tube. Closed at one side, the other end leads off via small tubing to a diaphragm. On the diaphragm rests a pen which, when adjusted to a smoked-paper kymograph, will yield a tracing of the pressure changes in the enclosed air column. The breathing records can then be analyzed with respect to the series of stimuli presented each subject.

In addition to the respiratory components of affective reactions, we arrange a sphygmograph to give us a record of the rate and form of the pulse. A sphygmomanometer, the device that the physician employs for obtaining blood pressure, may also be contrived to record the variations that occur. It would also be possible to enclose a leg or an arm in a cylinder containing water. By means of rubber tubing, a small opening at one end could be connected with another writing pen. Large shifts of blood volume from the viscera to limbs and back again would thus cause a rise and fall of the writing pen and give an indication of what was occurring in this constituent part of the affective response. Incidentally, this apparatus is known as a "plethysmograph."

Perhaps more important than the last instrument is the galvanometer which measures the galvanic skin response. We connect our subject to this apparatus by means of two electrodes, one taped to the palm of each hand. An imperceptible current then passes through the circuit of which the organism is a part. It so happens that when the sweat glands of the skin are active (not necessarily perspiring though), they show a decrease in resistance to the tiny current impressed upon the subject. These increases and decreases can then be amplified and studied in relation to the stimuli presented to the subject.[6]

---

[6] There is no need to be mystified by the electrical activity of the skin any more than that of muscle or nerve, since all living tissues appear to show such changes as one phase of their physiological functioning.

Having prepared the subject, we continue with our procedure. We now present the "suspects" with a list of 100 words. Of them, 80 are "neutral," but scattered throughout are 20 "critical" words. This is what we mean by critical. The neutral words may be assumed to have no particular affective significance, but the 20 critical ones have been selected from among the objects and situations of our "crime." Thus, we include such words as chicken, tongue, ether, pigeon, and so on. Our rationale here is that such words will inevitably serve as substitute stimuli for affective reactions which we hope were performed in the "crime" just committed. In other words, it is by this means that we hope to elicit *implicit affective action* and other behavioral indices of complicity.

We instruct each subject to respond as quickly as possible with the first word that occurs to him and present him with the 100-item list, keeping a careful record of his reaction time. We also observe what happens with respect to breathing, blood pressure, and galvanic skin reactions as an aid in diagnosing an affective reaction from a "neutral" one. For expository purposes, let us assume a series of exaggerated affective reactions on the critical words. This is an indication that these words are functioning properly as substitute stimuli. They successfully connect that person *now* who was involved in the *original* "crime" less than an hour ago. It was he who must have performed affective reactions in the crime situation that we designed to call out these responses, for it is he who now is reacting thus in a vestigial or remnant fashion. It is one subject who shows this implicit affective reaction and not the other two. It is he, therefore, who is implicated in the "crime."

But there are also other indices of complicity. For one thing, one subject shows long reaction times on the critical words as compared with the neutral ones. We may infer that again our choice of words was successful. Not wishing to give himself away, he tries to think of some substitute for the word that occurs first— but this takes time, and we find him out in this fashion when we average the noninvolved words versus the crucial ones. Occasionally, he shows his complicity by *significant responses*. For example, to the stimulus word, "chicken," we get the following three responses: "soup," "fowl," and "head." It is only necessary to put two and two together here in order to get the right answer. Com-

plete blocking (in one instance lasting 2 whole minutes!), perseveration of the same response, laughing, blushing, shifting, and the
like, are other indications.

Regardless of whether one uses instrumental techniques or
word reactions, the essential feature in the psychology of lie detection lies in contriving such substitute stimuli as will behaviorally
relate the person in an effective way *after* the "crime" is over to the
crime situation itself. This relation is such that the person so related performs in some slight form an affective response or some
connected verbal response. In this section, our primary interest
has been in the vestigial or remnant affective interactions.

VI. THE EFFECT OF KNOWLEDGE OF THE SITUA-
TION UPON JUDGMENT OF EMOTION [7]
IN FACIAL EXPRESSIONS [8]

N. H. Pronko

The purpose of this experiment was to study influence of the observer's knowledge of the situation upon his judgment of emotion
from facial expressions. Knowledge of situation means that the
judge sees the face, the whole bodily posture, and the general surroundings.

The materials consisted of a set of slides made from photographs which had been selected from back issues of *Life* or *Look*.
These pictures, taken at various times and places by candid cam-
eramen, were all unposed photographs of people expressing some
emotion. The pictures were of relatively unknown people and
were taken from those issues of magazines old enough so that the
subjects in the experiment would have no memory of them. All
the photographs showed clearly the facial expression. The final
set selected consisted of fourteen photographs. One of these sets
showed only the face of the individual; the other showed everything which had been photographed originally.

The data were collected under two different conditions. In
one group of ninety college students, the faces were shown one

---

[7] Again, we remind the reader that the term "emotion" is synonymous
with our use of the term "feelings."

[8] MUNN, N. L. The effect of knowledge of the situation upon judgment of
emotion from facial expressions. *J. abnorm. soc. Psychol.*, 1940, 35, 324–338.

week, and a week later the entire situation was shown. Each time they recorded their judgment of the emotion being expressed. For the other group of sixty-five students, the experimenter compiled a list of the most frequent judgments made by the first group, and then asked the students to check the emotion most nearly depicted by the photograph.

In general, the judgments in both groups were quite similar; for some facial expressions, such as joy, sorrow, distress, pain, and fear, the amount of agreement was about the same. This was true whether the face alone was exposed or the entire scene. For other expressions, the amount of agreement was higher after the entire situation was seen. Thus, picture No. 3, with face alone exposed, was judged to be strain by 10 per cent of the students, determination by 32 per cent, pain by 9 per cent, anger by 11 per cent, and hate by 11 per cent. However, when the entire picture was shown, 36 per cent judged it strain and 55 per cent determination. (Not all responses are included in these figures.)

For still other expressions, the exposure of the entire picture resulted in a significant shift in judgment. For example, one picture of an athlete in action was judged as sorrow when the face alone was exposed but as determination when the entire picture was shown. The total result was the creation of more agreement when the situation was shown than when the face alone was shown, though in many individual cases showing the face alone seemed to suffice. The author mentions no cases in which the total situation reduced the agreement in judgment. Hence, we may conclude that the general effect of seeing the entire situation rather than the facial expression alone will create greater uniformity of judgment among people concerning the emotional behavior which they are witnessing.

13

EMOTION

FAILURE OF A STIMULUS-RESPONSE COORDINATION [1]

I. INTRODUCTION
Harris Hill

Unlike any other type of behavior, the emotional reaction is not a positive response to a stimulus but rather a failure of a stimulus-response coordination to operate. What happens is that the organism is left in a crucial situation (in the most striking cases) without certain expected or desirable means of adaptation, either because of not having a response system for the particular stimulating circumstances or because of some failure of such an acquired response system to operate. Emotions are therefore essentially "no-response" activities.[2]

According to this description of typical emotional behavior, the precurrent reaction systems of attending and perceiving operate as they do in all organized actions; contact is established between organism and stimulus object, the stimulus functions for the organism. That is, the organism sees or hears the stimulus, but, owing to the particular conditions of the situation, no final or consummatory response occurs. The organism will perform some activity with respect to the stimulus object, it may be apparent or

---

[1] KANTOR, J. R. An attempt toward a naturalistic description of emotion. *Psychol. Rev.*, 1921, **28**, 19–42, 120–140.

[2] While, traditionally, the terms "feelings" and "emotions" have been used almost synonymously, we are using the word "emotion" to label a distinctly different behavior than that designated by the term "feelings." In this chapter, it will refer to a failure to perform a final adjustment, or a disruption of response.

inapparent, but this activity will not be correlated with a specific stimulus function.

If emotion is to be analyzed, we must ask, "What are the conditions that may be responsible for disruption of behavior?" In great measure, of course, the answer will only be found in observation of particular individuals, with their unique behavioral histories, behaving in specific situations. Generally, however, the most influential factors in any breakdown of behavior are localized around certain areas of the behavioral event. The first of these is composed of specific stimulus conditions. Equal in importance with stimulus conditions is the responding organism. Is the individual injured, drugged, or otherwise in a condition that may interfere with response?

The readings in this chapter illustrate and exemplify conditions under which breakdown of the individual's behavioral equipment may occur. As the experimental and observational studies are examined, it will be noted that each is so designed or occurs in such a way that pressure is brought to bear on the organism to respond. We need not cite a special experiment to show that this "motivational" factor must be present before breakdown occurs, because each of the cases presented illustrates this principle; in some instances, it is presentation of electric shock or some such noxious stimulus; in others, social pressures; while in still other instances, simultaneous presentation of two stimuli, each of which has been correlated with specific responses, may result in disruption of psychological activity. The essential feature of all is that an organism who has previously acquired a response to a particular stimulus object does not react with that response. Instead, it "goes to pieces," "freezes on the spot," faints, or "passes out." In every instance, too, momentarily or longer, there is a psychological paralysis or gap during which, of course, there may be physiological functioning of the organs of the organism.

II. PRESENTATION OF UNFAMILIAR STIMULI

The phase of conditioning in which generalized struggle to the conditioned stimulus often occurs may be used as an example of the type of situation in which unfamiliar stimuli result in momentary breakdown of behavior. This action is well illustrated by the Kellogg and Wolf [3] study of escape conditioning in dogs. The design of this conditioning experiment allows the subject to escape the injurious unconditioned stimulus by lifting his foot to the conditioned stimulus.

The animals which were conditioned were placed individually in a small sound-proofed room, in which they could be observed through one-way-vision windows. They stood within a heavy wooden framework or stock which was bolted on top of a table. Each foot was strapped to light balanced levers which permitted a vertical movement of 4 inches. . . . The conditioned stimulus was either the sound of a doorbell or a pure tone. In either case its duration was 2 seconds. The buzz was sounded alone for 1.8 seconds before the presentation of the unconditioned stimulus, and it coincided with the latter for the final 2 seconds. The unconditioned stimulus was either an a-c or d-c shock delivered through stainless steel electrodes securely taped to the anterior and posterior surfaces of the foot just above the tabs. The intensity of the shock stimulus was in all cases adjusted so as to be just strong enough to elicit an unconditioned flexion reflex of 4 inches. . . . The apparatus used for most of the subjects permitted the obtaining of simultaneous graphic records of the movement of all 4 feet, the respiration, and buzz, shock and time for every trial. It therefore gave a fairly good picture of the behavior of the whole organism [p. 589].

In Figure [45] are plotted a series of 4 learning curves, one for each foot of subject F13, as that subject made a sudden and "successful" change from struggle to non-struggle conditioned responses. The percent frequency of responsiveness given in this figure is the percent of CRs in each daily group of 20 stimulations. Although the RR foot only was shocked, conditioned responses were counted for any foot providing that foot was lifted at all during the period of the buzz stimulus. The graphs of the left front, right front and left rear feet may hence be considered as "error" curves since they depict unnecessary or incorrect responses. But the graph for the right rear foot is an increasing-score curve of efficiency of learning [pp. 597–598].

During early conditioning, it will be noted that the subject responded with all four feet in about 70 per cent of the trials. But soon the frequency rose to 100 per cent. In other words, this dog

---

[3] KELLOGG, W. N. & WOLF, I. S. "Hypotheses" and "random activity" during the conditioning of dogs. *J. exp. Psychol.*, 1940, **26**, 588–601. (Reproduced by permission of the authors and the American Psychological Association.)

struggled or lifted every foot randomly or in a disorganized, violent fashion on every trial. After 140 trials, the dog ceased this widespread, all-out activity and continued to react only with the right rear foot almost 100 per cent of the time. At this point, he developed a more organized and discrete response and continued to use it as a stable adjustment in this conditioning situation.

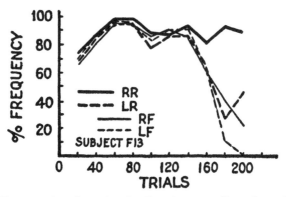

FIG. 45 Here are plotted a series of 4 "learning curves," one for each foot of the subject. The per cent frequency of responsiveness on the ordinate is the per cent of CRs in each daily group of 20 stimulations. Although the RR foot only was shocked, CRs were counted for any foot providing that foot was lifted at all during the ⅘ seconds of buzz preceding the unconditioned shock stimulus. The sudden dropping out of the CRs from the 3 non-shocked feet after 140 trials, is evidence of the phenomenon of insight, or a change in "hypotheses." (Kellogg, W. N., & Wolf, I. S., "Hypotheses" and "random activity" during the conditioning of dogs.)

Changes in behavior like these, which are so far-reaching and significant to the organism that they include violent effort from the whole body at one time, and complete removal of the violence immediately afterwards require some explanation other than "change," "random activity," or "trial-and-error." During the struggle behavior the subjects engage in a kind of behavior which, although definitely circumscribed by the experimental situation, is vastly different from that which follows [p. 598].

Apparently, behavior is disrupted when organisms are compelled to respond to noxious stimuli or to an unfavorable situation for which they have never acquired an organized response. After an organized response is firmly established, the disrupted action ceases.

III. STIMULI TOO NUMEROUS TO PERMIT EFFICIENT RESPONSES [4]

It was my desire to create for the subject problematical combinations of stimuli, to which he could not have been accustomed by practice and to which he could not respond in habitual modes. The subject was to react to visual stimuli by pulling levers and pushing pedals. He sat on a stool before the apparatus. At the level of his hands were five long levers, numbered from left to right, 1-2-3-4-5. His feet rested each on a pedal, the left pedal designated A, the right B. In a slot before him, in large type, appeared combinations of the signals—B-4-1-2, A-5-B-4-3-1, and the like. He was to respond by manipulating—all at once—the designated levers and pedals. Immediately upon completion of a correct response a new signal appeared in the slot, and it was the subject's task to react to a series of 24 such signals in the shortest possible time. The reaction apparatus had one notable advantage: it called for extended visible bodily movements, which could be very readily observed and studied. . . .

We made one discovery that came as a surprise to us, for it was found that the subject of the experiment frequently lost coordination completely under the stress of the conditions imposed on him. The preparatory process would get under way—and suddenly disintegrate. It is the kind of thing that often happens to people when learning to drive an automobile. The individual "gets rattled," "loses command of himself," and works his controls at random, in a flurry of blind excitement. We observed many instances of such loss of control, in our experiments, before it occurred to us that these states were emotional in character. . . .

Our observers reported, also, that the blurs cleared up, sometimes suddenly, sometimes gradually, as the adequate response emerged. . . .

"When the blur dissipates," one observer told us, "the feeling of relaxation is quite marked." Another said, "The feeling of uncertainty and the lack of clearness passed away when the stimulus was seen in its true relationship, and I was prepared to respond" [p. 133].

Although the subjects were capable of responding efficiently when stimuli were presented singly, or perhaps, in pairs, the de-

---

[4] HOWARD, D. T. In *Feelings and emotions: the Wittenberg symposium* (ed. REYMERT, M. L.) Worcester, Mass.: Clark Univ. Press, 1928, pp. 454. (Reprinted by permission of the author and publisher.)

mand for very complex action as response to multiple stimuli proved to be too great a strain on the individual's behavioral equipment. Consequently, the relationship between organism and stimulus objects lost its essential psychological characteristics. Frequently, the subject's final responses to a stimulus presentation showed no predictability and no tightly knit integration with the demonstrated functions of the stimulus series.

IV. STIMULI PRESENTED IN SUCH RAPID ORDER THAT ORGANIZED RESPONSES ARE PREVENTED

Harris Hill

An early study by Roback [5] shows the effect of imposing too rapid adjustment on the subject. By means of a revolving drum, he presented a stimulus series of eighty-five green dots and red crosses.

The specific instructions were to react to the stimuli flashed on the screen in front of the subject. Exposure of the red crosses required a double up-down movement of a telegraph key, while the green dots called for a double side movement of the same key. Only the forefinger of the left hand was to be used for tapping the key.

The stimuli were presented at increasingly shorter intervals so that the subjects had to keep constantly increasing their speed of reaction in order to keep up. Intervals between stimuli were such as to require 2 to 3.18 movements per second.

RESULTS. The results showed the usual emotional response. Mutual, inhibitory effects were common. There was also confusion and omission of response. The task was often abbreviated so that the more difficult movements suffered more than the simpler ones. With one subject, the interference effect showed itself not in omissions so much as in the inclusion of extra, haphazard movements.

In addition, Roback observed a number of other interesting things. Sometimes a second stimulus, coming closely on the heels of the first, would completely inhibit the response to the latter. There were also complete breaks in responding, additional taps after an

---

[5] ROBACK, A. A. The interference of the will-impulses. *Psychol. Rev. Mono.*, 1918, 25, pp. 158.

omission, and rhythmic activities when the subject could not respond in the manner required. These consisted of apparently automatic repetition of previous reactions, repetition of the same error in succeeding series, the creation of spontaneous tapping rhythm regardless of stimuli, and utter confusion lasting over a series of stimuli after a single error. In general, we can note a breakdown in the final adjustment of organisms who were asked to react faster than their behavioral equipment permitted.

V. PRESENTATION OF AMBIGUOUS STIMULI

Several of Pavlov's [6] experiments with dogs resulted in breakdown of behavior; the one quoted below is typical. The usual procedure is to establish a salivary conditioned response to a specific conditioned stimulus. This type of response is referred to in the following excerpt as "an alimentary conditioned reflex." After this is thoroughly established to some originally neutral stimulus and occurs upon each stimulus presentation, differentiation is attempted between the specific conditioned stimulus and a similar stimulus. In the following study by Pavlov, a salivary response to a luminous circle was first established by employing food as the unconditioned stimulus. Then, by always rewarding this response to a circle and not rewarding any responses made to an ellipse, discrimination between the two stimuli in terms of a salivary response was definitely established. The interest of the moment is in the conditions that bring about breakdown of this discrimination.

Experiments with regard to differentiation of shapes were continued by Dr. Shenger-Kristovnikova. An alimentary conditioned reflex was established in a dog to a luminous circle which was projected onto a screen placed in front of the dog. After the reflex had attained a constant strength the animal was able to differentiate from the circle a number of ellipses of equal surface and luminosity. In the first of the ellipses the ratio of the semi-axes was 2:1 and differentiation was established with ease. This was followed up by a series of ellipses which gradually approximated to the circle in shape, and so required a finer and finer differentiation. The ellipse with ratio of the semi-axes 9:8

[6] PAVLOV, I. P. *Conditioned reflexes. An investigation of the physiological activity of the cerebral cortex* (tr. ANREP, G. V.). Oxford, London: The Clarendon Press, 1927. Pp. 430. (Reprinted by permission of the publishers.)

proved to be the limit at which differentiation just failed. Some indication of differentiation appeared at first, but on repetition it gradually disappeared, and with it disappeared also all the previously established coarser differentiations. To renew these it was necessary to work up carefully from the very beginning, starting with the first ellipse with a ratio of semi-axes 2:1. When all the coarser discriminations had again been obtained, the ellipse with the 9:8 was tried once more. Its first application showed a complete discrimination, giving a zero secretion of saliva. Further tests, however, led to the same results as before. Not only was it impossible to obtain the differentiation again (if the first trial can be regarded as a real differentiation at all), but all the earlier, coarser differentiations disappeared as well . . . when the stage of minute differences between stimuli is reached, analysis of itself appears still feasible, but the relations . . . seem to present an insurmountable obstacle to its continued and permanent utilization by the animal for an appropriate response activity [p. 133].

Dogs which had previously stood quietly in the conditioning apparatus would now struggle and howl. In other similar experiments, such failures in discriminations as those described above have resulted in struggling, biting, defecating, urinating, and other disruption of behavior. This has been called experimental neurosis. Such dogs would often be behaviorally useless for further experimentation, so devastating and permanent was their behavioral breakdown.

VI. SIMULTANEOUS PRESENTATION OF STIMULI THAT CALL FOR RESPONSES THAT ARE PHYSICALLY INCOMPATIBLE
Harris Hill

Experiments that might be used as examples of this type of interference are usually said to be studying the effects of distraction. Two responses might conceivably be performed at the same time (for instance, a left-hand movement and a right-hand movement), but because the individual has not learned to behave in this way or because of the intrinsic difficulty of the responses, disorganization of one or both actions may occur. The following quotation from Boder [7] shows various effects that may be expected under certain of these conditions. Briefly, the subject's task was to push a bar forward or pull it back with one hand when certain stimuli appeared, while at the same time tapping as fast as possible with the other hand. This is not too far different from the difficult co-ordination called for in patting one's head with one hand and at the same time circularly massaging his abdomen with the other.

The subject was instructed . . . when the red light appears, pull the rheostat handle backward until the bell rings. When a green light appears, push it forward until the claxon sounds. In both cases you must return to the original position as soon as you hear the bell or the claxon. The stimuli will follow one another in quick succession. Watch carefully and respond as fast as you can, tapping at top rate all the time. Refrain from remarks until the experiment is over.

Several practice trials for the left hand were given, but with light stimuli being presented at a slower rate, so as to make definitely certain that the problem was well understood. Then several regular trials were given, but for practice purposes only. Following these, two experimental series were given. . . . Four stimulus-response situations in balanced order were completed in each series.

PERTINENT RESULTS. It has been found that if a concomitant choice reaction to light involving an intensive motor activity is to be performed with the left hand while tapping at top speed with the right, the rate of tapping is markedly reduced in speed *between* the concomitant reactions, and to a still greater extent during the concomitant response itself. In addition to a marked decrease in speed during such concomitant motor response, the tapping pattern itself is frequently broken up in the form of relatively long or excessively short stops at the reversals, or in the form of blocks in which the subject "loses his bearings. . . ." However, this disorganization of rate and pattern lasts in all cases less than a second, showing a recuperation frequently still within the space of time devoted to the concomitant motor response [p. 34].

The situation described above clearly shows the partial or complete disruption of response that occurs when the organism is "on the spot."

---

[7] BODER, D. P. The influence of concomitant activity and fatigue upon certain forms of reciprocal hand movement and its fundamental components. *Comp. Psychol. Monogr.*, 1935. 11, Pp. 121. (Reproduced by permission of the author and the American Psychological Association.)

VII. SIMULTANEOUS PRESENTATION OF STIMULI THAT DEMAND INCOMPATIBLE RESPONSES

In the experiment of Sears and Hovland [8] is found a partial explanation of what was described earlier in this chapter as factors that force or compel the response of an organism to a stimulus object. In every disruptive situation, some such conditions must be present. Those dealt with here are electric shock and instructions. In this experiment, we are mainly interested in these "pressures" or "motivational conditions" in conjunction with simultaneous presentation of stimuli that call for incompatible responses.

The hypothesis is advanced that frequency of blockage increases as the strengths of the conflicting responses approach equality.

The chief experimental problem involved in testing this hypothesis is the measurement of the relative strengths of the conflicting responses. In the first of the two experiments described . . . it was assumed that avoidance reactions established with the aid of electric shock punishment were stronger than ones established by instructions alone. In both experiments the conflicts were between incompatible avoidance responses . . . [p. 280].

In the first experiment, the subjects were seated on a high stool directly in front of a boxlike apparatus. From the top of the box protruded a lever that could be moved in any direction 3 inches from the center. The lever was so wired that an electric shock could be administered to the subject as the experimental conditions required. Light bulbs mounted on each side of the top surface of the box provided the stimuli for the required responses. A hundred and fifty men divided into three groups constituted the subjects.

GROUP A. . . . The subject was instructed to grasp the handle of the lever firmly and when either light flashed on to move the lever away from the light as quickly as possible. Nothing was said about shock nor was shock given on any trial. After ten reactions away from the light, in random order, both lights were flashed simultaneously for the 21st trial.

---

[8] SEARS, R. R. & HOVLAND, C. I. Experiments on motor conflict. II. Determination of mode of resolution by comparative strengths of conflicting responses. *J. exp. Psychol.*, 1941, **28**, 280–286. (Reproduced by permission of the authors and the American Psychological Association.)

GROUP B. . . . The subject was instructed as above except that he was told he would feel a shock when one of the lights flashed on and that moving the lever in accordance with the instructions would stop the shock. For half the subjects . . . the shock was associated with the left light, and for the other half with the right light. . . . The subject was told in advance with which light the shock would be associated. After 10 trials to each light, in random order, both lights were flashed simultaneously for the 21st trial. No shock was given on this conflict trial.

GROUP C. . . . The instructions and procedure for this group were the same as above, except that the subject was told there would be shock accompanying each light. No shock was given on the final conflict trial.

The influence of different relative strengths of conflicting responses on the mode of resolution of the conflict can best be described in terms of four classes of response. . . .

1. S—single reaction only; i.e., moving the lever directly away from one light and toward the other.

2. D—double reaction; i.e., first going to one side and then to the other.

3. C—compromise movements. . . . Some of the C resolutions were a circular spinning of the lever and others involved movements toward apparently irrelevant parts of the field.

4. B—blocking; either no manual response whatever, or one so slight that with the present apparatus the lever failed to move more than one inch from its original central position.

In Table 16 are given the proportions of subjects in each group who resolved the conflict by each of the four modes [pp. 281–282].

Table 16 *

The Proportion of Cases in Each Group Responding with Each of
Four Modes of Resolution

Group	Description		Mode of Resolution, Per Cent			
		N	S	D	C	B
A	No shock on either side . . .	50	28	6	2	64
B	Shock on only one side	50	46	12	14	28
C	Shock on both sides	50	40	2	2	56

*Modified from Sears and Hovland.

As is predicted by the hypothesis, the number of blockages for Group B (unequal strength) is far less than the number for either

A or C (equal strengths). A statistical analysis of the results indicated that the differences between A and B and between B and C would arise by chance less than once in 100 times.

In addition to providing an opportunity to study the effects of various motivational conditions, this experiment illustrates acquisition of behavior and also its disruption. The Sears and Hovland discussion has thrown some light on the motivational aspects of the problem; however, we are mainly concerned with behavioral breakdown.

The C and B modes of resolution given in Table 16 fall under our category of disrupted action, since none of these activities was the response acquired in the nonconflict situations. Throwing the C and B percentages together gives the following totals of disrupted responses: Group A, 66 per cent; Group B, 42 per cent; Group C, 58 per cent. Thus, even excluding the D-type responses, many of which could also be classified as disorganized, it is found that a predominance of disrupted responses may be expected when stimuli are presented that call for incompatible responses.

VIII. SITUATIONAL SETTING FACTORS THAT MAY BE PARTIALLY RESPONSIBLE FOR DISRUPTION OF BEHAVIOR

Illustrated materials given previously in this chapter were mainly concerned with disruptive situations in which the chief source of difficulty could be localized in the specific stimuli to which responses were to be made. The present section deals with situations in which unfavorable conditions are not directly the specific coordination of stimulus and response that is demanded. Rather, the disturbing element may be considered as situational, since it provides a background or setting for the specific stimulus and response. The effects of unfavorable situational influences are frequently breakdown of behavior that would otherwise occur in an organized manner. A condensation of a study by Patrick [9] will illustrate the adverse effects of several penalizing conditions.

---

[9] PATRICK, J. R. Studies in rational behavior and emotional excitement. II. The effect of emotional excitement on rational behavior in human subjects. *J. comp. Psychol.*, 1934, 18, 153–175. (Reproduced by permission of the author and the American Psychological Association and the Williams & Wilkins Company.)

The apparatus used in the investigation was a roomlike enclosure with an entrance door, which closed and locked itself upon the subject's entrance, and four exit doors. A narrow hallway led from the entrance door to the room part of the enclosure. The four doors giving exit from this room could be locked or unlocked at the discretion of the experimenter. His position was outside the enclosure, yet unobscured observation of the subject's actions in the experimental chamber was provided.

Three sources of disturbing situational stimuli were provided from which the subject could not escape when they were applied during his stay in the experimental room: (1) The top surface of the floor was inlaid with fine copper wire from which the experimental subjects could be given the desired electric shock. (2) A claxon horn projected from the wall into the room as the source of a loud noise. (3) A cold shower as the third type of disturbing stimulus, had triple-nozzle sprays projected from the ceiling in such a manner as to cover the entire room when turned on by the experimenter. After entering the room, the subject was to make his exit from it as quickly as possible by discovering one door of four that was unlocked. The order of selection of doors to be left unlocked was apparently randomized and changed for each subject. With Group B, the only one to be discussed in the present condensation, the subjects made ten test trials a day for ten consecutive days without application of the disturbing stimuli. This constituted the control series of trials.

Immediately following the series of runs of the first ten-day period, the same subjects were put through their second ten-day period of ten trials a day, which constituted the experimental series. . . . It was during this second series, while each subject was finding his way out of the situation through the ever-varying system of unlocked doors, that each subject was subjected to one of the types of emotional stimuli. . . . In order not to damage clothing, and also to keep conditions uniform, the experimenter had each subject change his clothes at the beginning and at the end of a day's run. A brown "union-all" suit furnished the wearing apparel while the experimentation was in progress. Thus, barefooted and bare-headed and with only a "union-all" suit on, each subject ran through the second series [p. 160].

Reactions of the subjects in the various situations were recorded. These reactions fall into five types of responses: (1) a single definite effort to open one of the three doors that might be unlocked; (2) trying all four doors once (the useless response here would be trying to open the immediately previous unlocked door); (3) the adoption of stereotyped modes of action, e.g., always attempting to gain exit by trying a certain sequence of doors; and (4) attempt and immediate reattempt to open one door. (5) The last type of behavior included several different sorts of action which have a common characteristic, i.e., automatism; the subject behaved in a relatively implastic, unadaptive manner. ("It is the unmodified primitive tendency to repeat an activity.")

In Table 17 and Fig. 46 are presented Patrick's results that are pertinent to the present discussion. The trend toward Type E reaction in the experimental situations is evident.

Table 17 *

Distribution of Classifiable Reactions by Each Subject during
Each Series of 100 Trials

Subject	Number of Classified Reactions	Type of Response (Per Cent)				
		A	B	C	D	E
		Control Series				
1	35	54	37	3	0	6
2	28	50	36	14	0	0
3	30	53	27	20	0	0
4	34	62	32	6	0	0
		Experimental Series				
1	37	22	16	3	8	51
2	57	11	14	19	2	54
3	52	8	13	12	2	65
4	52	27	13	2	4	54

*Modified from Patrick.

Under emotionally exciting conditions the same subjects who manifested a preponderance of Type A reactions under normal conditions manifested a preponderance of Type E reactions. In fact, under the influence of the emotional stimuli Types A and E relatively changed places when compared with their respective positions under normal conditions. Type E became the dominant type under exciting conditions. Certainly the results reveal a marked reduction in efficiency in the quality of the types of reaction . . . made by normal adult human subjects while operating under the influence of emotional stimuli . . . the perseveration tendency, Type E, has a tendency to manifest itself predominantly [p. 189].

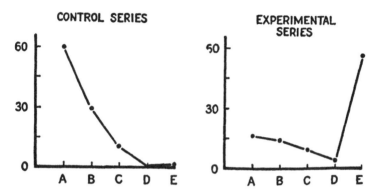

FIG. 46   Curves of the classified reactions. (Modified from Patrick, J. R., Studies in rational behavior and emotional excitement.)

IX. A FURTHER EXAMPLE OF SITUATIONAL SETTING FACTORS IN EMOTION

The "Luria technique" for studying emotions consists of having the subject perform complex responses in a control situation of favorable conditions. These same or very similar responses are then demanded of the subject under very unfavorable conditions. If extraneous variables have been controlled, a comparison of the responses given in the control and experimental situations furnishes an estimate of the adverse influence on behavior of the penalizing conditions.

An investigation by Hill [10] examined behavioral disorganization and disruption through recording speech and finger movements that were performed first under favorable and then under unfavorable conditions.

During a practice situation, 30 subjects learned to execute three responses simultaneously. These were the performance of particular right-hand and left-hand movements in conjunction with prepared

---

[10] HILL, H. Investigations of response disorganization: I. Speech and finger movements (in press).

speech responses. The finger movements were recorded on a fast-moving polygraph, and speech on a magnetic wire recorder. After the subjects had learned to perform in a well-integrated manner and control recordings had been taken, penalizing conditions were introduced in the form of strong electric shocks presented simultaneously with the stimuli for speech and finger movements. Several blocks of test trials were run immediately with stimulus conditions the same as in the control situation. Comparisons between responses performed before penalty with those performed following the penalty showed the disrupting influence of these specific unfavorable conditions.

Disorganization of behavior was scaled according to criteria of response efficiency. The scale extended from 0 to 10, 0 representing very efficient behavior and 10 representing disrupted actions.

When considering overt responses, this author found that generally the manifestation of situational disruption of behavior (i.e., response to an immediate situation as opposed to a recurring, unsolved difficulty) appear to be quite similar. The behavior of the individual loses its normal characteristics as measured by comparison with past behavior. Responses may be performed very slowly, e.g., they may be prolonged; or they may be very fast and powerful, having perseverative characteristics. They may be of a fragmentary nature, where a part of the normal response occurs or where the whole response is performed in a disjointed, stilted manner. Or the normal response may be omitted entirely while some seemingly irrelevant action is substituted. Thus, for various degrees of penalizing situations, depending upon the situation and the particular individual's behavioral background, there may be a progression of increasing disorganization ranging from efficient behavior through fragmentary action to completely substitutive activities.

X. EPILEPTIC BEHAVIOR AS AN EMOTIONAL INTERACTION
N. H. Pronko

There is a continuous gradation of intensity of behavioral disruption ranging from the rather mild form in which one has a gripping feeling in his intestines during a near collision to the most violent form to be observed during an epileptic fit. Since epileptic behavior is such exaggerated action, it shows better than do lesser degrees of emotionality the essential features of emotional behavioral segments. It will be remembered that this is an atypical behavioral segment in that the behavioral event is begun but not completed. The organism both attends and perceives the stimulus object (let us assume in some dangerous situation), but beyond this point there is a psychological disorganization in the sense that there is a gap during which there is no behavior going on. There is only physiological activity which consists of violent and chaotic explosive reflex action. The person in an epileptic fit sees what the dangerous object is but because of either suddenness or intensity of the stimulus object or because of failure to build up appropriate reaction, he does not complete the behavioral segment with a final reaction system. Instead he "passes out of the picture," psychologically speaking, and is reduced to helter-skelter "firing off" of separate organs and systems.

It is readily admitted that such a gap in the continuity of the individual's behavior may follow a serious interference with the organism's physiological functioning as from brain-tumor growth or abnormal biochemical conditions.

Thus, the epileptic, during this phase, fails to maintain posture and to orient himself properly. His gravitational responses cease to operate during the psychological gap. He falls to the ground with a scream, this scream occurring simply as a reflex spasm of the muscles of lungs, diaphragm, and vocal cords. Unless precautions are taken to prevent it, he may bite his tongue. Other muscles in the arms, legs, face, and eyes may also twitch reflexly so that the organism gives the appearance of "throwing himself about." Perhaps more interesting yet is the fact that salivation, urination, and defecation reflexes assert themselves during this psychological "gaposis." It may be reasonably assumed that in the short space of time immediately before and during the emotion, the glandular, bladder, and rectal conditions were much the same, nevertheless these systems were kept "in brake" as long as the organism operated in a behavioral way, i.e., as long as his action showed the six essential characteristics of differentiation, integration, variability, modifiability, delayability, and inhibition. As soon as he ceased "behaving," he immediately became the locus of a bundle of independently operating physiological stimulus-response units.

Naturally, such a condition as has been described is difficult to reproduce experimentally. For that reason, we include, by means of the following selection, a "field observation" of this dramatic action. Actually, the source is a literary one but is nonetheless a faithful description of epilepsy because it was derived from self-observation. Since Dostoyevsky [11] was himself an epileptic, he reports with clinical accuracy the behavior of the character, Myshkin, in the story.

The staircase up which Myshkin ran from the gateway led to the corridors of the first and second floors, on which were the rooms of the hotel. As in all old houses, the staircase was of stone, dark and narrow, and it turned round a thick stone column. On the first half-landing there was a hollow like a niche in the column, not more than half a yard wide and nine inches deep. Yet there was room for a man to stand there. Dark as it was, Myshkin, on reaching the half-landing, at once discovered that a man was hiding in the niche. Myshkin suddenly wanted to pass by without looking to the right. He had taken one step already, but he could not resist turning round.

Those two eyes, *the same two eyes*, met his own. The man hidden in the niche had already moved one step from it. For one second they stood facing one another and almost touching. Suddenly Myshkin seized him by the shoulders and turned him back towards the staircase, nearer to the light; he wanted to see his face more clearly.

Rogozhin's eyes flashed and a smile of fury contorted his face. His right hand was raised and something gleamed in it; Myshkin did not think of checking it. He only remembered that he thought he cried out, "Parfyon, I don't believe it!" Then suddenly something seemed torn asunder before him; his soul was flooded with intense *inner* light. The moment lasted perhaps half a second, yet he clearly and consciously remembered the beginning, the first sound of the fearful scream which broke of itself from his breast and which he could not have checked by any effort. Then his consciousness was instantly extinguished and complete darkness followed.

It was an epileptic fit, the first he had had for a long time. It is well known that epileptic fits come on quite suddenly. At the moment the face is horribly distorted, especially the eyes. The whole body and the features of the face work with convulsive jerks and contortions. A terrible, indescribable scream that is unlike anything else breaks from the sufferer. In that scream everything human seems obliterated and it is

11 Dostoyevsky, Feodor. *The idiot.* New York: Random House, 1925. Pp. 586. (Reproduced by permission of Random House.)

impossible or very difficult, for an observer to realise and admit that it is the man himself screaming. It seems indeed as though it were someone else screaming from within the man. That is how many people at least have described their impression. The sight of a man in an epileptic fit fills many people with positive and unbearable horror, in which there is a certain element of the uncanny. It must be supposed that some such feeling of sudden horror, together with the other terrible sensations of the moment, had suddenly paralysed Rogozhin and so saved Myshkin from the knife with which he would have stabbed him. Then before he had time to grasp that it was a fit, seeing that Myshkin had staggered away from him and fallen backwards downstairs, knocking his head violently against the stone step, Rogozhin flew headlong downstairs, avoiding the prostrate figure, and, not knowing what he was doing, ran out of the hotel.

Struggling in violent convulsions, the sick man slipped down the steps, of which there were about fifteen, to the bottom of the staircase. Very soon, not more than five minutes later, he was noticed and a crowd collected. A pool of blood by his head raised the doubt whether the sick man had hurt himself, or whether there had been some crime. It was soon recognized, however, that it was a case of epilepsy; one of the people at the hotel recognized Myshkin as having arrived that morning. The difficulty was luckily solved by a fortunate circumstance [pp. 221–223].

It is important to note that Myshkin's failure to deal with his attacker was not due to a failure to see him. He did see him, but instead of reaching for the dagger, he stops behaving but passes out and falls headlong down the stairs. These characteristics are exactly those that permit subsuming his action under emotions.

XI. AN EMOTIONAL BEHAVIORAL SEGMENT AS DESCRIBED BY A NEWSPAPER REPORTER [12]

Frequently, the severity of an emotional response is determined by the immediately preceding actions. Often, the very suddenness of the presentation or appearance of the disturbing stimulus accounts for much of the disruption, while under other circumstances, the sudden appearance plus the shocking stimulus function of the occurrence determine the severity of the emotional action.

---

[12] Broadcast by Robert Stimson, British Broadcasting Corporation correspondent, London, Jan. 30, 1948.

No matter how severe the action is that occurs in the shocking situation, it is always terminated by a response to some succeeding stimulus. To a certain extent this new stimulus frees the individual from the no-response phase of the situation, and a response may then be instigated that is an effective coping with the situation.

In the following news-service eye-witness account of Mohandas Gandhi's death will be found examples of these various phases of the emotional behavioral segment. The preoccupation of the audience with Gandhi's attire and actions as he entered the garden, the disrupting stimulus of Gandhi being shot, the no-response period, the new stimulus in the form of the American, and the frenzied reaction of the crowd combine to trace the sequence in a typical emotional action.

Robert Stimson, British Broadcasting Corp. correspondent, broadcast the eyewitness account of the assassination of Mohandas K. Gandhi:

> At three minutes past 5 o'clock, Mr. Gandhi came out of Birla House and, because he was a little late for evening prayers, he stepped more briskly than at any time since his recent fast.
>
> He was wearing his usual white loin cloth and a pair of sandals. He had thrown a shawl around his chest, as it was getting chilly.
>
> His arms were resting lightly on the shoulders of two companions and he was smiling.
>
> There were only 200 or 300 people in the garden, and they pressed towards him as he climbed the steps leading to the small raised lawn where the congregation had gathered.
>
> As he got to the top of the steps and approached the crowd, he took his arms from the shoulders of his friends and raised his hands in salutation. He was still smiling.
>
> A thick-set man, in his 30's I should say and dressed in khaki, was in the forefront of the crowd. He moved a step toward Mr. Gandhi, took out a revolver and fired several shots at almost point-blank range. It did not sound like a revolver but like a chinese cracker a child might have let off. Mr. Gandhi fell.
>
> GRABBED BY AMERICAN. For a few seconds no one could believe what had happened; every one seemed dazed and numb, and then a young American who had come for prayers rushed forward and seized the shoulders of the man in the khaki coat.
>
> That broke the spell.

There was a terrible cry of anguish—a wailing lament—from the crowd. Half a dozen people stooped to lift Gandhi. Others hurled themselves upon the attacker. I saw flailing arms beating his head and shoulders, and soon there was blood on his face. He was overpowered and taken away.

Meanwhile, Gandhi was carried tenderly back to the house across the main lawn that is brightly decked with flowers. I walked beside him. Those who were carrying him covered him with his own shawl; but his head was uncovered. His eyes were closed and there was a look of peace on his face.

He was taken into the house, into a bedroom on the ground floor, and there about a half-hour later he died as a member of his household read verses from Hindu scriptures.

For the sake of clarity, we must point out that when the crowd was described as "numb and dazed," this was the emotional or "no-response" phase of their behavior. However, the lifting of Gandhi and the aggression against his attacker are obviously co-ordinated and adjustmental (i.e., nonemotional) behaviors.

XII. STUTTERING: RECURRENT SPEECH DISRUPTION [13]

Harris Hill

An emotional behavior segment is a slice of an organism's behavior that shows the organism attending to a stimulus object and hearing it or seeing it but doing nothing further in an organized way as required by the situation. For example, when I have seen a gunman threatening me, I should grapple with him, run away, yell or something of the sort. If instead of doing something like that, I see him and faint or "freeze to the spot." I have just illustrated an emotional behavior segment. In this section, we consider how disrupted speech may fit into emotional activity.

The effects of mild behavior disorganization may have but little disturbing influence on other actions. Severe disruption, especially if it occurs several times under similar circumstances, may produce permanent or semipermanent results. That changes in

[13] HILL, H. An interbehavioral analysis of several aspects of stuttering. *J. gen. Psychol.*, 1945, **32**, 289–316. (Reproduced by permission of the author and the publisher.)

behavior due to severe disorganization are deleterious were shown in studies by Pavlov. Discrimination not only failed when the circle and the ellipse became very nearly the same figure, but failed as well at proportions that had previously been distinguished with ease.

A similar but much more complex form of behavior disorganization may be used to illustrate speech breakdown. A consideration of stuttering will illustrate several of the psychological factors that may be responsible for disruption when a response, that has failed in the past, must be attempted again. The diagram accompanying the following excerpt illustrates only one of the many forms of stuttering. The details are relatively simple in that no anticipation of difficulty occurs; the individual blocks without expecting interruption. Nevertheless, it must be emphasized that past instances of blocking exert their influence in breaking up the stimulus-response coordination. Although we may be sure that physiological activities take place during severe stuttering, the following paragraphs are only concerned with breaks in otherwise organized speech responses.

The following diagram shows perhaps the least complex type of blocking which involves an emotional behavior segment. The disruptive segment occurs after the initial sound of a word has been uttered.

Emotional Behavior Segment without Anticipation

There is the ba-	E.B.S.	ba-ba-ball.
	(A—P—?)	

Association or conditioning has invested the process surrounding the production of this word with fear or strong feeling responses, or the block may be a product of auditor or total situation precipitating factors. After the tonic block disappears the word is completed either as an integrated action or with accompanying clonic reactions.

Psychological stasis, except in severe natural surroundings, is no longer than a few milliseconds. Usually emotional activities are initiated by sudden, unexpected stimuli without anticipation of any kind. At other more infrequent times in normal experience, and at more frequent intervals with the stutterer, they come at an unexpected time but with anticipation. In the latter case, that with anticipation, there is usually some preparation for a definite type of action when the particular stimulus appears. With the normal speaker, and the stutterer in non-speaking situations, the pre-determined behavioral sets, or more technically psychological, the implicitly correlated stimulus-response functions, ordinarily operate; i.e., through consideration of the situation, the person determines a course of action, and this action takes place when necessary. Here there is no emotional behavior segment because the person has behavior equipment which is adequate to the situation and which precludes disruptive reactions.

The stutterer cannot provide himself with predetermined behaviors which will function in speaking situations to insure intact language interactions. He may attempt to do so by verbalizing to himself that when speech is demanded he will talk easily, that he will not be disturbed by the auditor, or that he will not think about the feared words beforehand, yet when the time comes for action, although infrequently there may be some slight, favorable change, introspection has added to his difficulty. In attempting feared words orderly progression is disrupted or entirely broken off and no consummatory response immediately occurs which is correlated with the specific stimulus situation. This is the typical emotional behavior segment. We make this statement concerning stuttering by reason of the character of anticipation and the nature of the ensuing speech behavior segment in which no orderly response patterns occur. This view is also held in part on the basis of the repetitive vocal activities which substitute for the smooth, final response of saying a word.

We do not wish to say that all stutterers' speech abnormality is of this nature, as apparently a considerable amount of it has been learned and conditioned, but we do wish to point out that during the emotional behavior segment, or in the disruptive period which may succeed it, any available behavior which is in any manner appropriate, and much which is not, is adopted during the disorganization or emotional phase. If such conditions held for a great number of situations, or intensely for fewer situations, specific patterns of post-emotional behavior segment acts might be established through conditioning. Disparity of symptoms between individual stutterers could thus be partially accounted for as well as the specificity of each individual's reactions.

If the emotional behavior segment is not too severe, a perseveration of the activity which was proceeding when it appeared may continue until either a new stimulus organizes behavior, or until the individual becomes aware of what is occurring and voluntarily does something to stop it. In either case, the stutterer has issued forth out of an emotional behavior segment into orderly, satisfactory (non-emotional) adjustmental speech. He is no longer "hung-up" [pp. 307–308].

XIII. AN EMOTIONAL BEHAVIORAL SEGMENT
Butcher Stops Auto on Tracks; Fails to Heed Warning Shout [14]

Joseph J. Landis, 69, of 1011 Mary's Drive, was killed at 10:01 A.M. Wednesday when the car he was driving was struck and dragged over 300 feet by the Santa Fe streamliner No. 15 at Twenty-second and Broadway.

Landis, a butcher for the Razook Finer Foods market, 2901 West Central, had been to the Cudahy Packing company to buy meat. He was driving west, leaving the plant, when struck.

The streamliner was going north. David F. Sharp, engineer, of Route 2, Emporia, told Traffic Investigator George London he was going between 28 and 30 miles an hour when he saw the car stop on the tracks. He was unable to bring the heavy train to a stop in the 120 feet he had after first seeing the car.

Auto Smashed Badly

The automobile, owned by Landis' employer, Sam J. Razook, was smashed completely on the left side, but did not overturn. It was draped around the front of the giant diesel locomotive and had to be rocked free.

Richard Oliverson, 54, of 3010 Maple, was a witness to the accident.

For the past 15 years a watchman for Cudahys, and since 1938, day watchman at the west gate, Oliverson said he shouted, "Streamliner coming!" to Landis and the car just ahead of him as they went through the gate.

The car ahead, Oliverson said, crossed the tracks and stopped before going onto Broadway. To his horror, the 1935 car driven by Landis stopped on the tracks.

"I ran to the car, opened the door, and told the man he'd better get off the tracks, that a train was coming," Oliverson said. "He looked at me and looked toward the train. I thought he was ready to move. He could have gone either way—back or forward—and cleared the train" [*sic*].

Stepping back, expecting to see the car move to safety, Oliverson said he stood by helplessly. By this time the train was so close he couldn't

---

[14] The Wichita Eagle (Evening Edition), Wichita, Kan., Feb. 25, 1948, Vol. 21, No. 286, pp. 1, 4. (Reproduced by permission of the publisher.)

get back to the vehicle again, and in a second the locomotive went grinding into the car.

The watchman said he believed the motor of the car Landis drove was running when he stopped on the tracks, but couldn't be certain. He said he did not know whether or not Landis stalled the motor after the warning.

Rushed to St. Francis hospital by Cochran ambulance after being extricated from the smashed auto by bystanders, Landis was pronounced dead on arrival.

Landis had driven just a few feet inside the city limits when the fatal crash occurred, according to the police. It is the first 1948 traffic fatality for the city, and it occurred on the city's sixtieth day without a fatal crash. . . .

The preceding item is a news story of what appears to be a typical emotional behavioral segment. It would be far better to observe such events in the laboratory, but, since it is morally impossible to stage them in the drastic way in which Landis' accident occurred under natural conditions, we do the best we can with the facts as reported. One test of the validity of the reported incident is: How well does it fit the description of other kinds of emotional behavioral segments?

The outstanding feature of the accident as observed by the watchman is the time element. Apparently, if Oliverson had sufficient time to run to Landis' car and warn him to get off the tracks because the streamliner was coming, Landis had time in which to carry out some act. It is not failure to see the train that was the apparent cause of the accident, for Oliverson informs us that Landis looked both at him and the train as he (Oliverson) stepped back fully expecting Landis to move to safety. Although Oliverson believes that the motor of the car that Landis was driving may have been running at the time of the accident, that is not important because there was adequate time for Landis to jump out of the car and save his life.

Although the very specific details of Landis' behavior can never be known, first, because he was killed, and second, because there was no observer inside the car who might have lived to tell the story, we may reconstruct the events as follows. We may be certain that a typical behavioral segment was initiated when Landis heard the watchman's warning and attended to the train. There is also sufficient evidence to warrant the inference that he perceived or "saw" the train. So far, this is a typical behavioral segment, but it is quite atypical beyond this point because whereas an ordinary behavioral segment is followed by a final reaction system as in the case of the driver of the car ahead of Landis', Landis does not drive the car ahead or back nor does he leap out. Apparently, he does nothing in the way of an overt psychological reaction such as the situation demands.[15] It is reasonable to suppose that, during the time he should have been acting psychologically, he was in a condition of psychological inactivity or "paralysis." In everyday terms, he might be described as being "frozen to the spot."

XIV. THE STARTLE RESPONSE

N. H. Pronko

The newborn infant performs some types of activity that have puzzled psychologists. Among them is the startle reflex which is elicited by sudden or intense stimuli of any sort but particularly by sudden, sharp noises. High-speed motion-picture analysis shows that some of the components of this reflex act are blinking, closing of eyes, quick forward thrust of head and neck, and a contraction of the abdomen that involves forward movement of the trunk and pronation of the arms.

The question is: How can the newly born infant perform such action? Older psychologists called it an "innate response" and let it go at that. Even the behaviorists explained it in this simple fashion. We believe that a more painstaking analysis is necessary.

One of the important features of the reaction we are considering is its lack of differentiation with respect to the stimulus objects that call it forth. Cold water, loss of support, loud sounds, intense lights—all indiscriminately call out such disorganized action as has been described above. Furthermore, this is a highly invariable response, showing uniformity from time to time in the same

---

15 This merely means that reactions showing the characteristics of psychological events were not observed for a time. Landis failed to show the specificity called for in his seeing the streamliner as well as in hearing Oliverson's warning. The differential or discriminatory as well as the integrated, variable, modifiable, and other features so commonly seen in his behavior (e.g., starting and operating the car) were not apparent in his activities during the phase we have labeled "emotional."

individual as well as from one individual to another. In other words, it is as universal as a knee jerk or a swallowing or sneezing reflex, occurring in Turks, Britishers, Americans, Mohammedans, and Protestants alike. It cannot be delayed or easily inhibited but occurs rather "automatically." Essentially, what we have said amounts to this—that the startle response lacks the usual characteristics of psychological interactions to which we have repeatedly alluded. In other words, if we grant that there is a continuum of acts distinctly physiological at one end of the scale and definitely psychological at the other end, we are forced to place this reaction closer toward the physiological than the psychological pole. At best, it is behavior at a most elementary level only.

Perhaps at later stages of behavioral development, through conditioning and so on, we may study it as a definitely psychological response. The adult who is reading a mystery and is startled by the cat moving in the next room or is "surprised" by someone in a passageway furnishes convenient examples of an act which may at this stage be inhibited, delayed, modified, and so on, within certain limits. But an organism cannot inhibit a knee-jerk or the vomiting reflex of a "sick stomach." This is the essential difference between the infantile and the adult startle response. The adult's behavior shows characteristics not found in tissue-excitation situations; the infant's "startle" comes closer to such specifications.

One last problem remains. How shall we account for the origin of the startle response? Is this an exception to the hypothesis of the reactional biography which states that all behavior is acquired during the individual's life history? We think not. In order to understand the development of the startle reaction, we need only take account of the organism's prenatal development. For 9 months, beginning at the point of conception, the organism is maintained in a remarkably constant and stable environment. Sheltered within the insulating walls of the mother's abdomen, the fetus enjoys a milieu of remarkably homogeneous stimulation. Light stimuli do not enter. Sounds are muffled. Temperature variation is negligible. Touch, smell, and taste stimuli do not exist in the ordinary sense. Being anchored, there are no sudden or large displacements of the organism through space. "Falling" or "being dropped" are experiences that are barred to the organism during the first 9 months of its existence.

Small wonder that certain psychoanalysts talk about a birth

trauma, for compared with its prenatal existence, the child, following birth, enters a new and uncertain world. In place of the constant food supply, there are intermittent meals and hunger to deal with. The bath water may be too hot or too cold, or the infant may stay wet and cold a long time unattended. Loud noises and intense lights are now experienced for the first time. Worse still are the sudden displacements by those who handle the child, as well as the accidental falls from perambulators, cribs, and high chairs. Although he has lived and developed for 9 months, he has had no opportunity for building up reactions to such situations.

Under the circumstances, being unequipped with an organized behavioral repertoire, he does only one thing. On the occasion of his first fall, the reaction called the startle reflex is performed and becomes organized with such general stimulating circumstances as a stable response. This is a case of "immediate-behavior origin" similar to the action of an infant in first contact with a hot radiator. A complex series of responses is not necessary to acquire such a primitive response. The very first contact guarantees an instantaneous origin of one or another reaction. Obviously, if no organized response was built up during the preceding 9 months, one can expect only the all-out, uncoordinated act called the "startle reflex."

The formulation of the startle reflex here proposed suggests the hypothesis that, should the prenatal circumstances permit a gradual increase in dosages of noise, light, and other intense stimulation, the organism would gradually build up responses of an organized sort. If the fetus could be made to fall through space from conception on, in line with other behavioral development, it is reasonable to suppose that some more organized adjustment might evolve. Under the circumstances, it is difficult to test such a hypothesis. Therefore, the validity of our interpretation must be judged by its conformity with general behavioral principles.

14

REMEMBERING

I. REMEMBERING AS A FORM OF DELAYED ACTION
John Bucklew, Jr.

Science thrives on making distinctions, and the science of psychology, with its specific and varied data, is especially dedicated to this task. To ignore the concrete differences among phenomena in favor of generalities is to introduce confusion and disorder into the psychological household. Psychology often employs the terms of popular speech for its vocabulary, but invariably these come to have specific or restricted meanings which differ considerably from popular usage. *Remembering* is one such word which in ordinary language stands for several different, though related, kinds of behavior. In one sense, it refers to the direct repetition of a previously learned act, as when the man *remembers* the poem he learned as a schoolboy. In another sense, it refers to any implicit action, as when I *remember* how the gymnasium was decorated for the dance last night. The looseness of popular usage becomes apparent when we change the above to read, "I think of how the gymnasium was decorated." Thinking and remembering are given different definitions in science; in popular speech, they may be used interchangeably.

Remembering, as a psychological category, can be made to include a type of activity having several distinct characterizations. For one thing, it is activity pointed toward the future, not the past. This morning I wish to remember to mail a letter I wrote last evening, therefore I arrange my morning walk to the office so that I will pass a mailbox. Later, the sight of the mailbox stimulates me to perform the action I had planned earlier.

Remembering, in this sense of the word, is a delayed action. It cannot be concluded immediately but must be postponed to some future time and place where a substitute stimulus will operate to bring about its completion. For this reason, it has a distinct value in a well-ordered life, for it serves to coordinate earlier behavior with later. An orderly routine of living is most conducive to the successful performance of these protracted segments of behavior, and one of the first symptoms of disorganized personality is failure to perform remembering behavior effectively.

In the morning when I arise, if I do not happen to see the letter I have written, the remembering-behavior segment may not be initiated at all. Later I will say I have *forgotten* to mail the letter. Or if I do not take the proper route, or am engrossed in conversation with a friend when I pass the mailbox, it has no chance to operate as a substitute stimulus. In this case, the behavioral segment fails of completion, and another form of forgetting has occurred. Later, a glimpse of the unmailed letter in my coat pocket may stimulate me to initiate the final action, but in this case, fruitlessly, for the essential mailbox is not in my immediate surroundings. Here the final phase of the remembering action has been displaced so that it cannot be completed. It has been initiated by a substitute stimulus other than the one planned. Only too often the final phase of our remembering occurs before or after it should!

Remembering-behavior segments may be delayed over considerable periods of time with many other activities interpolated between the beginning and the end. How is it possible for people to perform such delayed activities? Although they have reached no complete agreement on it, psychologists have been investigating the delayability of response for over a third of a century. Experimental techniques have been developed which permit the investigation and comparison of delayed responses in several species of animals, one of the earliest experiments making comparisons among children, apes, dogs, rats, and other animals. The techniques of experimentation vary, but the following is typical. The subjects are placed in an apparatus or room in which one of several doorways leads to some reward (such as food). The correct doorway is varied from one trial to the next in random arrangement but will always have a light shining above it. After the subjects have learned always to go to the lighted doorway, the delayed response is introduced. This is accomplished by lighting the correct doorway momentarily and then holding the subjects behind a barricade for a definite length of time after the light has gone out. When they are released, will they be able to go to the correct door? For organisms which can handle objects, such as chimpanzees or humans, the technique may be varied by concealing the reward in view of the subjects under one of several boxes. The distinctive cue for the correct box may be its position, color, shape, or size, or combinations of these.

Two generalizations have emerged from delayed-response experiments.[1] First, there is some relationship between the length of delay possible before the correct choices become only a matter of chance, and the position of the animal in the phyletic scale. Chimpanzees, for example, can endure longer delays than can rats. Secondly, the higher organisms seem capable of a variety of activities during the delay period without interfering with the accuracy of choice, whereas lower organisms bridge the delay period most efficiently by maintaining a postural set toward the correct doorway. A rat that may properly delay a response when he is permitted to face in its direction, may not be able to do so if he is turned in the opposite direction during the delay period. The change in postural orientation may disrupt the performance of the delayed response, although even this condition has not always interfered with the completion of a delayed response.

These principles of delay of response relate the remembering-behavior segment to the increasing complexity of organisms in the evolutionary scale. The typical remembering-behavior segments of human adults differ from the delayed response in several respects. For one thing, they are usually contrived and executed by the person himself and are not accomplished through experimental manipulation. The human must learn how to perform remembering behavior, as the mother who sends her child to the store for the first time can testify. Secondly, the typical remembering-behavior segment differs from the delayed-response experiment in the manner in which it is initiated. In the example of letter mailing, the action is initiated in absence of the mailbox itself. The individual responds to it implicitly through substitute stimuli.

---

[1] For a more complete discussion of the delayed response, the reader is referred to Moss, F. A. (ed.). *Comparative Psychology.* Chap. 10. New York: Prentice-Hall, 1942. Pp. 404.

In the delayed response, the action is initiated in the same situation, in the presence of the stimulus to which the final adjustment will later be made. Finally, human remembering is undoubtedly more complexly organized through the use of language behavior and other forms of implicit or semi-implicit responses.

One more characteristic of remembering needs to be mentioned. It is usually temporary, very often being performed once and never again. This characteristic separates it from the more permanent behavioral equipment resulting from ordinary learning. The temporary nature of remembering behavior, as contrasted to more permanent learning equipment, is well appreciated by the student who plans various memory aids to help him on tomorrow's examination. The reader who expects to find an explanation of the stability of learning is referred to the chapter on learning where such a discussion properly belongs. As will have been noted in the above, remembering technically refers to facts other than behavioral acquisitions. One does not need to acquire reactions in order to remember.

It is highly probable that most of our remembering acts involve delaying responses which have already been acquired in the past. However, when I must learn a formula to "give back" on an exam, then we have learning and remembering interrelated. Such a situation shows all the more clearly the need for distinguishing between the two.

II. SOME CHARACTERISTICS OF DELAYED RESPONSE: I. IMPORTANCE OF THE DISTANCE BETWEEN THE CHOICE OBJECTS

Delayed-response experiments with human and infrahuman animals show the essential, triphase characteristics of remembering actions. In fact, they might well be described as rudimentary remembering events. The action is "forward looking"; it is initiated when the experimenter brings the animal into visual contact with a stimulus object such as a bit of food (phase one), then a period of delay is introduced with the food object out of sight—perhaps placed under one of two or more boxes (phase two), and the event is completed if the animal succeeds in going to the box under which the food is placed, the box serving as the substitute stimulus (phase three).

In the first experiment to be described, by Harrison and Nissen,[2] certain features of the substitute stimuli were studied. These features were the spatial relationships between the objects under which the food was placed. For example, in a two-choice situation, could the animal more successfully respond after the interval of delay if the food were under one of two objects separated by only a few inches or by several feet? Further, what would happen if the food were presented (phase one) in one of two objects widely separated, but if these were brought close together before the animal was allowed to complete the response (phase three)? Lastly, what would happen in the reverse of the immediately preceding procedure?

Eight adult and near-adult chimpanzees served as subjects. A slice of banana was used as a lure on each trial.

The subject worked in an outdoor cage, and the apparatus was set up just outside one side of the cage. It consisted essentially of a board 66 inches long on which were mounted four hinged food covers 3 by 2 by $2\frac{1}{2}$ inches. On any one trial only two covers were in place. The spacing of the covers is illustrated as follows:

$$a \qquad\qquad b \quad c \qquad\qquad d$$

The distance from *b* to *c* was 5 inches, center to center, and from *a* to *d* it was 60 inches, center to center.

In the initial phase of some trials, covers *a* and *d* were in place, and the chimp observed food placed under one or the other. During the interval of delay, the apparatus was screened, covers *a* and *d* were removed, and *b* and *c* were substituted. If food had been placed under *a*, it was now under *b;* if it had been under *d,* it was now under *c.* Thus the cover with the food was in the same spatial relationship with the cover without the food in the initial and final phases of the delayed response, but the distance between the covers was much less in the final phase.

On other trials, the above procedure was reversed, and the choice objects were initially close together and finally far apart.

Two other variations were made in the procedure. Covers *a* and *d* were used in both phases, and the same was true in the case of covers *b* and *c.*

2 HARRISON, R. & NISSEN, H. W. Spatial separation in the delayed response performance of chimpanzees. *J. comp. Psychol.*, 1941, **31**, 427–435.

In the delayed-response experiment, the animal observed the experimenter place the food under one of the pair of covers; then the board was drawn back and screened from the cage. After a measured time interval, the board was pushed forward so that the animal could reach through the cage and secure the food from under the food cover.

Since the experimenters were interested in the relative accuracy of performance in the four situations, it was necessary to keep the general level of performance below perfection (100 per cent successes in all situations) and above the 50 per cent level of success. This was done by varying the length of the period of delay or by distracting the animal by tossing him a peanut during the delay.

Seven of the eight subjects performed better when the boxes were far apart in both initial and final phases (*a* and *d*) than they did when the boxes were close together (*b* and *c*). Furthermore, when the distance separating the food boxes was changed during the delay, successes were more frequent when food was presented under *a* or *d* and offered after the delay under *b* or *c* than when the initial phase employed *b* or *c* and the final phase *a* or *d*. In brief, greater separation of the food boxes at the initiation of the delay was conducive to greater accuracy than was greater separation at the time of the completion of the response; a greater distance between the choice objects throughout the delayed trial was more effective than a lesser distance.

Change in the absolute positions of the food covers was generally detrimental to success, suggesting that the animals, in performing delayed responses to spatially separated objects, react to both the "relative" and the "absolute" positions of the objects.

This can be concluded from the general nature of the results: (1) When food was presented under *a* or *d* and tested under *a* or *d*, responses were 87 per cent correct. (2) When *b* or *c* was used in both phases, the per cent of correct responses was 74. (3) When food was presented under *a* or *d* and tested under *b* and *c*, 73 per cent of the responses were correct. (4) When food was presented under *b* or *c* and tested under *a* or *d*, only 56 per cent of responses were correct.

Consider numbers 1 and 3. The same distance relationships are used in each case in initiating the delay but not in the completion of the response. And when the distance relationships change during the delay, the level of successes decreases. Successes are frequent (73 per cent) under these changed distance relationships, indicating that "relative" relationships of the objects of choice are responded to, but the decrease testifies to the significance of the "absolute" relationships existing between the objects of choice and other objects in their surroundings. "Absolute" refers to the distance between the objects, the position of the covers with respect to the board upon which they were placed, and other spatial relationships. The experiment which follows this one investigates further the details of "absolute" and "relative" factors in spatial types of delayed responses.

The experimenters draw the following conclusions regarding the significance of the distance between objects of choice in this sort of delayed reaction.

1. Eight mature chimpanzees made significantly higher scores in spatial delayed response when the food containers were 60 inches apart than when they were 5 inches apart.

2. The effectiveness of spatial separation was much greater at the time of baiting or presentation of the cue than at the time of response, at the end of the delay interval.

3. The results suggest that the animals responded to both the "relative" and "absolute" positions of the food containers.

4. Shifting the position of the food containers between baiting and response lowered the accuracy of the performance [p. 435].

III. SOME CHARACTERISTICS OF DELAYED RESPONSE: II. "RELATIVE" AND "ABSOLUTE" RELATIONSHIPS BETWEEN CHOICE OBJECTS

In a follow-up of the preceding experiment, Harrison and Nissen [3] analyzed in more detail the ways in which the substitute stimuli for delayed responses operated. The present experiment was designed to find out more about the "relative" and "absolute" features of the spatially separated objects of choice (food containers).

---

3 HARRISON, R. & NISSEN, H. W. The response of chimpanzees to relative and absolute positions in delayed response problems. *J. comp. Psychol.*, 1941, 31, 447–455. (Reproduced by permission of the American Psychological Association and the Williams & Wilkins Company.)

The problem is illustrated in the following way. Three food boxes might have these spatial relationships:

$$x \quad\quad y \quad\quad z$$

If only x and y are presented to the subject and he witnesses food being placed under y, and then, during the delay, the food cover x is removed and z is put into place, how will the subject respond after the delay to the situation y—z? An "absolute" response would be defined as a reaction to y, to the original object, in spite of the changed relationships of the objects of choice. Note that the food containers are identical in appearance, and this "absolute" response would be based upon the positions of y with respect to the board holding the food containers and other objects in the setting. A response to z would be a "relative" reaction, a response to the same spatial relationship between the objects of choice that existed when the delayed reaction was initiated.

Basically, this is the procedure that was employed by Harrison and Nissen. However, in different experimental settings, the distance separating the two food containers was varied. The apparatus was similar to that employed in the preceding study. The different settings were:

Setting 1 (food under c, distance 5 inches):			
Initial position	b	c	
Final position		c	d
Setting 2 (food under d, distance 5 inches):			
Initial position		d	e
Final position	c	d	
Setting 3 (food under b, distance 15 inches):			
Initial position	a	b	
Final position		b	e
Setting 4 (food under e, distance 15 inches):			
Initial position		e	f
Final position	b	e	

A 20-second interval of delay was used, and, after the subject observed the food being placed under the cover as indicated, the food containers were shifted while the board carrying them was screened from the subject. Actually, a slice of banana was placed under *both* food covers,.or under neither, for the test at the end of the delay to avoid training the animal to respond on either an "absolute" or "relative" basis. The experiment was not performed to discover whether or not chimpanzees could build up either or both types of delayed responses but to find out how they would respond at the time of the experiment.

EXPERIMENT A. Three adult chimpanzees served as subjects and were given 256 delayed-response trials with 128 trials on Setting 1 and 128 trials on Setting 2. All subjects responded predominantly to the "relative" positions of the food containers. That is, in Setting 1, they responded after the delay to *d* and in Setting 2 to *c*. About 80 per cent of the responses were of this "relative" sort.

EXPERIMENT B. Two of the chimps were given 640 trials on all four settings in mixed order, 160 trials on each. For Settings 1 and 2, responses again were predominantly "relative." However, with Settings 3 and 4, where the food covers were far apart, the majority of the responses were "absolute." Here the animals more often reacted to the original container in which food had been placed. It appeared that the distance separating the objects of choice was an important feature in determining whether or not responses were "relative" or "absolute."

EXPERIMENT C. With two chimpanzees serving as subjects, Settings 1 and 2 (smaller distance between food boxes) and Settings 3 and 4 (greater distance between food boxes) were presented in alternate sessions for a total of 256 trials with each pair of settings. Again, responses to Settings 1 and 2 were primarily "relative" and to Settings 3 and 4 predominantly "absolute."

EXPERIMENT D. This experiment was designed to see whether or not primarily "relative" responses (Settings 1 and 2) would be influenced by some obtrusive and constant landmark. A "barber pole" 7 inches high, painted with red and gray stripes, was fastened to the front edge at the center of the board carrying the food containers. When food covers *b* and *c* were presented in beginning a delayed trial, the barber pole was to the right of *c*. Then, when *c* and *d* were presented after the interval of delay, the pole was between the objects of choice.

Each of the three chimpanzees used in Experiment A received 64 trials with each of Settings 1 and 2 with the barber pole added to the stimulus setting. Responses were still predominantly to the "relative" positions of the objects, but the dominance of "relative" over "absolute" responses was much less than in Experiment A, being 67 per cent as compared with 80 per cent.

The results of the four experiments are summarized thus:

Seven adult chimpanzees were given a total of 3456 trials in spatial delayed response. By shifting the boxes during the delay interval, the experimenter gave the subject opportunity to respond to either relative or absolute position—that is, to the box which had the same position relative to the second box, or relative to stable features of the experimental situation, as had the container which was baited at the beginning of the trial.

The results show clearly that the type of response made was a function of the distance between the boxes. When the containers were close together, response was predominantly to relative position; when they were farther apart, response to absolute position was dominant.

The addition of a conspicuous and stable landmark to which the position of the baited container could be related somewhat increased the percentage of responses to absolute position. The data suggest, also, a possible generalization or interference of reaction tendencies to absolute *versus* relative position [p. 455].

IV. ANOTHER TYPE OF DELAYED RESPONSE IN THE CHIMPANZEE

The two preceding studies of delayed response required the chimpanzees to respond, after an interval of delay, to a spatial relationship between two objects of choice. In the experiment which follows, selected from a series of studies by Riesen and Nissen,[4] the initial phase of the delayed reaction brings the animal into contact with a colored light (either red or green). To complete the action satisfactorily the animal must, after a delay, respond to a second light of the same color as the original. Thus, the first light serves as a substitute stimulus for the second. (This is called the matching-from-sample technique.)

APPARATUS AND PROCEDURE. A box 27 inches wide, 15 inches high, 15 inches deep, was mounted on tracks so that it could be pushed against the wire netting of the animal cage or be withdrawn, out of reach, a distance of 10 inches. The side of the box facing the subject was a panel containing three windows of flashed opal glass, each 5 inches wide

---

4 RIESEN, A. H. & NISSEN, H. W. Non-spatial delayed response by the matching technique. *J. comp. Psychol.*, 1942, 34, 307-313. (Reprinted by permission of the authors, the American Psychological Association and the Williams & Wilkins Company.)

and 8 inches high; a space 5½ inches wide separated adjacent windows. Behind each window a 150 watt G. E. red or green bulb could be flashed on or off. These bulbs, being protected from extraneous illumination, could not be seen through the opal glass. The middle window was in fixed position; the two side windows could be moved back by the subject reaching through the cage netting with its fingers.

The animal was first trained to push that one of the two side windows the color of which (red or green) matched the color of the middle window. All the windows were lighted and the box was moved against the cage. If the subject pushed the window of matching color, a small piece of orange or banana automatically dropped down in front of the window. Incorrect choice was not rewarded. Correction in case of error (i.e., a second choice) was permitted only during the early part of training. After this problem was learned, the following changes in procedure were introduced in order: (1) The middle window was lighted first and the side lights were not turned on until the apparatus was in place for response. (2) The middle light was turned off just as the side lights were turned on. (3) The middle light was turned on for 5 seconds, then turned off. After a measured interval of time the side lights were turned on, ending the delay period, and, simultaneously, the apparatus was pushed forward into response position.

RESULTS. The time available for this experiment was limited (July 6 to Aug. 10, 1938). Training of Kambi, a nine-year-old adolescent female, was discontinued after 520 trials, that of Wendy, an adult female, after 460 trials. Neither animal had mastered the problem of responding to the matching color at the end of this training.

The third subject, Bimba, a preadolescent female, nine years old, completed all preliminary training in 640 trials. Step 3, as described above, was then introduced. The results of the delayed response tests may be summarized as follows: There were 40 trials (two sessions of 20 trials each) at each delay interval; percentage of correct responses at each of the delay intervals of 2 sec., 4 sec., 8 sec., 15 sec., and 20 sec., was 83 per cent, 90 per cent, 88 per cent, 78 per cent, and 75 per cent respectively. Each of these scores is reliably above chance (exceeding 50 per cent by 3.1 or more times the sigma$_p$ of 50 per cent) and perhaps would have been higher if the delays could have been lengthened more gradually.

It may be noted that of the 3 subjects Bimba alone had previously had extensive training in non-spatial delayed response. Other factors, however, may have been responsible for the individual differences observed. Kambi was in rather poor health during the course of the present experiment. Wendy's interest in the problem may have been attenuated by separation from her infant which was effected soon after the beginning of training [pp. 307–309].

V. AN ANALYSIS OF CERTAIN CUES IN THE DELAYED RESPONSE

J. W. Bowles, Jr.

In the experiment here summarized, MacCorquodale [5] analyzed some of the features of the stimulus for the delayed response in rats.

The apparatus consisted of a boxlike arrangement with four doors, each door being marked with a symbol—a cross, a vertical bar, a diagonal bar, or a horizontal bar. The rat was placed in the center on a false floor separated by a gap from the box. The rat had to jump this gap. During training, the size of this gap was increased until it equaled 20 centimeters. The rats became accustomed to jumping the gap through a doorway where the experimenter was tapping a food cup.

A hardware-cloth cylinder was placed over the rat on the jumping platform to prevent him from jumping until it was so desired.

As the animals learned to jump the increasing gap, the door was left less and less wide open so that they became adapted to hitting the door with their heads.

Delayed trials were then introduced. A rat was placed on the jumping platform inside the restraint cage. After about 30 seconds, the experimenter opened the door to be used far enough to get the food cup under it. He tapped on the food cup for about 15 seconds to attract the rat's attention. During this time the rat could see not only the food cup but also the symbol on the door.

The delay was timed from the closing of the door in front of the food cup to the raising of the restraint cage to permit the animal to respond. Delay also was measured from the lifting of the cage to the time when the rat jumped.

LENGTH OF DELAY.   Intervals of 5, 10, 15, and 30 seconds and

⁵ MacCorquodale, Kenneth. An analysis of certain cues in the delayed response. *J. comp. Physiol. Psychol.,* 1947, **40,** 239–253.

1, 2, and 4 minutes were tried. Even at the longest interval, there was no significant decline in the percentage of correct responses. The rats continued to jump to the door behind which the food had been placed about 50 per cent of the trials. (With four choices "chance" expectancy would be 25 per cent.) The best-performing rat was tried with longer intervals of delay, and successes were at the 50 per cent level with a 6-minute delay, at the 45 per cent level with an 8-minute delay, and again at the 50 per cent level with a 10-minute period of delay. In this last instance, the animal was returned to the living cage for 9 of the 10 minutes, obviating any possibility of gross postural orientation being a factor in the delay.

In no case was postural orientation observed in this experiment, contrary to the findings of the pioneer investigator in this field, W. S. Hunter. Rats did not assume an orientation toward the correct opening. Instead, they typically ran around the cage clockwise, counterclockwise, or both.

IMPORTANCE OF THE SYMBOLS. It had been claimed that various symbols on the doors might be important factors in determining success in the delayed response. This was not found to be the case. The door with the diagonal stripe was responded to more frequently than any others (total number of correct and incorrect responses), but there was no evidence that the door was better "structured" in Gestalt terminology. It did not form an inherently better perceptual field. Actually, the mechanism working the apparatus was behind this door, and the animals' attention was attracted by noises from it and the experimenter.

When a test was made of the number of *correct* responses to each door, no differences were found, i.e., no door was correctly responded to a disproportionate number of times. These and other tests strongly suggested that choices were not influenced by the markings on the doors. No door was "better" in this respect than any other, nor did any animal build up a preference for one door over another. The evidence indicated that the painting on the doors was not operating as a stimulus or a part of a stimulus complex.

In a second phase of the experiment, some modifications were introduced. After determining that an opaque hood dropped over the cage during the delay did not decrease the accuracy of the responses, the correct door was interchanged with one of the other three during the delay. Thus, if the food had been placed in the door with the horizontal bar, that door and the food might be moved to the space occupied by the door with the vertical bar, and the vertical-bar door placed over the originally correct opening. If the animal were differentiating the symbols, he should respond to the old door in its new position; if he were responding to the spatial relationships of the doors, he should jump to the old position with its new door.

On the first trials, it was found that 58 per cent of the responses were to the originally correct *opening* (a percentage consistent with the findings earlier in the study), indicating that the delayed responses were performed to the positions of the doors, and that the animals were not discriminating the symbols. This was further verified by the finding that approximately one third of the responses were to each of the other doors. The correct door in its new position was not responded to any more frequently than either of the other two. On succeeding trials, "reinforcement," i.e., food, was given if the rat responded correctly to a doorway whose position had been changed during the delay interval. Unless such successes were accidental, they would require that the animals respond to the various symbols and not to positional relationships of the doors. However, during the series of twenty trials, they never learned to perform delayed responses to the symbols.

In summary, the MacCorquodale experiment revealed that, at least in delayed-response experiments of this sort with rats as subjects, the conditions on the part of the stimulus which are of primary importance are the positional relationships among the objects of choice. Possible cues such as differential marking of the doors do not operate as stimulus variables if the rat has an opportunity to build up delayed responses on the basis of spatial relationships. It further indicated that gross postural orientations such as observed by Hunter are not essential for delayed responses in the rat.

VI. POSTHYPNOTIC SUGGESTIONS AND REMEMBERING

N. H. Pronko

When an individual ties a string around his finger in order to help him remember to do something and later looks at the string and remembers, "memory" [6] is not so difficult to understand. Almost everyone has been in situations in which he may have remembered to mail a letter, yet he could not say *what* made him remember. It is the manner of the operation of the more subtle substitute stimuli that we wish to explore in this section.

For our purposes, we may take a post hypnotic suggestion as a suitable illustration. During the hypnosis, which the subject has entered in a cooperative fashion from the moment he agreed to serve in that capacity, the subject's relationship to his surroundings are such that he is in excellent contact with certain stimuli at the expense of his contact with others. From the very beginning, at the suggestion of the experimenter, he attends to certain stimuli within very narrow limits, but, at the same time, he loses hold on certain others outside of the limits specified by the experimenter. Therefore, during the hypnosis, the subject is less active, less alert, and, consequently, not so critical or appreciative of happenings about him or even involving him as he normally is.

With this background, we are prepared to go ahead with a discussion of posthypnotic suggestion. Let us take the case of a person who, while in the hypnotic situation, is told that "when he wakes up" and hears the experimenter clear his throat, he will leave the room and get himself a drink of water from a certain fountain but he will not remember what made him do it. Note what we have done in this situation. Actually, we have designated a definite stimulus object (the water fountain) for the subject to react to in the future. At the same time, we have organized a definite water-drinking action to be performed in connection with the specified object. Furthermore, we have indicated the exact time at which the act should go off (i.e., when the experimenter

---

[6] The term "memory" is not meant to imply a stuff, substance, or function. Psychologists are becoming increasingly aware that in a scientific sense this word can be used to refer only to remembering *acts*.

clears his throat). All three variables have been related in such a way that the act is "primed" in advance of its occurrence.

According to expectations, after the hypnosis is over, our subject is talking with others when the experimenter clears his throat. He gets up somewhat hesitantly, leaves the room, is observed to do as directed, and returns. A remembering-behavior segment was completed, as indicated by his trip to the water fountain. Essentially, what happened was an organization of an action to be performed with a certain stimulus object as a substitute stimulus. Prearrangements for the functioning of these interrelated variables constitute the basic feature of remembering acts.

Incidentally, the subject's forgetting of the original suggestion is due to the different setting factors in the hypnotic and posthypnotic situations. The subject is in more or less discrete behavioral conditions in the two circumstances. And because the "remembering" goes from a less effective to a more effective behavioral condition, it is more likely to be consummated than the *recall* of the suggestion given to the subject by the experimenter (when the subject was in the hypnotic condition) after the hypnosis. In conclusion, neither hypnosis nor remembering need be considered mystical, since both can be understood in terms of all the variables involved, i.e. from empirical study.

VII. OTHER BEHAVIORS COMMONLY CALLED "REMEMBERING"

N. H. Pronko

The preceding sections have dealt with a reaction the essential features of which have been a continuity that has a beginning point, an interpolated time interval, and a completion at some time future to the beginning point. This *temporally integrated* behavior might well be represented as follows: Response initiated (interpolation of time interval or delay)—response completed.

As indicated early in this chapter, traditionally, other reactions than those with the characteristics described for remembering have been included under this category of behavior. As a help to the student, we include in the following sections an account of some studies of this type. They are intended for purposes of comparison and contrast. Regardless of his conclusions, the student will profit from a careful analysis of the reactions called forth in the situations to be described. We suggest that memorizing requires only a reperformance of previously acquired action, as when I ask you how much is two times two. Immediately, compare this with your action when I ask you *now* to meet me for dinner (not now) but *later* this evening. This will serve as a paradigm for the suggested "dissection" of the materials in the remaining sections.

VIII. A STUDY OF "ROTE MEMORY"

D. T. Herman

How rapidly can the order of a series of disconnected materials be memorized? Does variation in the conditions under which the individual works influence his speed of memorizing? Ebbinghaus, in 1885, began a series of studies centering about the questions. In addition, a large number of psychologists [7] since his time have found in these questions numerous interesting problems of both practical and theoretical importance.

Herman, Broussard, and Todd [8] attempted to determine the number of trials it would take to memorize a series of twelve pictures of common objects. Each picture (a chair, bucket, gun, dog, tree, and so on) was exposed on a screen one at a time for 0.1 second with a 2.9-second interval between exposures. College students were used as subjects. The subject was told, on the first time through the series, to notice each picture exposed and its order. On the second trial through the series, he was *to anticipate* each picture. Thus, when the experimenter said the word "ready," the subject was to name the first picture (if he could); when he saw the first picture, he was to name the second; when he saw the second, he was to name the third picture, and so forth. The procedure of the study was to go through the series of pictures as many times as was necessary for each subject to anticipate the entire series of pictures without error.

---

[7] McGEOCH, J. A. *The psychology of human learning.* New York: Longmans, 1942. Pp. 633.

[8] HERMAN, D. T., BROUSSARD, I. G. & TODD, H. R. A study of the effect of intertrial interval upon the rate of learning serial order picture material. *J. gen. Psychol.* (in press).

At first thought, the problem seems easy. Let us look at the results. Twenty subjects were used. On the average, 9.5 trials were taken to memorize the series, but college students show decided *individual differences* in memorizing the series. One subject memorized the series in 3 trials, while another took as many as 17 trials.

Would it be easier or harder to learn the series if it were in printed words rather than in picture form? Another randomly selected group of comparable college students was used in the same manner as the first group, but with this difference. The printed word for the object was used instead of the pictured object. This group showed an average of 12.2 trials to memorize the series. This is a significantly greater number of trials than was required by the group learning the picture series. Again, here *individual differences* were found. One subject took only 3 trials and another took as many as 19 trials.

Does it make any difference what the individual does between trials? At the end of each trial, that is, after the twelfth picture of the series was flashed, the group that averaged 9.5 trials to learn the series was told *"to rest"* for 20 seconds before the next trial. What if they were told to rehearse, to go over the series "in mind" for the 20-second interval? Would this help speed the memorizing? Herman, Broussard, and Todd ran tests on another comparable group under these conditions and found no reliable difference in the number of trials necessary to learn the series. Does this mean that the "rest" subjects actually used the 20-second interval to rehearse? The investigators concluded that they did.

Still another question was raised to throw light on the conditions of memorizing. What if the subjects were prevented from using the 20-second interval at the close of each trial for rehearsal? This could be effectively done by requiring a group of subjects to read aloud from a book for each 20-second interval. A test run in this manner showed a reliable increase to an average of 13.5 trials to memorize the picture series. And here again, marked individual differences were found. The fastest subject learned in 6 trials, while the slowest subject took 23 trials. It appears clear from these findings that speed of memorizing is subject to a number of variables. As with other questions in psychology, when we ask, "How fast can a person memorize?" the answer is, "Under what conditions?"

IX. SPEED OF MEMORIZING AND COMPLEXITY OF LEARNING MATERIALS

D. T. Herman

Herman and Broussard [9] sought to determine the effect of progressively increasing the complexity of the material to be learned upon speed of memorizing. Simultaneously with the exposure of each of a series of twelve pictures, subjects had a tone of high or low pitch sound in their ears through earphones. Subjects were instructed that, after the first time through the series of pictures and tones, they were to "anticipate" (see the preceding selection) both picture and tone until they could "anticipate" the entire series without error. Under these conditions, subjects took 18.8 trials on the average to memorize the series of picture and tone stimuli. How many trials would it take for pictures alone and for tones alone? Two groups of subjects tested under the conditions took 9.5 trials and 8.3 trials, respectively. Would the same be true if subjects learned the picture series alone or the tone series alone while they were given both the picture and tone stimuli? Under these conditions, pictures were memorized in an average of 10.9 trials, and tones were memorized in an average of 8.8 trials.

Interesting findings result from these data. Learning of pictures and tones together takes 18.8 trials on the average. Learning pictures alone and tones alone *totals* 17.8 trials on the average. Learning each series alone while the other is presented *totals* 19.7 trials on the average. The two figures for totals, 17.8 and 19.7 trials, approximate very closely the trials taken to memorize the two series together, 18.8 trials. Does this mean that the number of trials taken to learn the two series together is merely the sum of the trials taken to learn the two series separately? The data of this study would seem to support such a proposition. Would the same be true for other series? The investigators leave the answer to this question to further research.

9 HERMAN, D. T. & BROUSSARD, I. G. A study in the learning of two types of serial order materials presented simultaneously. *J. gen. Psychol.* (in press).

X. STUDIES IN THE RETENTION OF MEMORIZED MATERIALS

D. T. Herman

Once a subject has learned a list of discrete materials, how long does he retain it? For how long a period afterward, without intervening contact with the materials or practice of them, will he be able to reproduce the responses he learned? In the main, Ebbinghaus' pioneer work on these questions has been confirmed by subsequent experiments. Ebbinghaus used nonsense syllables (in German). He learned lists of syllables and, at varying periods subsequent to the learning sessions, he would relearn each list. Thus, 24 hours after training list A, he would relearn it. On original learning, it took him 15 trials and on relearning it took him 4 trials. Ebbinghaus assumed a savings, that is, a retention, as indicated by the 6-trial difference for the two learnings. Thus, a 60 per cent "savings" is a measure of the amount retained in this case.

Ebbinghaus learned a large number of lists of syllables. For each, he gave himself a definite time interval before he relearned it. He did this in order to determine the savings as a function of the interval before relearning. For some lists, he relearned after a few minutes; for other lists, he relearned after a longer period, stretching for as long as 31 days after original learning. On the basis of these studies, Ebbinghaus developed his classic "curve of retention."

The curve (for meaningless syllables) showed that soon after learning the forgetting was rapid. Thus, about 42 per cent was forgotten within the first 19 minutes after learning. After 24 hours, about 64 per cent was forgotten, and after 48 hours, about 73 per cent. But after this, less was forgotten per unit of time. After 3 days only slightly more than 73 per cent was forgotten; after 6 days approximately 75 per cent. After 31 days, the longest period that Ebbinghaus used, 75 to 80 per cent was forgotten. It is this *decreasing rate of forgetting* per unit of time that characterizes the so-called "curve of retention." Other investigators have found the same to be true for retention of nonsense-syllable learning.

Whitely and McGeoch [10] used poetry instead of nonsense syllables. Six stanzas of unfamiliar poetry were studied for 15 minutes. The amount learned in 15 minutes of study was taken as 100 per cent. After 15 days, 26 per cent was forgotten. Another group of subjects were tested for retention after 30 days, and approximately 58 per cent had been forgotten. But after this, up to 120 days, forgetting was at a slower rate. In 90 days, 60 per cent had been forgotten, and in 120 days, 70 per cent.

Dietze and Jones [11] showed retention curves of much the same sort for the important content of an article which they read just once. After 1 day, they forgot about 25 per cent; after 10 days, about 40 per cent was forgotten, and after 30 days, about 50 per cent; after 150 days only very slightly more than 50 per cent was forgotten. Jones [12] showed that the retention curve of students on the content of college lecture material was much the same in form as that found by Ebbinghaus and others.

XI. A STUDY IN RETENTION OF HUMAN MAZE LEARNING

Tsai [13] studied the retention of a learned maze pattern over a period of 9 weeks after learning. Subjects were blindfolded and with a stylus traced through a complex pathway. At many points, the pathway led into blind alleys from which the subject had to retrace his movements to get back onto the correct pathway to the goal. Through trial-and-error learning, subjects eventually reached the criterion of 3 successive, errorless trials. At varying intervals, from 1 to 9 weeks after learning, subjects were asked to trace through the pathway again to determine how well they retained the responses. A curve of retention similar to that for verbal responses was found. Subjects tested after 1 week showed

10 WHITELY, P. L. & McGEOCH, J. A. The curve of retention for poetry. *J. educ. Psychol.*, 1928, 19, 471–479.

11 DIETZE, A. G. & JONES, G. E. Factual memory of secondary school pupils for a short article which they read a single time. *J. educ. Psychol.*, 1931, 22, 586–598, 667–676.

12 JONES, G. E. Experimental studies of college teaching. *Arch. Psychol.*, N.Y., 1923, 10, No. 68.

13 TSAI, C. A comparative study of retention curves for motor habits. *Comp. Psychol. Monogr.*, 1924, No. 2, 29 p.

approximately 5 per cent errors, those tested after 3 weeks showed approximately 15 per cent errors, but subjects tested from 3 to 9 weeks after learning continued to show approximately 15 per cent errors.

XII. THE AMOUNT RETAINED DEPENDS UPON HOW RETENTION IS MEASURED

As with other forms of psychological activity, the amount of learned material that is retained depends upon specific conditions. To the question, "How much can one remember?" the answer of the psychologist is, "Under what conditions?"

Luh [14] had several groups of subjects learn a list of twelve nonsense syllables by the method of anticipation. He tested them for retention at intervals of from 20 minutes to 48 hours after learning. Five methods of testing for retention were used: (1) *recognition,* by which the subject was given new syllables which he had not learned as well as those he had learned, and he was asked to select those that he had learned; (2) *relearning,* by which the subject was to relearn the list and calculate retention from the savings; (3) *reconstruction,* by which the subject arranged mixed-up syllables in their proper order; (4) *written reproduction,* by which the subject wrote in proper order all the syllables that he recalled; and (5) *anticipation,* which was the method used in the original learning. The following figures show the amount forgotten after 48 hours as determined by each method of studying retention.

Method	Amount Forgotten (Approximate, per cent)
Recognition	25
Relearning	48
Reconstruction	58
Written reproduction	80
Anticipation	90

This article does not imply that it is impossible to determine the stability of learned reactions. Rather, it means that the answer always depends upon which of the operations listed above was employed. Different methods give vastly different answers.

[14] Luh, C. W. The conditions of retention. *Psychol. Monogr.,* 1922, **31**, No. 3, 87 p.

15

LEARNING

I. LEARNED REACTIONS VERSUS WHAT?
N. H. Pronko

Psychologists of a bygone era grew excited over the problem of which reactions were "acquired" or learned and which were "inherited." Either long, intermediate, or short but variable lists of responses which he considered "native" were compiled by each writer. It is suggested that these early workers fell into the error of their ways through failure to arrive at a distinction between behavioral and physiological data in the manner indicated in the early chapters of this book.

Without going into lengthy discussion at this point, we simply indicate that the contents of physiology books are nothing like those of psychology textbooks. The former deal with such topics as respiration, circulation, digestion, and excretion. The latter are typically concerned with learning, remembering, forgetting, hating, loving, imagining, reasoning, and so on. The subject matters are, therefore, distinct. Should one identify them in his *interpretation* of the different data, the validity of such a procedure can be empirically checked.

As developed here, all behavior (i.e., reactions showing the six characteristics of modifiability, delayability, variability, integration, differentiation, and inhibition) can be traced back to a beginning point for every individual. Without exception, none of the complex psychological reactions that the reader now possesses was performed as such at birth or in the uterus. For each, there was a point of origin and elaboration. Therefore, since we find no inherited *psychological* action and can furthermore operationally account for all evolution of behavior during the in-

373

dividual's reactional biography, the term "learning" loses the meaning that was attached to it in bygone times. As a matter of fact, a thorough study of the field of learning is as broad as psychology itself. We can use the term meaningfully, however, for certain techniques for bringing about the coordination or connection of stimulus with response.

Obviously, for every organism there are objects which, before he is confronted with them, do not function as stimulus objects. Either rapidly (one-trial learning) or more gradually, responses become elaborated so that they operate when the organism is brought into contact with such stimuli. The degree and manner of coordination between stimuli and responses are, of course, dependent upon many variables. It is apparent that the age and species of the organism, its health status, condition of fatigue, hunger, thirst, disease, injuries, and the like, will play a role in determining how thoroughly stimulus-response coordinations occur and are reperformed after their coordination.

Other variables may be located on the side of the stimulus object. These include size, shape, intensity, or number of presentations of the stimulus objects. Setting factors such as illumination, air, temperature, objects, or persons in the surroundings comprise still another set of conditions.

In recent years, laboratory studies of human and infrahuman animal learning have proceeded apace and have contributed richly to our understanding of the many variables operating in acquisition of behavior. It is with the special intent of calling attention to the complexity of behavioral events that the following studies of learning are included in the present chapter.

II. THE EFFECT OF SURROUNDINGS ON MAZE LEARNING [1]

J. W. Bowles, Jr.

In order to determine the effect of maze surroundings upon maze learning, Walthall arranged a setting in which the extramaze features were radially symmetrical about the center of the maze. This was accomplished by placing around the maze a "dome" 18

[1] WALTHALL, J. WILSON, JR. The influence of different maze surroundings on learning. *J. compar. and physiol. Psychol.*, 1948, 41, 438–449. (Reproduced by permission of the author and the American Psychological Association.)

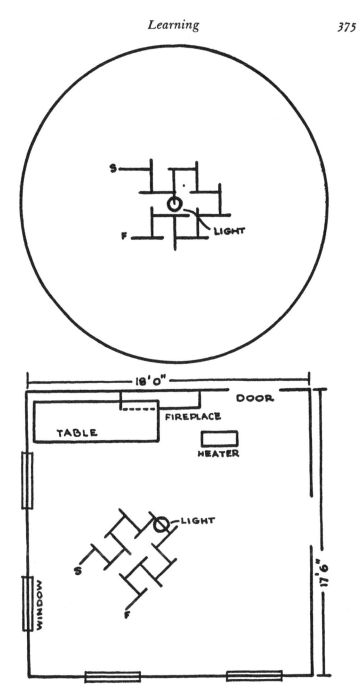

FIG. 47 *Top.* Position of the maze in the dome. *Bottom.* Position of the maze in the room. (Walthall, J. Wilson, Jr., The influence of different maze surroundings on learning.)

feet in diameter which arched to the center so as to rise to a maximum height of 8 feet above the maze. Another setting, a heterogeneously structured environment, was furnished by the experimental room, the arrangement of which is indicated in the figure. A comparison of the two surroundings is thus made possible.

Animals (white rats) were given one trial per day. They were first transferred from the home cage to another similar cage which was placed on the floor just beyond the start of the maze. Only the cage of animals being run was in the experimental room at any one time. The home cage, with twenty-four hours' ration of Purina Chow in it, was placed on the floor just beyond the finish point of the maze. The animals were placed on the maze one at a time. As soon as they reached the finish point they were lifted from the maze and placed in the home cage containing food pellets. Retracing was prevented by the withdrawal of a preceding maze unit if the animal started to retrace, and only one entrance into any one cul was counted for a given trial. An error was scored if the experimenter estimated that the animal's snout had reached a point midway between the choice-point and the end of the cul, and the record for each trial indicated the individual culs entered by each animal. Both the groups and the individuals within groups were run in random order from day to day.

There were two general groups of animals. For one group, designated D, the maze was placed in the dome; for the other group, designated R, the maze was placed in the room. The two general groups were composed of sub-groups, each sub-group consisting of sixteen animals. One sub-group of each general group was given three successive tests of eight trials each without having had any previous experience with the maze. Each remaining sub-group of the general group was given an eight-trial test prior to which it had run on the maze eight, sixteen, or thirty-two times in the other environment [p. 441].

Table 18 shows the average number of errors per animal per day for each of the test periods as well as the averages for the dome and the room general groups. These points stand out. The animals that were run in the dome surroundings, with or without previous experience in the same maze with room surroundings, made a higher number of errors both as individual animals and as a group. This difference is a statistically significant one. Both the means of the dome tests as well as those of the room

Table 18

Schedule of Tests and Mean

		Mean
Do	Eight-trial test in dome, no previous experience with maze	5.02
Dr8	Eight-trial test in dome, 8 prior runs in room	3.58
Dr16	Eight-trial test in dome, 16 prior runs in room	3.10
Dr32	Eight-trial test in dome, 32 prior runs in room	3.00
Dd8 *	Eight-trial test in dome, 8 prior runs in dome	2.95
Dd16 †	Eight-trial test in dome, 16 prior runs in dome	1.42
Ro	Eight-trial test in room, no previous experience with maze	4.62
Rd8	Eight-trial test in room, 8 prior runs in dome	2.86
Rd16	Eight-trial test in room, 16 prior runs in dome	2.68
Rd32	Eight-trial test in room, 32 prior runs in dome	2.28
Rr8 ‡	Eight-trial test in room, 8 prior runs in room	1.61
Rr16 §	Eight-trial test in room, 16 prior runs in room	0.77
Mean dome		3.18
Mean room		2.47

* Same animals as DO.
† Same animals as DO and Dd8.
‡ Same animals as RO.
§ Same animals as RO and Rr8.

tests run in a descending order corresponding to the previous maze running of the animal. Furthermore, the average of each dome group is higher than that of the corresponding room group. The assertion seems justified that variation of the room-dome variable definitely affected the stimulus-response integration of the two groups of animals. According to Walthall, this hypothesis is supported by (1) difference in the averages of the test scores, (2) qualitative differences in the form of the test learning curves, and (3) differences in the factors determining the order of cul difficulty. These three probable effects may be most parsimoniously attributed to the heterogeneity of structure of visual stimuli in the room.

CONCLUSIONS. Under the conditions of this experiment, it appears probable that the following conclusions are justified.

1. The experimental variable which is a function of dome environment *vs.* room environment is a matter of symmetry *vs.* heterogeneity of the extra-maze visual stimuli.

2. Variation between symmetry and heterogeneity of the extra-maze visual stimuli is accompanied by:

    a. Quantitative differences in the means of test scores;

    b. Qualitative differences in the form of the test learning curves;

  c. Differences in the factors determining the order of difficulty of the culs.

 3. The transposition of practice effect is greater when transposition is from symmetrical to heterogeneous than when it is from heterogeneous to symmetrical extra-maze visual stimuli [p. 448].

The significance of this experiment lies in pointing out the importance of surroundings in learning. Rats are sensitive to setting factors, as indicated by the differences in learning results. There is no reason for thinking that it would be different with a roomful of pupils instructed to learn a spelling list. Teacher-in-the-room does not give the same results as teacher-out-of-the-room. Both groups of subjects show a sensitivity to their surroundings.

III. AN ILLUSTRATION OF THE SPECIFICITY OF LEARNING

J. W. Bowles, Jr.

A maze learning experiment performed by Grice [2] illustrates the specificity of learning. He used 23 albino rats as subjects, and the apparatus consisted of the simple T-maze. In the preliminary training period, the subjects were first deprived of water for 20 hours and then placed in one of the goal boxes, which had been removed from the apparatus, and allowed to drink for 15 minutes. On the second day, following another 20 hours of water deprivation, the animals were given four trials in running an alley to a goal box and were allowed to drink for 10 seconds upon entering the goal box. Each goal box was employed twice in this training.

 Following this preliminary training, the animals were introduced to the experimental maze. They were given four trials per day for 12 days, always under 20 hours of water deprivation. Food was always available in their cages to eliminate hunger as a variable. The daily trials were run in this order: Trial 1 was a free choice; the animal was allowed to enter either goal box at the end of the T-maze. In the second trial, by means of closed doors, the animal was forced to go to the side opposite his first choice. Trial 3 was again a free choice. In Trial 4, the rat was forced to the side

---

 [2] GRICE, G. R. An experimental test of the expectation theory of learning. *J. comp. physiol. Psychol.*, 1948, 41, 137–143. (Reproduced by permission of the author and the American Psychological Association.)

opposite that chosen on the third trial. This procedure resulted in an equal number of runs to each side every day.

Both goal boxes were fitted with water bottles. The entire floor of the left goal box was covered with food; the animals had to walk over the food to get to the water bottle, and they stood on the food while drinking. None of the animals picked up or nibbled the food, but most of them sniffed at it and pushed it with their noses. There could be no doubt that the rats had visual, olfactory, and tactual contacts with the food each time they entered the left goal box. During these experimental sessions the subjects were allowed to drink for approximately 5 seconds before being removed from the goal box.

After the 12-day training period under thirst conditions, the animals were satiated for water and shifted to a 24-hour food deprivation. Water was constantly available in the cages, but the water bottles were removed from the goal boxes. For one half of the rats the food was left in the left goal box as it had been during the original training series; for the other half it was shifted to the right goal box.

There were four trials per day in this training series, all trials being free choices. Training was continued until the rats ran seven out of eight consecutive trials to food. The animals were allowed to eat for 10 seconds when they entered the box containing food, or to remain for 10 seconds in the incorrect box if they entered that one.

The first trial after the shift to 24-hour food deprivation was regarded as a test trial for the subjects. Notice that up to this time the rats had all been subjected to the same conditions. They had been running the maze under water deprivation for 12 days and had been forced to walk across the food in the left-hand box to get to the water bottle two times each day. How would they react to the maze now that they were deprived of food? (The shift of the food to the right goal box in the case of half the subjects would not influence the running of this first trial under food deprivation.)

On the first trial after the change to the hunger condition, 12 of the 23 animals (52 per cent) took the left-hand path which had led to food during the training under thirst conditions, while 11 subjects (48 per cent) took the right path which had led only to water. The difference in the two percentages is, of course, insignificant. Here the specificity of stimulus-response connections is clearly illustrated. The animals, in running the maze under water deprivation, had failed to build up responses to the food stimuli so that, when deprived of food, they did not run to the goal box that had contained food during the training under thirst conditions. If such "incidental" learning had taken place, 100 per cent of the rats should have gone to the left goal box on the first trial under food deprivation.

That no learning had taken place with regard to the food stimuli was further demonstrated by the finding that the learning of the correct response to food under hunger conditions was no more rapid for the subgroup for whom the food remained in the left-hand goal box than it was for the subgroup that had to learn to run to the right goal box.

In summary, when rats were "exposed" to food objects while running a T-maze under water deprivation, they failed to acquire responses to the food objects. When running the maze under food deprivation, of course, they quickly learned the correct response to the goal box containing food. Stimulus-response connections are thus shown to be specific to the conditions of the learning situation.

IV. HUNGER AND THIRST AS CONDITIONS INFLUENCING LEARNING
J. W. Bowles, Jr.

Kendler [3] has investigated the effect of hunger and thirst on learning in rats by comparing the relative performances of hungry and thirsty animals with satiated ones in learning the simple T-maze. The question put to experimental test was this: Will two groups of animals, one hungry and thirsty and the other satiated, learn a T-maze with equal facility if they both have the same experience with food and water? Or will food and water in the goal boxes work in such a way as to speed up the learning of the hungry and thirsty animals?

Thirty-two white rats served as subjects. On their first contact with the maze, they were allowed to explore it freely for 1

---

[3] KENDLER, H. H. A comparison of learning under motivated and satiated conditions in the white rat. *J. exp. Psychol.*, 1947, **37**, 545–549.

hour. No food or water was available in the maze during this time. On the second day, the animals were given two trials under the same conditions, except that as the animal passed through the maze, doors were lowered so that retracing was impossible.

After these initial contacts with the maze, the subjects were divided into two groups. One group of 20 rats (Group M) was both hungry and thirsty, having been deprived of both food and water for approximately 21 hours. The second group (Group S) of 12 rats was satiated for food and water. Food and water were constantly available in the living cages of this group, and additional food and water consumption was encouraged an hour before the daily trials. This was accomplished by placing a different food and additional water in the living cages. That this group was satiated is indicated by the fact that none of the subjects attempted to eat while in the maze.

During the training trials for both groups, M and S, food was present in one goal box of the T-maze and water in the other. Approximately one half of the animals in both groups had food in the left goal box and water in the right. For the other rats this was reversed, as a check on positional effects.

The training series consisted of four runs in the maze each day for 7 days. The training for both groups was the same except for the difference in conditions of hunger and thirst. The first trial on each day was a free choice; the animal could turn into either of the two goal boxes. The second run was a forced trial; by means of a closed door the animal was forced to go to the box opposite the one that he had gone to on the first trial. Trial 3 was a repetition of Trial 1, while Trial 4 was again a forced trial to the side opposite that selected in Trial 3.

Group M animals were allowed to eat for 20 seconds in the goal box containing food and to drink about 10 swallows of water in the goal box containing water. The rats in Group S were kept in either goal box for about 30 seconds, although they neither ate nor drank. Since food was scattered about the floor of the food box and the Group S animals were brought into contact with the nozzle of the water bottle before removal from the water box, all animals definitely came into contact with food in one box and water in the other. The forced trials made these contacts the same in number for all animals in both groups.

The questions to be answered were: Would the satiated

animals, given the same number of trials with the food and water boxes when they were not hungry, go to the proper box when they were subsequently deprived of food or water? Would they, when hungry, go directly to the food box and when thirsty to the water box, as a result of their incidental experiences before? How would they compare with the group which had learned to run the maze under conditions of hunger and thirst? If learning the positions of the food and water was merely "incidental," a function of having come into direct contact with these objects in their respective boxes, there should be no difference between Groups M and S. On the other hand, if hunger and thirst were organismic setting factors influencing learning, Group M should be decidedly superior.

The test trials contrived to answer these questions consisted of one run per day for 4 successive days. Animals in both groups were treated in the same manner. On the first and third days, some rats in both groups were hungry when put into the maze, and some were thirsty. On the second and fourth days, rats that had run the maze under conditions of hunger now did so under thirst, and vice versa.

The results of these test trials showed marked group differences. Subjects trained under conditions of hunger and thirst learned much more than the other group. The average number of errors for the subjects of Group M was 0.60. Group S subjects showed 1.33 average errors. This difference was found to be statistically as well as behaviorally significant. Furthermore, 50 per cent of Group S rats made 2 errors in the test trials, but only 20 per cent of Group M animals made this many errors. Of the Group M rats, 60 per cent made no errors, but only 17 per cent of the rats in Group S made 4 errorless runs. It must be concluded that, in the learning here investigated, hunger and thirst definitely influenced the efficiency with which maze-running reactions are acquired. Operationally, they can be said to constitute variables in a psychological situation.

V. A STUDY OF PROACTIVE AND RETROACTIVE INHIBITION
N. H. Pronko

Learn task A, then learn task B. You will find that because B was learned after A, there will be an interference effect of B on A. This interference of a second task on a previously acquired one has been called "retroactive inhibition." The term "retroactive" relates the inhibition to previous learning.

It has also been shown experimentally that the *prior* learning of a task will have an interference effect on the learning of another task. This forward interference has been called "proactive inhibition." Except for the present or future time involved, they are essentially the same and show that S-R units are not acquired in isolation. In fact, they affect each other. These, then, are also variables in learning situations.

In an experiment by Underwood,[4] subjects were presented with lists of pairs of adjectives (paired-associates), e.g., happy-purple, wicked-fruitful, and so on. They were to learn which pairs of adjectives belonged together, so that upon subsequent test, when only "happy" was presented, the subject would respond with "purple," and so on down the list. These word lists were presented by means of a memory drum, a device for exposing a single word or word group at a time.

Both groups of subjects learned word lists that might be represented with the following pairs: happy-purple; happy-busy. That is, "happy" was used as the stimulus in both situations. But in Situation I, they were required to respond with "purple"; in Situation II, with "busy."

The subjects studied for proactive inhibition were put through Situation I and Situation II as described above. Following a rest interval, they were tested for the response they had learned in Situation II.

Subjects studied for retroactive inhibition went through the same procedure but after a period of time were tested for the retention of the response they had learned in Situation I. Testing for retention was by means of the method of recall and the savings

---

4 UNDERWOOD, B. J. Retroactive and proactive inhibition after five and forty-eight hours. *J. exp. Psychol.*, 1948, **38**, 29–38.

method. Recall consists in reproducing the response as previously learned. The savings method compares the number of trials necessary to achieve stable learning again with the number of trials required in the original learning of the material. Between the learning and test sessions, the experimenter used two different time intervals, one of 5 hours and the other of 48 hours.

Results showed that after a 5-hour interval, effects of proactive inhibition were less than those of retroactive inhibition. In other words, retaining the second set of responses was superior to the retention of the first. But, after the 48-hour interval, retention was essentially the same for both proactive and retroactive inhibition. This means that the list learned second could be recalled as well as the list learned first after this time interval.

In brief, Underwood found that after a short time interval between learning and recall, subjects had more trouble (greater retroactive inhibition) in recalling originally learned lists than they did subsequently learned lists. With longer rest intervals, this difference disappeared. These results show that the time variable and the conditions of learning and retention are important features of the interference effects labeled "pro-" and "retroactive inhibition."

Effects of proactive and retroactive inhibition can best be interpreted, perhaps, in terms of interference of reaction systems. In learning situations which have a rather close temporal relationship, and which require similar sorts of responses to similar or identical stimulus objects, reaction systems acquired for the first learning situation may interfere with later tests of learning of the second situation (proactive inhibition). Reaction systems operating in the second learning situation may later interfere with tests of retention of the first learning (retroactive inhibition).

Such interference effects will occur when reaction systems are not adequately organized with respect to the learning situations in which they operated. When stimulus-response coordinations are exceedingly well integrated, then pro- and retroactive effects of inhibition are minimized. This occurs when the subject "overlearns." At any rate, the study described above does show in an empirical way that the series of stimulus-response units in a learning situation are themselves variables in such situations. The results of this study have implications for such everyday situations as studying and training for a job.

VI. THE ROLE OF PUNISHMENT IN A
LEARNING SITUATION
N. H. Pronko

What result will punishment have on learning? If animals are put into a choice compartment and shocked on incorrect or correct responses, how effectively will they learn? If they respond to a lighted alley and receive food but also shock, will they learn better or worse than do those that are shocked when they enter a dark alley and are given food for entering a lighted alley? And how will these two groups compare with rats rewarded in the lighted alley and frustrated in the dark alley? Reduced to its simplest elements, this is what Wischner [5] did in a laboratory experiment which was designed to shed light on the effect of punishment on learning.

Group I, the shock-right group, then, received both shock and food on entering the choice alley that was lighted and received nothing in the dark alley. Group II received shock on entering the dark alley and food on entrance into the lighted alley (shock-wrong animals). The no-shock animals of Group III received food for entering the lighted alley but were frustrated in the dark alley. If all three groups learn with equal facility, then it may be said that punishment has no effect on learning.

RESULTS. The results of Wischner's experiment did, however, show different results among the three groups. Whether we consider the number of trials required to master the problem or the errors made during learning, the groups perform very differently. The shock-wrong group (food for entering light alley and shock for entering the dark alley) was superior to the others. The average number of trials required to learn was 104 and the average error was only 24.2. The group that received nothing in the dark alley and food in the illuminated one (the no-shock group) was next best in performance. It required 152 trials to learn and made 54.6 errors on the average. The shock-right group that received both shock and food on going to the illuminated alley did worst. The average number of trials here was 159, and the average errors rose to 71.3.

---

[5] WISCHNER, G. J. The effect of punishment on discrimination learning in a non-correction situation. *J. exp. Psychol.*, 1947, **37**, 271–284.

These results are interpreted as follows. Where food is connected with the "correct" response and shock with the "wrong" one, the corresponding approach and avoidant responses become easily connected with their clean-cut stimuli. That is what happened in the case of the shock-wrong group. The no-shock group had no distinctive response to perform to the dark alley but a clearly defined, food-approach reaction to the lighted compartment. Apparently, this was a more favorable situation than that of the shock-right group. The latter group was involved in a frustrating situation which *simultaneously* evoked food-getting and shock-avoiding reactions. It is remarkable that the group learned to make the correct response at all. The way in which it achieved the adjustment is interesting. Wischner's observations show that the rats of this group would typically get set before the lighted alley. Then, with a "hop, skip, and a jump," they would clear the electric grid with a single, quick contact and head for the food. Says the author: "It is highly probable that this acquired mode of adjustment lessened the pain stimulation and decreased the potency of the shock stimulus as a determining factor in the situation" [p. 282].

VII. AN EXAMPLE OF CONDITIONED LEARNING AND "SENSORY PRECONDITIONING"

N. H. Pronko

In a typical conditioning experiment, a shock to the organism calls forth a withdrawal response. If a tone is paired with the shock for a number of trials, conditioning is established so that tone alone, except for only occasional reinforcement with shock, will elicit the withdrawal response. Suppose, however, that before we do any conditioning, we simply present the organism with light and tone for 10 trials—no shock. Then we proceed to condition him as described above. After having conditioned the withdrawal response to tone, will the light also elicit this response?

This is essentially what Karn [6] did. He worked with two groups of 12 subjects each. The experimental group was brought

[6] KARN, H. W. Sensory pre-conditioning and incidental learning in human subjects. *J. exp. Psychol.*, 1947, **37**, 540–544.

into a dark room and seated before a panel. An electric light and a buzzer were mounted on this panel. Each subject was asked to sit before the apparatus and to look at the light. Light and buzzer were presented simultaneously for 2 seconds. Fifty such presentations were given, and the subjects were told when to come to the laboratory for a second (the conditioning) session.

Of course, it is understood that the control group did not take part in the procedure described above. Now both groups were submitted to a conditioning procedure. The light-buzzer panel was used. In addition, an apparatus for conditioning a finger-withdrawal response was used. This consisted of a diaphragm upon which the subject placed his middle finger, with the palm of his hand resting upon an electrode. The electrode delivered an adequate, but not intense, shock. The subject could avoid it by lifting his finger.

Conditioning of the finger withdrawal was then begun by presenting the sound 1 to 3 seconds before the shock. When the subject gave 5 successive responses to buzzer alone (without a shock), conditioning was discontinued. Then, without warning, both groups of subjects were presented with the light. Only the experimental group had experienced this light at the time it was pre-experimentally paired with the sound but without shock.

RESULTS. The number of trials necessary to reach conditioning was not essentially different. The experimental group that had had buzzer and light presented before conditioning required an average of 15 trials. The control group average was 14.7. Karn does not believe that conditioning was affected by the experimental group's preliminary experience with buzzer and light in combination.

The most interesting point is the difference in the way the two groups responded to the 10 presentations of light alone following conditioning. Table 19 shows that the experimental group of 12 subjects reacted to the light stimulus (never associated with shock) a total of 75 times out of a possible maximum of 120 responses. Compare this performance with that of the control group that had *not* experienced the light-buzzer combination before the conditioning sessions. There were only 9 responses to the light out of a possible total of 120 responses. Out of 12 subjects in this group, 8 failed to respond at all during the 10 test trials. It is important to point out, too, that of the 4 control subjects who did respond to light alone, 3 gave this response toward the end of the series. Without exception, every experimental subject responded on the first trial if he responded at all.

Table 19

Results Obtained from Experimental and Control Subjects

	Experimental Group			Control Group	
Subject	Trials to Condition	Responses to Light (Maximum Possible, 10)	Subject	Trials to Condition	Responses to Light (Maximum Possible, 10)
Male	12	10	Male	11	0
Male	17	0	Male	16	2
Male	21	2	Male	31	4
Male	8	10	Male	13	0
Male	16	6	Male	10	0
Male	22	8	Male	9	1
Female	9	7	Female ...	13	0
Female	8	0	Female ...	26	0
Female	16	10	Female ...	12	0
Female	13	6	Female ...	12	2
Female	27	6	Female ...	12	0
Female	11	10	Female ...	12	0
Total		75	Total		9

This experiment shows in a definite, operational or empirical manner some of the ways in which responses and stimuli get connected. If two stimuli are experienced together in some fashion, and later a different response is performed to one of those stimuli, there is a similar relationship established between the latter response and the second stimulus. The following diagram is an attempt to present this interconnection graphically.

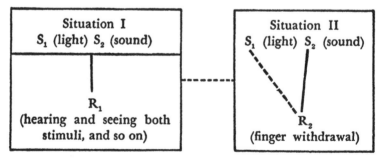

Situation I
S₁ (light) S₂ (sound)

R₁
(hearing and seeing both stimuli, and so on)

Situation II
S₁ (light) S₂ (sound)

R₂
(finger withdrawal)

The first situation represents the discriminatory, attitudinal, and other possible reactions to the light-sound stimuli. Situation II represents the definite withdrawal response connected with the sound stimulus. The dotted line shows the somewhat indirect relationship of this withdrawal response to the light stimulus. This relationship is intersituational rather than intrasituational. The response connection to the two stimuli in Situation II is a function of the connection of these two stimuli in Situation I.

In our opinion, the important point of this study is the insight it gives into the apparently intricate relationship between the various stimuli on the one hand and responses on the other, as well as between stimuli and responses in accounting for stimulus-response connections in learning.

VIII. LEARNING WITH AND WITHOUT INCENTIVE
J. W. Bowles, Jr.

From the introductory remarks to this chapter and the preceding sections, one should be able to predict that learning may be facilitated through the operational manipulation of the many factors present in the learning situation. This means, then, that such variables would operate to connect response and stimulus more readily, more effectively, or for a longer period of time than when they are absent.

The study [7] here reported investigated the retention of nonsense syllables learned under two different experimental conditions. Two groups of subjects, students in two different elementary psychology classes, were used. Both groups were presented with the following list of twenty nonsense syllables:

1. MOF	6. KIV	11. HIF	16. BOF
2. POB	7. JAT	12. DEJ	17. VAD
3. MEF	8. WOX	13. BIW	18. TUD
4. FUB	9. FOV	14. VAW	19. NAX
5. YAF	10. YIL	15. LAJ	20. ZAH

[7] HEYER, A. W., JR. & O'KELLY, L. I. Studies in motivation and retention: II. Retention of nonsense syllables learned under different degrees of motivation. *J. Psychol*, 1949, **27**, 143–152. (Reproduced by permission of the authors and the publisher.)

However, different instructions were read to the two groups during original learning.

One group (the experimental group) was instructed as follows.

In this course we have continuously emphasized that the facts we discuss are derived from experiments. It seems reasonable, therefore, to expect that you, as students, participate in certain experiments and be graded on the basis of your performance. We are going to ask you to learn a list of twenty nonsense syllables, standard material for the study of learning. Since the ability to learn this type of material is not related to such things as intelligence, previous education, or background, but is definitely related to, and as a matter of fact, determined by, how hard you try, or how well *you* are motivated, grading you on how well you learn this material represents one measure of your participation in the course. Your grade on this exercise will *count a full 10 per cent of your quarter's grade.* Ready? [p. 145].

The following instructions were read to the control group.

We want to present to you today some material that we have had prepared for use in the experimental study of learning. Since this material is new we have to find out how well suited it is for our purposes. I am going to show you twenty cards that have nonsense syllables printed on them. We wish to know whether some of these are easier to learn than others, part of the tedium of preparing for experimental work. I will show you the twenty syllables in the same order five times. You will then be asked to write down *in order* those syllables you can remember. Thanks for your cooperation. Ready? [p. 145].

The experimenter then presented the list of nonsense syllables to each group five times, following which the subjects were given 10 minutes to recall and record the twenty syllables in order.

Exactly 1 week later and without any previous warning that another recall test would be given, the following instructions were read to both groups.

You will remember that a week ago you were shown a list of nonsense syllables. We are interested in finding out how well you remember those syllables. I will pass out the answer sheets and the styli. Write down as many as you can of the syllables in the order which they were shown to you. Even though this has no bearing on your grade, do the best you can. Remember, you are to write down as many as you remember of the nonsense syllables in their correct order. You will be allowed 10 minutes for this exercise [p. 146].

The following table shows the results for both immediate recall and recall 1 week later. The groups are compared in three different ways: (1) *total errors,* including errors of omission, improper order of placement of the syllable, and production of syllables not in the original list; (2) *correct syllables,* the total number of correct syllables regardless of their order; and (3) *total number of syllables recorded* whether right or wrong.

Table 20

Performances of "High-motivation" and "Low-motivation" Groups
Immediately after Learning Nonsense Syllables and
One Week Later

Experimental Group (High Motivation)		Control Group (Low Motivation)
	Average Number of Errors Produced	
6.87	Original learning	8.72
12.52	One week later	15.25
	Average Number of Correct Syllables Reproduced	
14.65	Original learning	13.89
9.41	One week later	7.28
	Average Total Number of Syllables Reproduced	
17.67	Original learning	16.71
13.89	One week later	10.69

Owing to the relatively easy learning task assigned, the two groups were not differentiated in their performance when they were required to reproduce the nonsense syllables immediately after learning. Nevertheless, the reader will note a sharp discrepancy in their performance 1 week later. These numerical results yield a statistically significant difference and show that the kind of arrangement utilized here which relates the behavior to be performed to the individual's grade in the course is an effective technique for coordinating stimulus-response units, as measured by retention tests 1 week later. It is suggested that the above experiment is analogous to everyday life situations. Those students who have interest and enthusiasm in a course probably learn better than those who merely pay their tuition and "sit through" a course.

IX. THE ROLE OF REINFORCEMENT IN LEARNING
N. H. Pronko

Skinner has done striking experiments with rats and pigeons. Many other workers have preferred to work with what Skinner has called *respondent behavior,* where such a stimulus as shock to the foot of a dog will call out a foot-withdrawal response. Then, by conditioning it to a piano note, the same definite reaction will in time be elicited by the piano note as well as the shock. This is particularly true if the response to the piano note is occasionally reinforced with shock. Such reinforcement facilitates the connection between the foot withdrawal and the piano note.

Skinner has also been interested in *operant behavior.* Besides reflexes, a living organism shows a certain degree of spontaneity in its stances, turnings, posturings, and so on. The way these looser, less discrete reactions have become connected with stimuli has engrossed Skinner and his students. They have published many ingenious, rigorous, and quantitative studies of such behavior. The way in which an accidental or incidental (operant) response of a pigeon became connected to a stimulus, and how this response was *reinforced,* is shown in the following experiment reported by Skinner.[8]

A pigeon is brought to a stable state of hunger by reducing it to 75 per cent of its weight when well fed. It is put into an experimental cage for a few minutes each day. A food hopper attached to the cage is periodically swung into place so that the pigeon can eat from it. A solenoid and a timing relay hold the hopper in place for five sec. at each reinforcement, after which it disappears to reappear again whenever the experimenter chooses.

If a clock is now arranged to present the food hopper at regular intervals *with no reference whatsoever to the bird's behavior,* operant conditioning usually takes place. In six out of eight cases the resulting responses were so clearly defined that two observers could agree per-

---

[8] SKINNER, B. F. "Superstition" in the pigeon. *J. exp. Psychol.,* 1948, **38,** 168–172. (Reproduced by permission of the author and the American Psychological Association.)

fectly in counting instances. One bird was conditioned to turn counterclockwise about the cage, making two or three turns between reinforcements. Another repeatedly thrust its head into one of the upper corners of the cage. A third developed a "tossing" response, as if placing its head beneath an invisible bar and lifting it repeatedly. Two birds developed a pendulum motion of the head and body, in which the head was extended forward and swung from right to left with a sharp movement followed by a somewhat slower return. The body generally followed the movement and a few steps might be taken when it was extensive. Another bird was conditioned to make incomplete pecking or brushing movements directed toward but not touching the floor. None of these responses appeared in any noticeable strength during adaptation to the cage or until the food hopper was periodically presented. In the remaining two cases, conditioned responses were not clearly marked.

The conditioning process is usually obvious. The bird happens to be executing some response as the hopper appears; as a result it tends to repeat this response. If the interval before the next presentation is not so great that extinction takes place, a second "contingency" is probable. This strengthens the response still further and subsequent reinforcement becomes more probable. It is true that some responses go unreinforced and some reinforcements appear when the response has not just been made, but the net result is the development of a considerable state of strength [pp. 168–169].

The experiment might be said to demonstrate a sort of superstition. The bird behaves as if there were a causal relation between its behavior and the presentation of food, although such a relation is lacking. There are many analogies in human behavior. Rituals for changing one's luck at cards are good examples. A few accidental connections between a ritual and favorable consequences suffice to set up and maintain the behavior in spite of many unreinforced instances. The bowler who has released a ball down the alley but continues to behave as if he were controlling it by twisting and turning his arm and shoulder is another case in point. These behaviors have, of course, no real effect upon one's luck or upon a ball half way down an alley, just as in the present case the food would appear as often if the pigeon did nothing—or, more strictly speaking, did something else.

It is perhaps not quite correct to say that conditioned behavior has been set up without any previously determined contingency whatsoever. We have appealed to a uniform sequence of responses in the behavior of the pigeon to obtain an overall net contingency. When we arrange a clock to present food every 15 sec., we are in effect basing our reinforcement upon a limited set of responses which frequently occur 15 sec. after reinforcement. When a response has been strengthened (and this may result from one reinforcement), the setting of the clock implies an even more restricted contingency. Something of the same sort is true of the bowler. It is not quite correct to say that there is no connection between his twisting and turning and the course taken by the ball at the far end of the alley. The connection was established before the ball left the bowler's hand, but since both the path of the ball and the behavior of the bowler are determined, some relation survives. The subsequent behavior of the bowler may have no effect upon the ball, but the behavior of the ball has an effect upon the bowler. The contingency, though not perfect, is enough to maintain the behavior in strength. The particular form of the behavior adopted by the bowler is due to induction from responses in which there is actual contact with the ball. It is clearly a movement appropriate to changing the ball's direction. But this does not invalidate the comparison, since we are not concerned with what response is selected but with why it persists in strength. In rituals for changing luck the inductive strengthening of a particular form of behavior is generally absent. The behavior of the pigeon in this experiment is of the latter sort, as the variety of responses obtained from different pigeons indicate. Whether there is any unconditioned behavior in the pigeon appropriate to a given effect upon the environment is under investigation.

The results throw some light on incidental behavior observed in experiments in which a discriminative stimulus is frequently presented. Such a stimulus has reinforcing value and can set up superstitious behavior. A pigeon will often develop some response such as turning, twisting, pecking near the locus of the discriminative stimulus, flapping its wings, etc. In much of the work to date in this field the interval between presentations of the discriminative stimulus has been one min. and many of these superstitious responses are short-lived. Their appearance as the result of accidental correlations with the presentation of the stimulus is unmistakable [pp. 171–172].

X. STIMULUS SURROUNDINGS AND EFFECTIVE-
NESS OF LEARNING [9]

J. W. Bowles, Jr.

It would seem reasonable to suppose that if certain aspects of a stimulus situation stand out, then stimulus-response units will be easily connected. This was implied in the "dome versus room environment" maze experiment discussed earlier.

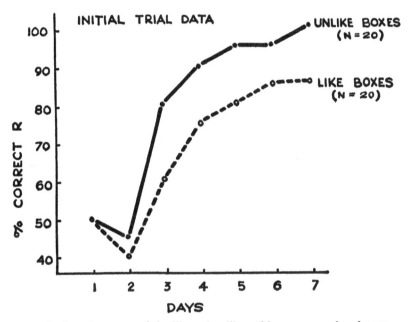

FIG. 48 Learning curves of the like and unlike end box groups as based upon the per cent of correct responses on the initial trial of the day. (Denny, M. Ray, The effect of using differential end boxes in a simple T-maze learning situation.)

The present experiment illustrates how such variables on the side of the stimulus may operate in facilitating or retarding learning. The investigator, in this instance, used a simple T-maze with interchangeable end boxes. Some were the same size and color

[9] DENNY, M. RAY. The effect of using differential end boxes in a simple T-maze learning situation. *J. exp. Psychol.*, 1948, 38, 245–249. (Reproduced by permission of the author and the American Psychological Association.)

as the alleys. These will be referred to as the "like end boxes." Unlike end boxes were 1 inch taller and 2 inches wider than the alleys, and they were constructed differently. The box leading to the goal was painted white and had a floor made of hardware cloth, while the negative box was painted black and had a beaver-board floor.

Twenty animals were run in the mazes with like end boxes at the ends of the alleys and twenty with unlike end boxes substituted. Four trials were given per day. The subjects were trained for a period of 6 days and tested on the seventh.

Results were computed in two ways: (1) for the percentage of correct responses on the first trial of the day and (2) for percentage of correct responses of the first two trials on each day from day 2 to 7. The two groups gave different results in both instances, a difference which was more striking in the averages for the first two trials. These are shown in the accompanying figure. (Fig. 48).

CONCLUSIONS. The above experiment shows definitely that stimulus-response connections do not proceed the same way when two groups of rats are run in mazes with different end boxes. When end boxes are different from the alleys, connection of response and stimulus is more effective, as shown by the higher percentage of correct response. Apparently, when end boxes are similar to the rest of the maze, they are not so easily discriminated; thus, a differential response does not so readily become built up. However, Denny prefers to interpret these results in terms of secondary reinforcement.

XI. DOES LISTENING TO THE RADIO INTERFERE WITH STUDYING? [10]

N. H. Pronko

Many college students insist that music does not "bother" them and that they can study effectively with the radio on. An experiment was designed to test this common presupposition. If music is used as a distraction, will it interfere with reading efficiency?

---

[10] HENDERSON, M. T., CREWS, ANNE, & BARLOW, JOAN. A study of the effect of music distraction on reading efficiency. *J. appl. Psychol.*, 1945, **29**, 313–317.

And what, if any, difference will there be between the distracting values of classical and popular music? Henderson and his collaborators took fifty subjects and divided them into three equally matched groups. These three groups showed comparable averages on their entrance psychological examination and their reading-test scores.

The subjects were first required to fill out a questionnaire in which they were asked specific questions about their study habits. Did they usually study with the radio on? Did they think that such listening cut down their study efficiency? How much studying did they do with the radio on? And what type of program did they listen to?

As a measure of reading proficiency of the three groups, the experimenters used the Nelson-Denny Reading Test. This test has a paragraph-comprehension section and a section on vocabulary. These students had taken Form A of the same reading test when they entered college a year earlier.

One of the three groups was a control group. It simply took the reading test without any distraction. The first experimental group of fourteen freshmen women took the reading test while listening to popular music. The other, made up of nineteen subjects, took the test with classical music as distraction.

MUSICAL RECORDINGS: POPULAR MUSIC (order of presentation): 1. "Two O'Clock Jump" (Harry James); 2. "That's What You Think" (Gene Krupa); 3. "Sunday, Monday, or Always" (Frank Sinatra); 4. "Mr. Five by Five" (Harry James); 5. "Prince Charming" (Harry James); 6. "Tuxedo Junction" (Glenn Miller); 7. "Idaho" (Benny Goodman); 8. "Crosstown" (Glenn Miller); and 9. "Close to You" (Frank Sinatra). *Classical Music: Symphony in D Minor* by César Franck (Philadelphia Symphony Orchestra, Victor Recording, 6726–6730).

Table 21 shows the averages for the no-distraction, classical, and popular groups, the differences in performance on the first and second reading test, and the significance of these differences. The paragraph-comprehension score of the group that studied while listening to popular music shows the greatest reduction. This score decreased 25.1 score points below the pretest score. Although the vocabulary scores showed an increase, these increases are not statistically significant.

Table 21

Nelson-Denny Averages and *t* Scores

	N	Pretest (Form A)	Final Test (Form B)	Differ-ence	*t* (Fisher)	P
No distraction ..	19					
Vocabulary ...	..	43.1	50.0	+6.9	1.260	0.20
Paragraph	..	45.3	49.2	+3.9	0.923	0.35
Classical	17					
Vocabulary ...	..	42.6	48.4	+5.8	0.906	0.35
Paragraph	..	47.3	46.1	—1.2	0.266	0.80
Popular	14					
Vocabulary ...	..	43.8	47.8	+4.0	0.605	0.55
Paragraph	..	48.0	22.9	—25.1	6.160	<0.001

Tables 22 and 23 compare results of subjects accustomed to studying with the radio and those not so accustomed. These results show that both groups perform alike. The paragraph-comprehension scores of the popular group show a significant drop whether or not they were accustomed to studying with the radio. The other changes were within the range expected by chance.

Table 22

Nelson-Denny Averages and *t* Scores of Those Who Use the Radio When Studying

	N	Pretest (Form A)	Final Test (Form B)	Differ-ence	*t* (Fisher)	P
No distraction ..	14					
Vocabulary ...	..	42.3	49.8	+7.5	1.089	0.30
Paragraph	..	44.1	48.9	+4.8	1.062	0.30
Classical	9					
Vocabulary ...	..	41.4	50.4	+9.0	1.341	0.20
Paragraph	..	47.8	46.9	—.9	0.134	0.85
Popular	8					
Vocabulary ...	..	45.5	50.5	+5.0	0.670	0.50
Paragraph	..	53.8	25.1	—28.6	5.485	<0.001

Why did the classical music not influence test results and why did the popular music not affect vocabulary scores? The authors suggest that the complex rhythm and melodies of classical music are difficult to grasp. Since this music is subtle and vague, it is likely to be listened to. It simply formed a background which did not dis-tract the subjects from their reading tasks. In other words, since they didn't care for it, they did not listen to it.

Table 23

Nelson-Denny Averages and *t* Scores of Those Who
Do Not Use the Radio When Studying

	N	Pretest (Form A)	Final Test (Form B)	Differ- ence	*t* (Fisher)	*P*
No distraction ..	5					
Vocabulary ...	..	36.8	40.6	+3.8	0.531	0.60
Paragraph	..	39.6	40.0	+0.4	0.042	0.95
Classical	8					
Vocabulary ...	..	43.3	46.1	+2.8	0.245	0.80
Paragraph	..	46.8	45.3	—1.5	0.201	0.85
Popular	6					
Vocabulary ...	..	41.5	44.2	+2.7	0.244	0.80
Paragraph	..	40.3	20.0	—19.7	3.849	<0.001

A possible explanation for the effect of popular music on the comprehension scores but its lack of effect on vocabulary scores is next considered. The experimenters believe that the nature of the reading test explains this difference. The vocabulary materials are intermittent and unrelated and require no sustained concentration. On the other hand, the paragraph-comprehension materials are meaningfully related and demand sustained effort. This implies that popular music interfered with the more complex of the two test sections.

In summary, then, whether or not music interferes with the kind of learning that goes on during study depends both upon the complexity of that music and upon the complexity of the test materials. In this experiment, classical music did not influence test results, and popular music affected only the paragraph-comprehension parts of the test. With older people or with serious students of music, the results might be still different.

XII. HOW DO ORGANISMS LEARN?

N. H. Pronko

How is it that, once organized, learning interactions persist and repeat themselves when the organism and the stimulus object that were originally involved are brought together? *Stated in this operational fashion,* the question has possibilities of solution, for it is possible to isolate the variables that operated in the original learning. The experiments reviewed in the preceding part of this chapter have actually succeeded in doing this, and we have seen that when end boxes in mazes are easily discriminated, rats learn more easily than when end boxes are the same as the rest of the maze. Other setting factors such as domes or room surroundings have also been observed to affect the learning built up in such surroundings. The introduction of extraneous stimuli was also seen to affect the stimulus-response connections as observed in the study situation. Relating the response to be learned with the individual's grade in the course also appears to facilitate learning, and so for the other variables explored. The important point is that the factors in a learning situation can be isolated and evaluated as to their relative importance so that our question as to how learning does or does not remain stable is answerable in such terms.

Not all psychologists have handled learning in the fashion described above. For many investigators, learning is assumed to be something that happens inside the organism rather than an event involving organism, stimulus object, and setting factors. Such formulations have led to a search for some "modification" of a hypothetical sort within the organism. Traditionally, the brain has been seized upon as this special tissue. Woodworth and Marquis illustrate this typical orientation in the following quotation:

RETENTION [11]

After considering . . . the process of learning or "committing to memory," we come now to the second of the three main divisions of our subject and ask how what has been learned can possibly be retained. Some have said that it is retained "in the unconscious." But what can this mysterious statement mean? It might mean unconscious activity or unconscious inactivity. Unconscious activity would mean that a boy who has learned the multiplication table must be continually reciting it to himself, though unconsciously, and that the same boy, since he has also learned to skate, swim, and climb a tree, must be continually going through all these activities, and singing all the songs he knows, remembering all the people he knows, etc., etc. Any theory of retention

---

[11] WOODWORTH, R. S. & MARQUIS, D. G. *Psychology.* New York: Holt, 1947. Pp. 677. (Reproduced by permission of the authors and the publisher.)

that demands continued activity of all learned responses breaks down from its own weight. But if retention is unconscious inactivity, the word "unconscious" is superfluous and misleading; for the meaning must be that learning modifies the structure of the organism, and that the structural changes persist though remaining inactive until aroused by some effective stimulus. Exercise and reinforcement produce changes in the brain structure, changes which are submicroscopic in size but sufficient to enable a person to do again what he has learned to do and to see things again as he has learned to see them [pp. 209, 284].

The modified structure which retains a given memory is called a memory trace. We do not know the exact nature of this trace but we have a right to assume that every learning process leaves some trace in the brain. These traces, persisting for some time at least, make it possible to remember what has been learned. We need not assume that an inactive memory trace will necessarily last to the end of a person's life. It may die out gradually with the result that what was once learned is finally forgotten [pp. 555–556].

There are obvious difficulties in such an interpretation. The reader will note that the "modified structure" mentioned is purely hypothetical. Is it necessary to point out that brain cells are as impermanent as fingernail or skin cells and that they are constantly being replaced through cell division? How could one then possibly remember an event in his latter years that he had not recalled since childhood? A stand opposed to that of Woodworth and Marquis is taken by Lashley and Wade [12] who state:

At the present time nothing whatever is known concerning the nature of the alterations in the nervous system which constitute memory traces. Knowledge of cerebral physiology is in fact so limited that it does not even lend greater plausibility to one than to another of the many speculations concerning the organic basis of memory with which the literature is burdened. Association with direction of flow of nervous excitation or with a ratio of excitation is neither more or less fantastic than is association between hypothetical conditioned-reflex arcs. The only relevant facts are those of psychology . . . [p. 86].

A progression toward a more objective handling of retention is illustrated in the following excerpts.

---

12 LASHLEY, K. S. & WADE, M. The Pavlovian theory of generalization. *Psychol. Rev.*, 1946, 53, 72–87. (Reproduced by permission of the authors and the American Psychological Association.)

XIII. RETENTION [13]

The term "memory" has been ill-advisedly used in the experiments upon the effect of intervals of disuse upon habit functions. The term "retention" has been employed in a static sense in this same connection, referring chiefly to the "persistence of modifications" in the nervous system. Both terms are ill-defined. It seems possible to keep the term retention and make its meaning more definite. In behavior the term retention covers this phenomenon; viz., that an object to which an animal has learned to respond in a definite way will for a more or less definite period in which the given response has been prevented (i.e., by not presenting the object) call forth in various degrees of perfection the old (or habitual) response. If the response is as definite at the end of the period of disuse as before we say that there has been no loss in retention or that retention was perfect. In most cases the response, after a period of disuse, is not perfect (i.e., there is excess effort). The effect of the period of disuse can be measured (in terms of time, distance, errors, etc.) by comparing the first trial after disuse with the last trial before disuse; or otherwise expressed, the last trial Z of regular training with the first trial *a* of retraining. If a certain length of time is over-stepped the excess effort of trial *a* may be as great as that of *A*, the first trial in the training series. In this case the habit appears to be lost. Only complete retraining will tell us whether this is really the case [pp. 241–242].

XIV. LEARNING AND THE NERVOUS SYSTEM [14]

Unless the reader has clearly grasped the conception of an independent science of behavior, it is not likely that he will be convinced by arguments. A purely descriptive science is never popular. For the man whose curiosity about nature is not equal to his interest in the accuracy of his guesses, the hypothesis is the very life-blood of science. And the opposition to pure description is perhaps nowhere else as strong as in the field of behavior. I cannot expect that a mere demonstration of the

---

[13] WATSON, J. B. *Behavior: an introduction to comparative psychology.* New York: Holt, 1914. Pp. 439.

[14] SKINNER, B. F. The behavior of organisms. New York: Appleton-Century-Crofts, 1938. Pp. 457. (Reproduced by permission of the author and the publisher.)

independence of a science of behavior will dissuade the reader from his willingness to let the two disciplines proceed together as closely enmeshed as they are at the present time. There are, however, arguments of a more positive sort that he should take into consideration. The first of these is hygienic. A definition of terms in a science of behavior at its own level offers the tremendous advantage of keeping the investigator aware of what he knows and of what he does not know. The use of terms with neural references when the observations upon which they are based are behavioral is misleading. An entirely erroneous conception of the actual state of knowledge is set up. An outstanding example is the systematic arrangement of data given by Pavlov. The subtitle of his *Conditioned Reflexes* is "An Investigation of the Physiological Activity of the Cerebral Cortex," but no direct observations of the cortex are reported. The data given are quite obviously concerned with the behavior of reasonably intact dogs, and the only nervous system of which he speaks is the conceptual one discussed above. This is a legitimate procedure, so long as the laws established are not turned to "explain" the very observations upon which they are based; but this is commonly done, as for example, by Holt. . . . Holt's procedure is especially interesting because he is clearly aware of the kind of fallacy of which he is the victim. In the early pages of the book cited he quotes Moliere's *coup de grâce* to verbalism—

I am asked by the learned doctor for the cause and the reason why opium induces sleep. To which I reply, because there is in it a soporific virtue whose nature it is to lull the senses!

He then proceeds to explain behavior with a conceptual nervous system! I can see little difference between the use of the term instinct, to which he objects, and his own explanation of learning in terms of "Pavlov's Law," except that a neural reference is assigned to the Law which is lacking for the instinct. The reference is not at present supported by the data.

A second argument for maintaining the independence of a science of behavior is that it is then free from unnecessary restraining influences. Behavior, as I have said, is far more easily observed as a subject matter than the nervous system, and it is a mistake to tie one science down with the difficulties inherent in another. A single reflex arc, identifiable as such and as the correlate of a reflex, is at present inaccessible. Even gross dynamic properties are equally obdurate. Although the neurologist may speak, for example, of an afferent discharge from the stomach or of some other process as the basis of hunger, no method has to my knowledge been devised to obtain measures of resulting cortical or sub-cortical states of the drive as delicate as the measures of behavior described in Chapter Ten. We shall accept too great a handicap if we are to wait until methods have been devised for the investigation of neural correlates in order to validate laws of behavior. It is especially necessary to avoid restricting the term reflex to correlations for which arcs have been located. The restriction is commonly urged by the neurologist who is perhaps justifiably dismayed by the so-called "units" of behavior which are featured in psychological work. But the isolation of an arc is not a useful criterion to appeal to in order to exclude the misuse of the notion of a unit. Other criteria are available which are based upon the lawfulness of the unit during various changes in its state.

The current fashion in proceeding from a behavioral fact to its neural correlates instead of validating the fact as such and then proceeding to deal with other problems in behavior seriously hampers the development of a science of behavior [pp. 426–428].

XV. DOES LEARNING OCCUR IN THE BRAIN? [15]

The attribution to the brain of the power to associate ideas is equivalent to endowing it with a middle type of psychological property. Not that connecting brain processes with ideas is less magical and mysterious than making the brain produce sensations, but rather, the whole procedure is more palpably verbal. As Herrick puts it: "Even though we do not know how the brain thinks, we know as surely as we know anything in biology that is does so."

In fact, psychologists and neurologists have written millions of words about associations and association centers, but all they amount to is translating into neural language the old associationistic type of psychic lore. Actually, not one iota of evidence is or can ever be proposed.

Though the attribution of learning powers to the brain appears less objectionable, it really is not. Psychologists who talk about brain-learning functions seem to hold mentalistic constructions in abeyance. However, to attribute psychological-learning functions to the brain is

---

[15] KANTOR, J. R. *Problems of physiological psychology*. Bloomington, Ind.: Principia Press, 1947. Pp. 398. (Reproduced by permission of the publisher.)

simply to echo the old mind-location assertions. If the learning is complex it is assumed the mind's cortical seat has the power to perform it. If the cortex is injured or removed, then the powers are shoved down to some subcortical region. The following quotation from Woodworth's *Experimental Psychology* admirably illustrates the indecisive treatment of psychological brain functions.

In learning, work is done by the organism; this work leaves after-effects which we may include under the noncommittal terms, *trace*. What is retained is this trace. The trace is a modification of the organism which is not directly observed but is inferred from the facts of recall and recognition.

The *explanatory concept* of association implies a direct connection within the organism, probably within the brain, between the mechanisms concerned with item A and B.

It seems almost certain that the locus of any practice effect is the cerebral hemispheres and that practice leaves behind some change in the neural structure or condition.

Typical of much psychological writing are the strong indications of belief in the powers of the brain with a coordinate neglect of it in later exposition and interpretation. A fine example is Marquis's statement in discussing the neurology of learning:

The ability of an animal to learn—the ability to modify its behavior on the basis of previous experience and to adapt successfully to new situations—depends upon the structure and organization of its central nervous system. The difference between an untrained dog and a dog which has been taught to "beg" when food is held out, is a difference in the brain. The dog's reaction of course, involves the functioning of receptors, sensory nerves, motor nerves, and muscles, but the modification produced by the training is a modification of brain function. The neural connections from the receptors to the brain, and from the brain to the muscles are fixed and unchangeable. When a man learns through long practice to aim and shoot a gun accurately, he has not trained the eye or the finger. He has altered the brain processes in such a way that the movements of the finger are more precisely related to the visual stimulation. The later exposition, of course, makes no pretense to substantiate such a statement.

It has become a cultural tradition that the psychological functions of the brain consist of behavior control by the development of complex synaptic connections. This autistic creation of psychological processes is based on no more adequate foundation than the anatomical fact of neural synaptic junctions. The operation of these junctions has been transformed into functions called engrams or neurograms. Lashley, however, has warned against the procedure of inferring changes in neural operation from behavior and then explaining learning in terms of the inferred engrams or functions.

The fundamental importance of the synapse seems a logical conclusion, yet we must bear in mind when evaluating theories of learning that the properties of the synapse are still entirely hypothetical. If we deduce its properties from the facts of learning we gain nothing by explaining learning in terms of these hypothetical properties.

The objection to *brain functions* is twofold. They not only are of no value in explaining learning or any other complex event, but they prevent all who place such faith in them from explaining behavior events in terms of all the numerous factors the events themselves make available for the purpose. In this connection it is interesting to note that Marquis, whom we have quoted above as espousing this faith, continues to believe it even though he appreciates its futility. Writing in collaboration with Hilgard, he says:

> In the present status of knowledge, neural theory is not basic to conditioning theory. The known facts of neural function cannot be utilized to predict or to limit the results of behavioral studies. . . . Even the basic law that a response varies in magnitude with intensity of stimulus would be equally true if the nerves were copper wires or pneumatic tubes. The facts of speed of conduction and synaptic delay cannot predict the latency of a conditioned response, for we have no idea what length of nerve or how many synapses are involved. . . . Many of the so-called neural facts, such as reflex inhibition, which seem most relevant to conditioning are in reality behavioral laws stated as relations between afferent and efferent nerve activity without direct observation of any intermediate neural event. This point of view of course does not preclude the possibility that on the basis of future work neurological prediction of behavioral facts may be achieved.

Whenever one wishes to emphasize the presence of biological activities in psychological situations or to consider biological and psychological actions in relationship, one must always differentiate between the two types of events. Anatomical organization, which provided the connections between sense organs and cortical terminals, also between cortical terminals and motor projection paths, is a biological fact. The actions of the biological structures—conduction, coordination, and other functions—are and remain biological and cannot be connected with psychological events except as participating factors. Psychological events may be regarded as the larger field situations of which the biological activities, howsoever essential, constitute only components. To localize psychological functions in the brain involves an enormous amount of interpretative and attributive construction deviating widely from an observational contact with events. At the least, the questionable commerce with neural constructions does not enrich psychology and makes physiology poor indeed [pp. 102–105].

Operationally, the term "learning" can only refer to a field event involving an organism under specific circumstances in the process of acquiring a response to a given stimulus object. Why? Because that is what everybody must start with. The *mutual interaction* [16] of organism and stimulus object is the empirical fact. The traditional view which treats learning as if it were something occurring *inside* the animal leaves learning unexplained. Stating it as a field event permits one to understand learning as well as any other class of action in terms of the variables involved in the given situation. Perhaps the future of psychology will be directed toward such study in regard to learning as well as other behaviors. Certainly, the progress gained in the study of learning data justifies such faith. The contemporary student appears to be in a transitional period with respect to this problem. The field is rife with theoretical and experimental business.

---

[16] The term "interaction" is here used to stress the mutuality of action of the two variables involved. Organism and stimulus object may be said to interact in a fashion similar to that of two chemical substances or gravitating objects interacting with one another. Of course, the details of the interaction differ.

16

INTERRELATIONSHIPS

BETWEEN PHYSIOLOGY AND PSYCHOLOGY

I. INTRODUCTION

N. H. Pronko

Before the student of psychology can learn to handle his subject matter adequately, he must sooner or later settle the problem of how physiological and behavioral data are related to one another.

An examination of textbooks in physiology and psychology, selected at random, shows that each field is concerned with different subject matters. Physiology may be said to study "part reactions." Digestion, excretion, secretion, circulation, and reproduction are typical classes of the actions studied. Portions of organisms, such as a heart-lung preparation, can be profitably studied. Even where total organismic function is considered, as in the physiology of exercise, it is studied as an interrelation of organs or systems or their excitation by such agents as oxygen or carbon dioxide.

Psychology has a different subject matter. The classes of data in its textbooks will include hearing, tasting, loving, hating, fearing, reasoning, judging, understanding, dreaming, inventing, and so on. How is it that one person understands someone speaking English but not Hungarian? Vice versa, another person understands Hungarian and not English, while still another understands both. Fundamental answers to these questions will be understood in terms of a history connecting a given individual and the language in question. Further examination will show extreme degrees of differentiation or discrimination, inhibition, variability, modifiability, integration, and delayability. Neither the history nor these six characteristics will be found as distinctive features of the physiologist's subject matter (see Chapter I for further discussion).

On this operational or empirical basis do we separate the two fields.

Next, we consider the explanation of psychological data. Imagining behavioral facts to be mental or psychic does not solve the problem but makes it even more mystifying. It is rather apparent that a framework which makes the two (body and mind) parallel but inexplicable events has not been very fruitful. It is our opinion that the materials brought together in this chapter suggest that physiological factors be considered as factors that participate in psychological events. That is, *when* an organism learns, it is true that there are nervous-system and other types of physiological functioning, but the action is simultaneous rather than cause or effect. Why? Because learning is a more inclusive field event than organismic functioning. Note that in a learning situation the living organism is only *one* of the variables involved, and that there are also a *something to be learned* (a stimulus object), presence or absence of people, radios, and other variables. It is the occurrence *between* the organism and stimulus object that is the essential behavioral datum. No less than that. The interbehavior of the *two* is the fundamental fact for investigation.

With such a formulation, nothing is left out of the picture. As a matter of fact, since the organism as one variable is a breathing, digesting, living thing, deterioration, disruption, or disorganization of its systems, organs, or tissues may play a role in his behavior. This role may be that of a negative factor which prevents the learning of certain behaviors because the necessary structure is lacking, such as absence of eyes for building up visual responses, or absence of legs for dancing.

Interference effects may be noted, as when a spastic's nervous (i.e., connective) system is injured in such a way as to *prevent* his bringing together appropriate patterns for making the proper speech sounds, or the more general defect preventing all speech, as in aphasia. Drugged conditions, infections, injuries, blood loss, fatigue, and fever are other physiological factors that may (or may not) play a role in a particular behavioral interaction.

The operation of the negative factors described above must be understood in a relative rather than absolute fashion—an individual born without arms or legs may nevertheless become a toy maker, and there have been armless artists, too, who have painted with their feet. The current press reports other cases of persons with two wooden legs who dance as entertainers, armless mothers who attend their babies by means of legs and feet, and so on. Thus, the psychological consequences of injuries are dependent on compensatory factors occurring during the individual's reactional biography. A Helen Keller rendered blind, deaf, and anosmic but by whom heroic efforts are made to compensate for such defects, achieves a higher degree of behavioral complexity than many so-called "biologically normal" individuals.

The person's biological make-up may serve in a more positive way as a locus of psychological stimulation. His dry throat, heavy breathing, or heartbeat may be reacted to in the same way as one may react to the belching or snoring of others. Furthermore, injuries, cripplings, and the like, may be reacted to by stimulating the acquisition of behaviors to elicit sympathy and attention from others. On the other hand, anatomic and physiological defects may arouse compensatory behavior. A Demosthenes overcomes a speech defect. A crippled child unable to compete on the athletic field is spurred on by his very defectiveness to build up reactions of an intellectual sort that permit him to surpass other children. A warranted generalization regarding the role of biological factors in behavioral acquisition seems to be that no one can say in advance what place these variables will have because they may stimulate different individuals in utterly different ways. Similarly, one may react to one's own shape, size, skin color, or deformity in various ways, but regardless of how the organism's tissue, organ, system, or total organismic functioning operated in a behavioral event, they must be given their proper place in the total event of which the organism is always only one variable in a situation involving many other variables.

II. THE PROBLEM OF MOTIVATION
John Bucklew, Jr.

A phenomenon readily appreciated from everyday life is the goal-directed behavior of people. In fact, the selection and achievement of goals are such ubiquitous occurrences in human behavior that their nature and explanation have long been subject matters for speculation. The ordinary citizen will explain it merely by saying that he has certain motives or purposes which he pursues. These determine his behavior. Further questions will, in all probability, uncover the implicit assumption that motives and purposes are the "mind" or "will" operating upon the body.

The origin of the theory of motivation reveals the same sort of interpretations which our ordinary citizen employs. Motives were considered to be internal, psychic springs of actions which governed what the organism did. This type of thinking corresponds to the mentalistic period of psychology. Even today, it is by no means extinct in scientific circles. The doctrine of instincts, considered in a previous chapter, was one part of this interpretative scheme. Instincts were conceived of as unlearned actions which achieved certain definite ends; motives were, at least in part, acquired.

Behavioristic psychologists, early recognizing the disadvantages of mentalistic explanations, attempted to remedy matters by transforming "psychic springs of action" into definite physiological processes within the organism. These processes, actual or assumed, were labeled "drives," and, in accord with available data, were localized in various bodily regions. Hunger drives, for example, became primarily an affair of contractions of the empty stomach. Sexual drive presumably sprang from tensions of the sexual apparatus, from internal secretions of the sexual glands, or from both. Motivated behavior, under this scheme, was explainable as (1) a source of energy supplied by physiological states operating on the organism in conjunction with (2) external stimuli which the organism had learned to recognize as leading to certain definite goals.

The theory of motivation in this form can be operationally examined, for it is expressed in terms of natural processes. If localized energy sources in the organism serve to motivate behavior, then it becomes possible to test this by trying to remove the alleged source of the drive. Without this, the motivated behavior should cease or should be significantly reduced. For hunger drive, the experiment of Tsang, summarized in the following section, was one of several such experiments which have been performed. Others have been performed on thirst and sexual drives with similar results.

Is it sound interpretation to say that goal-directed action springs from internal drives and needs, or is this a fictitious account of human behavior? Much literature now points to the conclusion that goal-directed activity varies with a host of factors which may operate in conjunction with, or in independence from, specific physiological states. This literature deals with the behavior considered to be biologically fundamental—such things as food ingestion or sexual activity. If more than physiological conditions are needed to account adequately for these motivations, then the topic of motivations becomes increasingly a stress on any factors— those of the organism, those of the stimuli, those of the general setting of behavior, those of the life history—which dispose the individual toward some goal action.

There is a very general issue, a type of social philosophy, at stake in the scientific determination of what motivation is or is not. Can complex social institutions, such as war, business, or art, be derived from biological determiners, or do these things operate with a great deal of independence of biological facts? If, for example, sexual behavior itself can occur with some independence of physiological states, then how much can be said for the current notion that artistic motivations are traceable to the fact of biological sex? The selections immediately following are chosen to illustrate some of the literature concerning the study of motivation. They, as well as subsequent items from the areas of sex behavior and the role of the nervous system, are meant to help answer the question: What is the relationship between physiology and psychology?

III. HUNGER MOTIVATION IN GASTRECTO-
MIZED RATS [1]
John Bucklew, Jr.

INTRODUCTION. There is no direct evidence that the motivational effects of food privation upon maze running are a result of stomach contractions. The contrast between the continuous activity of the animal in the maze and the intermittent character of the hunger contractions raises some doubt as to the importance of the latter in motivation. This experiment was a preliminary at-

[1] Adapted from TSANG, YU-CHUAN. Hunger motivation in gastrectomized rats. *J. comp. Psychol.*, 1938, 26, 1–17. (Reproduced by permission of the author and the publisher.)

tempt to control the gastric contractions in order to test the effect of food deprivation on motivation. The method was to perform a partial gastrectomy, eliminating the contracting part of the stomach, and to compare the learning of animals so prepared with that of normal controls during hunger motivation.

OPERATIVE TECHNIQUE. After experimentation, the technique was developed of cutting off the main bulk of the stomach and leaving a narrow strip of tissue along the lesser curvature of the stomach. The cut surfaces were sewed together to form a narrow passage between the esophagus and the duodenum. The tissue along the lesser curvature of the stomach is not active even in the normal stomach. The rest of the stomach contracts against it during hunger pangs. Thus, in cutting out the main bulk of the stomach, leaving only the lesser curvature, the experimenters eliminated that part of the stomach which moved during hunger contractions.

In the seven rats used in the operated group, from 90 to 95 per cent of the whole stomach was removed. Thus, gastric contractions should be clearly reduced, if not eliminated altogether. The rats were 3 months of age at the time of the operation. Two and one half weeks after the operation, the rats were back on their normal diet. When their body weight had returned to what it was before the operation, the experimental testing of the animals was begun. After the experiment was over, an autopsy was performed on the rats to determine how much of the stomach had been removed and how well it had healed from the effects of the operation (see figure 49).

PROCEDURE. The rats were tested in two kinds of apparatus. One of these was an alley-type maze of fifteen sections. The other was an activity cage in which the amount of activity which the rat displayed over any given period of time could be recorded and measured.

The procedure for the maze was as follows: first there was a preliminary feeding in the maze for 3 days; then on the first day after that, 1 trial was given. On the second day 2 trials were given, and thereafter 5 trials per day were run. The criterion for learning the maze was 10 consecutive errorless runs. The rats were allowed 150 trials as a maximum. At the end of each successful run the animals were rewarded sparingly with food. In addition to the data for the gastrectomized rats, the experimenter had data concerning

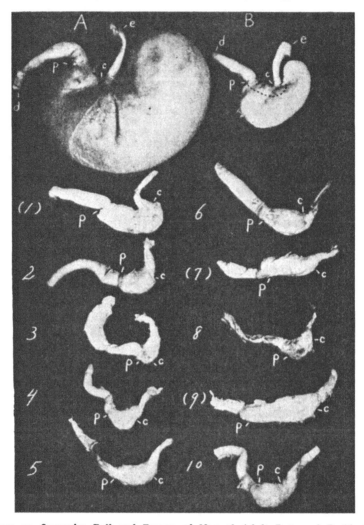

FIG. 49 Stomachs, Full and Empty, of Normal Adult Rats and Residual "Stomachs" of Gastrectomized Rats, X 1. A, stomach immediately after a hearty meal; B, stomach after fasting for 24 hours. 1–10 gastrectomized cases. c, cardia; d, duodenum; e, esophagus; p, pylorus. Cases 1, 7, and 9 are unsatisfactory operations and excluded from the group averages. Broken line in B marks the locus of the incision. For photography the specimens were fastened to a black cardboard by loops of thread which are visible in the pictures. (Adapted from Tsang, Yu Chuan, Hunger motivation in gastrectomized rats.)

normal rats; these data had been compiled in previous studies. Thus, the operated rats could be compared to a control group of normal animals.

RESULTS OF THE MAZE.   In comparing the operated group with the control group, the experimenter used the results of the first trial on each day. He considered that the animals were only comparable on the first trial because introducing even a small morsel of food into the residual stomach of those animals who had been operated on might change their hunger motivation to a much greater degree than if the morsel were introduced into the stomach of a normal animal. Table 24 shows the results in average time on the first trial and average number of errors on the first trial for the normal and gastrectomized rats.

Table 24

Average Time and Average Errors on the First Trial
for Normal and Operated Rats

	Average Time in First Trial		Average Errors in First Trial	
Days	Normal	Gastrectomized	Normal	Gastrectomized
1	165	55	4.6	3.1
2	58	40	2.4	2.7
3	31	17	1.3	0.3
4	12	15	0.3	0.3
5	12	14	0.4	0.4
6	9	59	0.2	1.1
7	10	10	0.0	0.1
8	9	12	0.0	0.1

The results in this table are for the first trial on each of the 8 days during which the rats were run. They show that there is little difference between the two groups either in average time or in the average number of errors made.

RESULTS OF THE ACTIVITY CAGE.   After the maze test, the gastrectomized rats were put into an activity cage in order to measure the relative activity before and after eating. This cage consists of a revolving disk which turns when the animal moves. Each revolution of the cage is automatically recorded. In each cage, the animal always had a supply of fresh water. Three activity records were taken each day: the total activity for the hour just before feeding, for the hour just after feeding, and for a total period of 21 hours.

One of the seven rats had to be dropped out of this part of the experiment, so the results for the operated group include only six rats. Table 25 shows the number of revolutions for each of the records on each of the six rats.

Table 25

Number of Revolutions

Rat	One Hour before Feeding	One Hour after Feeding	Total over 21-hour Period
1	172.9	61.0	1,428.1
2	411.9	152.9	5,427.1
3	1,231.1	434.0	13,358.5
4	204.9	76.9	1,700.4
5	549.1	120.1	4,710.4
6	292.1	246.0	4,493.9

The results of the activity cage are in harmony with previous results on normal rats. It had been found that activity in normal rats was highest in the hour before feeding, and, in this experiment on the operated rats, it was found that they were three times as active before feeding as after feeding. This would indicate that in the absence of a contractile stomach the animal is still capable of hunger which "drives" it to greater activity. On the whole, however, the operated rats were not so active as the normal rats had been in other studies. Perhaps gastrectomy has a depressing effect on general activity, but without relation to the hunger cycle.

CONCLUSIONS.   From the data of this experiment, Tsang concludes that the motivation of gastrectomized rats, as measured in maze running and the activity cage, is not essentially different from that of normal rats possessing a stomach. Hence, the motivational factors of hunger cannot be said to arise exclusively from contractions of the stomach.

IV. STIMULUS FACTORS IN FOOD PREFERENCE
John Bucklew, Jr.

That motivating factors include more than internal states of the organism is clearly illustrated by wartime experiences of the army in feeding its soldier population. Dove [2] has reported on some of these problems which arose during the war, and upon experimental work which has been undertaken as a result of them.

During World War II . . . each item of the ration had been carefully produced and prepared according to quality specifications, and each item had been tested to contain and retain through long periods of storage its quota of vitamins, minerals, protein, and calories. But when the soldier-consumer refused to accept some of these ration items, and when these items began to accumulate in storage dumps in various theatres of war, a new problem in supply, heretofore unrecognized, was raised to a major issue. To determine the causes of non-acceptance followed as an official directive.

Parallel with the refusals by the soldier-consumer, populations under economic stress, or belabored with a poor soil, or lost in the forest fringe or in marginal environments, or seduced in overspecialization, reveal similar conflicts over acceptance and non-acceptance of foods [p. 187].

Dove further explains that formerly families in our country selected, grew, and prepared their own foods in a manner acceptable to members of the family group. However this is no longer true. And, especially in military life, the food must now be selected and prepared ahead of time. This renders it necessary to have some means of testing ahead of time what foods will be acceptable and what ones will not. Tests carried out in various army camps indicate that it is expedient to eliminate some foodstuffs ahead of time because they will be rejected by the soldiers. Others are found suitable to only a part of the soldier population, and still others are very well liked and can be stocked immediately.

Dove adds that preferences for foods and prejudices against foods seem to be closely related to food habits which have been built up during the individual's lifetime. These food habits are, in turn, related to a variety of factors such as soil, climate, food crops, socioeconomic conditions, and even religious convictions of people.

The final evaluation of the food depends not only on its potential nutritional qualities but as well upon the acceptability

---

[2] DOVE, W. F. Developing food acceptance research. *Science*, 1946, **103**, 187–190. (Reproduced by permission of the publisher.)

which it possesses. This is determined by the per cent value per unit weight multiplied by the weight accepted.

Table 26 illustrates how varieties of a type of food, in this case, corn, can be ranked according to *palatability*. The figures for 1942 were taken from corn grown from the same seed on the same plot of land. Many factors, such as the maturity of the corn, may affect its preference rank.

In general, preference is shown for yellow varieties of corn over white varieties. Since yellowness usually indicates the presence of carotene and of Vitamin A, there would be a rough correlation between the palatability rating and Vitamin-A content. However, one variety containing carotene was rated low.

It is also known that the ranking of a particular variety is relative to the others tested. In one sample of several corns, one variety was generally rated as "sweet and tender," but when this same variety was placed in another group all of which were generally rated well, it was called "tasteless and flat."

Table 26 *

Preference for Four Varieties of Corn, as Shown by Average Ranking

Taste-tester Varieties	Average Placement in Palatability Rank in 2 Consecutive Years	
	1941 Tests	1942 Tests
Golden bantam	1.59	1.62
Early yellow sensation	2.93	2.16
Early Crosby sweet	4.10	4.80
Seneca "60"	4.93	5.40

* Taken from Dove, W. F. The relative nature of human preference: with an example in the palatability of different varieties of sweet corn. *J. comp. Psychol.*, 1943, 35, 219–226.

Apparently, the "hunger-motivating" properties of corn are not entirely described in terms of physiology and chemistry.

V. MOTIVATIONAL FACTORS IN GROUPS [3]
John Bucklew, Jr.

The question investigated by these experimenters was whether the members of a group who ranked low in some activity would have the same goals or levels of aspiration as those members who ranked higher. Subjects for the experiment were fifth-grade children of two schools of a Middle Western town. In all, there were seventy-seven children, of whom fifty-three were in the experimental group and twenty-four in a control group.

The task chosen was one which was unrelated to ordinary schoolwork and which did not correlate closely with intelligence-test scores. This task, the Woodworth Wells Cancellation Test, consists of a sheet with rows of numbers printed in haphazard arrangement. The task is to cancel out with a pencil all the examples of any one number which the experimenter chooses for cancellation in a given trial.

The cancellation test was given six times altogether, twice each week for 3 consecutive weeks. For the first trial, the same instructions were given to all children. They were told that the task was a diversion from their regular schoolwork and was not at all difficult. Then the procedure was explained to them.

For the following trials, the original group was divided into a control group and an experimental group. The children in the control group continued as in the first trial, but the children in the experimental group were first shown their scores and the class average from the previous trial, and then told whether their score was above or below the average. They were also allowed to look at a bar graph showing their relationship to the class average and to other individuals. However, this graph was so arranged that each child knew his own score but did not know the score of any other person. This was done by giving each child a number and using this number instead of his name on the graph.

When the child was given the card telling him what his score and the class average was, he was asked to put down the score he thought he would make that day. This was taken to be the child's

[3] Adapted from ANDERSON, H. H. & BRANDT, H. F. A study of motivation, involving self-announced goals of fifth-grade children and the concept of level of aspiration. *J. soc. Psychol.*, 1939, 10, 209–232.

goal, or level of aspiration, for that day's work. Table 27 summarizes the results showing the relationship of level of aspiration
to the child's standing in the group.

Table 27

Table Showing the Actual Scores and Announced Goals by
Quartile Groups for Each Day's Trial

	Trial	Score	Trial	Goal
Upper quartile	1	103.2	2	104.5
	3	115.7	4	108.0
	4	116.5	5	113.9
	5	121.5	6	107.7
Second quartile	1	86.4	2	91.7
	3	93.2	4	92.8
	4	95.0	5	97.1
	5	99.3	6	99.7
Third quartile	1	75.7	2	80.8
	3	82.3	4	86.6
	4	87.8	5	85.4
	5	88.4	6	87.1
Lower quartile	1	69.2	2	85.6
	3	73.5	4	85.3
	4	70.1	5	87.0
	5	74.2	6	83.4

The general results of this study can be seen most easily by
comparing the scores and the levels of aspiration of the upper 25
per cent of the group with the same figures for the lower 25 per
cent. In both cases, the actual scores showed an improvement from
the first to the last day. However, the significant fact is in the relationship between the scores and the goals to which they aspired.
For the upper group, it can be seen that the goal which they said
they would reach tends to fall below what they achieved on that
day's work. For the lower group, the goal which they announced
tends always to be above what they actually achieved. The central
conclusion of the study is, then, that irrespective of their achievement, the announced goals of the children tend to fall in toward
the middle of the group. This would seem to indicate that the level
of mediocrity is the level toward which the children in each case
are aspiring.

VI. GLANDS AND SEXUAL BEHAVIOR
J. W. Bowles, Jr.

Both past and present "popular psychology" have talked of glands "regulating" personality and otherwise determining behavioral happenings in which organisms are involved. Emphasis has been placed for the most part upon the endocrines. Perhaps "gland psychology" represents little more than a fad in the science of psychology that has developed with the growing interest of the biologist in the ductless glands. That this is true is suggested by the dearth of facts revealing glands as determiners or regulators of behavior.

The lack of correlation between glandular action and behavior is apparent in the following summary of Kinsey's [4] investigation of homosexuality in the human male.

Popular opinion has held and continues to hold that homosexual behavior is dependent upon some inherent abnormality. With the discovery of the sex hormones, this abnormality is often assumed to be glandular in origin.

Androgen and estrogen analyses of urine samples have been made with small groups of so-called "normals" and "homosexuals" to support this glandular theory of sexual behavior. However, differences between groups have not been significant. In fact, different samples from the same individual have shown extreme variation.

One is not warranted in concluding that the relatively small differences in averages (of urine samples) between two such small groups are significant when successive samples from single individuals show 7 to 50 times as much difference [p. 424].

A more serious error in studies of this sort is the assumption that heterosexual and homosexual behaviors are mutually exclusive phenomena derived from inherently different individuals. An analysis of the sex histories collected by the personal-interview technique of 1,058 males reveals that the "homosexual" or "heterosexual" classification of human males is not based on fact. In this large sample, 354, or 35.5 per cent, of the individuals, had been

---

[4] KINSEY, A. C. Criteria for a hormonal explanation of the homosexual. *J. clin. Endocrin.*, 1941, 1, 424–428. (Quoted by permission of the publisher.)

involved in one or more homosexual experiences. The sample included a large number of college students from 140 American colleges. In this subgroup, 30 per cent reported some homosexual experience. The incidence of homosexual behavior continues to increase throughout the early adult years, showing that these are not all early-adolescent activities.

In brief, homosexuality is not the rare phenomenon which it is ordinarily considered to be, but a type of behavior which ultimately may involve as much as half of the whole male population. Any hormonal or other explanation of the phenomenon must take this into account [p. 426].

Note that a large percentage of "normals" used as controls in such glandular studies may actually have a history of homosexual experiences some time in their lives!

In further analysis, Kinsey reports a wide range of individual differences in frequency of homosexual behavior; some cases had only one experience, others a few experiences, and so on to the other extreme of homosexual contacts several times per day over a period of years. In short, Kinsey states that, "we fail to find any basis for recognizing discrete types of homosexual behavior" [pp. 426–427].

Not only do individuals differ in the frequency of this sort of behavior, but there are many other striking differences. Some individuals have confined themselves to one partner, some have contacted thousands, some initiated homosexual behavior in preadolescence, some in later life. In some cases, homosexual behavior was limited to a brief life span; in some, it was continued up to 60 years; in others, it was discontinuous, being interspersed with heterosexual behavior. In some cases, homosexual behavior constituted a small fraction of total sex behavior. This varied continuously to the other extreme in which the individual rarely or never engaged in heterosexual relations. In general, a large number in the sample were exclusively heterosexual, a relatively large number reported a history of both hetero- and homosexual activities, and a small group gave an exclusively homosexual history. The "both" group might carry on both sorts of activity in the same or successive life spans, in the space of 1 day or even 1 hour.

Further, Kinsey found no sharp distinctions between "passive" and "active" homosexuals, which is a traditional classification.

Many played either role. Also, stigmata in the appearance of "homosexuals" was lacking. Some might be described as showing "effeminate" characteristics, others as being very "masculine." Thus, differences in sex behavior vary in complex ways and defy "typing." Actually, no two individuals could be found with identical sex histories.

In summary, then:

Throughout the case histories, the circumstances of the first sexual experience, psychic conditioning, and social pressures are obvious factors in determining the pattern of the behavior. It would appear that no similar correlation has as yet been shown between hormones and homosexual activity. It is, of course, not impossible that endocrines are involved; but in order to demonstrate that, it would be necessary to show a correlative variation in hormones and behavior which includes such gradations, combined patterns, and changes of pattern as have been described here [p. 428].

VII. THE LAYMAN'S CONCEPTION OF THE NERVOUS SYSTEM

The present excerpt [5] is included because it is excellent proof of how folklore about the nervous system conditions both people's illnesses and their interpretations, a pervasive feature of our civilization.

The importance of popular misconceptions in determining the character of one's complaints comes out nowhere more clearly than in relation to the muscles and the peripheral nerves. For although muscles actually develop innumerable fatiguing tensions, imbalances, pulls, droops and spasms, they are seldom accused of being defective or diseased by the hypochondriac, unless he has undergone unintentional but effective coaching by an interested therapist. It is true that backaches, headaches, pains in the neck, the thighs, the arms and the legs are exceedingly common complaints, but the complainer is far more likely to refer these directly to his nervous system than to the muscles themselves. Thus the peripheral nerves, although quite incapable of movement, are continually accused by laymen of quivering,

[5] CAMERON, NORMAN. *The psychology of behavior disorders.* Boston: Houghton Mifflin, 1947. Pp. 622. (Reproduced by permission of the author and the publisher.)

pulling, clenching, drawing or knotting up. Whereas the actual changes giving rise to most of these complaints originate in local striped or smooth muscle response, for the public it is the nerves that are tensed, taut, frayed, get on edge or go to pieces. It is the central nervous system which is referred to as exhausted, debilitated, broken down, deteriorated or diseased.

This widespread tendency to interpret freely the changes in striped or smooth muscle tonus and reactivity in terms of "nerves," nervousness, neurasthenia and central nervous system dysfunction represents a serious cultural lag. During the most of the nineteenth century so little was known about neurophysiology that any of the behavior disorders could be ascribed to hypothetical nerve disturbances with a clear scientific conscience. Thus even so advanced a thinker as Freud ascribed hypochondria, fatigue syndromes and anxiety neuroses to neural disorder, called them *actual neuroses* and excluded them from psychoanalysis. Indeed, until recent years so inadequate has been our recognition of the potentialities for behavior pathology in situational relationships and self-reactions that, even though no lesions or physiopathology could be demonstrated in the brains of neurotics or in two-thirds of psychotics, it was still maintained on all sides that neural defect, depletion, deterioration or disease was the only conceivable basis for behavior disorder. Popular thinking still persists in looking upon over-reactions to need, frustration, anxiety, guilt and disappointment as indications of nervous system disorder in spite of the large body of organized evidence to the contrary. Likewise, because of the inevitable lag in the dissemination and acceptance of new technical information, many persons today who discover in themselves conflicting or antisocial trends, who develop fear and tension symptoms, or whose thinking grows confused under stress, are left to conclude immediately that their brain is diseased, constitutionally inferior or deteriorating [pp. 199–200].

The next quotation [6] upsets another common notion about the brain as a "knowledge box."

Man's old belief that damage to the vital centers profoundly upsets the balance of the personality finds some support from careful psychiatric observation; man's common belief that *any* blow to these centres must produce far-reaching changes is not substantiated, but the

---

[6] ANDERSON, CHARLES. Chronic head cases. *Lancet*, 1942, **2**, 1–4. (Reproduced by permission of the publisher.)

notion dies hard. Patients commonly entertain the notion that the head is a fragile box filled with precious objects, such as thoughts and vaguely defined vital centres. After an injury the resulting change in the personality and capacity for work is attributed to damage to the contents of the box, and the complaint of headache is in many cases a response to the patient's discontent with his own emotional and intellectual capacities, though defects of these may have been present before the injury. Now he can explain why he has failed: "I have a headache" [p. 1].

It is important to point out that no one has as yet operationally "teased out" such variables as the patient's attitudes and folklore about the brain and the actual brain damage in cases of head injury.

VIII. BEHAVIOR AND THE NERVOUS SYSTEM

This excerpt from Skinner [7] considers possible relationships between behavior and the nervous system. Skinner appears to treat the two as independent fields.

If the reader has accepted the formulation of behavior given . . . without too many reservations, and if he has been reasonably successful in excluding extraneous points of view urged upon him by other formulations with which he is familiar, he has probably not felt the lack of any mention of the nervous system in the preceding pages. In regarding behavior as a scientific datum in its own right and in proceeding to examine it in accordance with established scientific practices, one naturally does not expect to encounter neurones, synapse, or any other aspect of the internal economy of the organism. Entities of that sort lie outside the field of behavior as here defined. If it were not for the weight of tradition to the contrary, there would be no reason to mention the nervous system at this point; but an analysis of behavior is rarely offered without some account of the neurological facts and theories supposedly related to it. Although I have no intention of dealing with such facts or theories in detail, I can scarcely avoid some discussion of the all but universal belief that a science of behavior must be neurological in nature.

[7] SKINNER, B. F. *The behavior of organisms.* New York: Appleton-Century-Crofts, 1938. Pp. 457. (Reproduced by permission of the author and publisher.)

The various forms of neurological approach are too diverse to be considered exhaustively. I have already mentioned the primitive and yet not altogether outworn view that the phenomena of behavior are essentially chaotic but that they may be reduced to a kind of order through a demonstration that they depend upon an internal fundamentally determined system. This is the view which most naturally presents itself as a materialistic alternative to a psychic or mentalistic conception of behavior. The sort of neural homunculus that is postulated as a controlling force bears an unmistakable resemblance to the mental or spiritual homunculi of older systems, and it functions in the same way to introduce a kind of hypothetical order into a disordered world. The argument rests historically (and depends logically) upon a demonstration that neurological phenomena are intrinsically more lawful than behavior. It is only recently that this could not be appealed to as an obvious fact. The science of neurology achieved a degree of experimental rigor long before a science of behavior could do so. Its subject matter was chiefly "physical" (in a somewhat naive sense) while the data of behavior were evanescent: it could adopt the methods and concepts of its relatives in the biological sciences: and it could more easily confine itself to isolated parts of its subject matter. But the historical advantage has not been conserved. It is now possible to apply scientific techniques to the behavior of a representative organism in such a way that behavior appears to be as lawful as the nervous system. I know of no experimental material, for example, concerning the central nervous system which consists of smoother or more easily reproducible curves than are illustrated in many of the figures of this book. Accordingly, if we are to avoid historical influences in arriving at a modern verdict, we must discount the priority of the science of neurology; and in recognizing that the two sciences are of, let us say, equal validity, we may no longer subscribe to a point of view which regards a chaos of behavior as reducible to order through appeal to an internal ordered system [pp. 418–19].

The very notion of a "neurological correlate" implies what I am here contending—that there are two independent subject matters (behavior and the nervous system) which must have their own techniques and methods and yield their own respective data. No amount of information about the second will "explain" the first or bring order into it without the direct analytical treatment represented by a science of behavior. The argument applies equally well to other sciences dealing with internal systems related to behavior. No merely endocrinological information will establish the thesis that personality is a matter of glandular secretion or that thought is chemical. What is required in both cases, if the defense of the thesis is to go beyond mere rhetoric, is a formulation of what is meant by personality and thought and the quantitative measurement of their properties. Only then can a valid correlation between a state of endocrine secretion and a state of behavior be demonstrated. Similarly, in the developmental sciences, no principle of development—part out of whole or whole out of part—will account for an aspect of behavior until that aspect has been independently described.

I am asserting, then, not only that a science of behavior is independent of neurology but that it must be established as a separate discipline whether or not a rapprochement with neurology is ever attempted. The reader may grant this and at the same time object that the neurological side should not be ignored. He may contend that the two fields are admittedly related and that much might be gained from exploring both at the same time, rather than in holding to the strict isolation represented by the present book. The arguments for this view are much less convincing than its general acceptance at the present time would seem to demonstrate.

Much of the tendency to look to the nervous system for an "explanation" of behavior arises from clinical practices where explanation has a relatively simple meaning. The discovery of a cerebral lesion as the "neural correlate" of, let us say, aphasia is doubtless an important step in the understanding of the condition of a patient. But the success in this instance of finding "what is wrong" with behavior by looking into the nervous system depends largely upon the negative nature of the datum. The absence (and in many cases the derangement) of a function is much more easily described than the function itself. "He speaks" is admittedly an inadequate description of verbal behavior, which demands great amplification. "He cannot speak" is a fairly complete description of the opposite case, so long as the unanalyzed notion of speaking is accepted. The significance of this difference for the present argument may be pointed out by comparing the correlation of aphasia and a lesion with the correlation of normal speech and the neural processes involved in it. It is not difficult to point to a mere damage to verbal behavior and a corresponding damage to the nervous system, but almost no progress has been made toward describing neurological mechanisms responsible for the positive properties of verbal behavior. This argument is provisional, of course; eventually a correlation of important properties may be reached. The point at issue is not the possibility of successful correlation but its significance. Although the discovery of a lesion may be of first importance for diagnostic or prognostic purposes, a description of the phenomena of aphasia, in their relation to normal verbal behavior, is aided very slightly if at all by this added knowledge. It is wholly a matter of the interests of the investigator, whether he makes this excursion into the nervous system. In general, a descriptive science of behavior can make little use of the practices of the clinician, except in so far as they are descriptive. Usually the descriptive side is neglected because of the pursuit of the neural correlate. Thus, to continue with the example of aphasia, the monumental work of Head is of little value to the student of behavior because his analysis of the nature and function of language is antiquated and obscure.

The clinical practice of looking into the organism is carried over in the widespread belief that neurological facts somehow *illuminate* behavior. If my statement of the relation of these two fields is essentially correct, the belief is ill-founded. It obviously springs from the ancient view of behavior as chaotic. If there is any illumination at all, it is in the other direction. Behavior is by far the more easily observed of the two subject matters, and the existence of an intermediate science dealing with a conceptual nervous system testifies to the importance of inferences from behavior in neurology. In any event, I venture to assert that no fact of the nervous system has as yet ever told anyone anything new about behavior, and from the point of view of a descriptive science that is the only criterion to be taken into account.

The same statement of the relation between neurology and behavior will serve to dismiss the claim that neurology offers a *simpler* description of behavioral facts. This view is again reminiscent of the belief that simplicity is not to be sought for in behavior itself; but aside from this it may be contended that different kinds of behavioral facts may eventually be found to spring from a single neurological source and that the number of terms required for description may therefore be reduced by resorting to neurological terms. Perhaps such a view lies behind the interpretation of "brain waves" as the basis of thought or endocrines as the basis of personality, since the physiological system is apparently simpler than the behavior to be explained. But just what kind of correspondence between behavior and physiology this implies I am not prepared to say. Either it is not a one-to-one correspondence, or there must be a common "simplifying" property in the behavior itself. If, for example, the discovery of a single kind of synaptic process is some day made to account for the various kinds of "learning" discussed in previous chapters, it can successfully account for them only if some common property between the several cases may be demonstrated at the level of behavior. It is toward the reduction of seemingly diverse processes to simple laws that a science of behavior naturally directs itself. At the present time I know of no simplification of behavior that can be claimed for a neurological fact. Increasingly greater simplicity is being achieved but through a systematic treatment of behavior at its own level [pp. 423–425].

IX. ON THE BEHAVIOR OF THE LUMBO-SPINAL DOG

The following article [8] shows that truncated organisms tend to react as organisms insofar as their injuries will permit them to do so. The list of possible reflexes observed in spinal animals is shown in the accompanying table. We should indicate that a spinal animal is one whose spinal cord is completely separated from the brain.

Unless one has actually worked with spinal animals, he is not likely to possess an adequate conception of the complex and coordinated responses which it is possible for them to make. Sherrington and his associates have described at least 15 different reactions in spinal preparation, including such comprehensive and elaborate acts as the shaking of the entire body as if to shake off water, and the making of alternating walking movements with the hind legs. Modes of locomotion in the spinal dog have more recently been discussed by Cate; and responses of greater specificity which change with the cutting of certain of the spinal roots have been noted by Shurrager and Culler. Considered as a whole, the activity of which these "paralyzed" organisms are capable is little short of remarkable.

PROBLEM AND METHOD

It is the object of the present paper to examine the behavior of the spinal animal from the point of view of the psychologist. The observations reported were obtained from six laboratory dogs whose

[8] KELLOGG, W. N., DEESE, JAMES, & PRONKO, N. H. On the behavior of the lumbo-spinal dog. *J. exp. Psychol.*, 1946, 36, 503–511. (Reproduced by permission of the authors and publisher.)

spinal cords were completely sectioned between the first and the third lumbar roots. These should be of especial interest, because—since the lesion was well down in the cord—the spinal segment was smaller than that usually studied, and the resulting activity would be expected to be more limited [p. 503].

Table 28 *

Reflexes Observed in Spinal Dogs with Lumbar Transections

	Nature of Reflex	No. of S's in Which Observed	Stimulus
Flexion Reflexes	(A) Unilateral flexion	6	Electric shock to homolateral foot
		6	Cold (running water) on homolateral foot
		5	Pinching toes of homolateral foot
	(B) Partial bilateral flexion (full flexion in stimulated limb—muscle twitch in contralateral limb)	5	Electric shock to one of the rear feet
	(C) Complete bilateral flexion (female dog assumes typical urinating posture)	1	Distension of bladder or act of micturition (in female animal)
	(D) Digital flexion	5	Palpation above paw
		5	Palpation of plantar surface of foot
Extension Reflexes	(E) Crossed-extension	5	Manual flexing or manipulation of contralateral limb
		5	Electric shock to contralateral limb
		1	Spontaneous (?) flexion of contralateral limb
	(F) Direct unilateral extension	4	Pressure on hind paw while limb is flexed
	(G) Bilateral extension (animal stands unaided)	6	Rectal pressure
		5	Stimulation of anus with stiff brush
		5	Undefined external manipulation of caudal region

Table 28 (Continued)

Nature of Reflex	No. of S's in Which Observed	Stimulus
(H) Micturition	5	Distension of bladder
	6	Squeezing of lower abdomen
(I) Defecation	6	Rectal pressure
	4	Stimulation of anus with stiff brush
	5	Squeezing of lower abdomen
(J) Erection of tail as in defecation (or urination for female)	3	Distension of rectum or of bladder (in female). Stimulation of anus with stiff brush
(K) Assuming of complete defecating posture of a normal animal, including bending of trunk, erection of tail and bilateral extension of 2 hind limbs (standing)	2	Rectal pressure produced by act of defecating
(L) Continuous tremor of muscles of hind leg	1	Stimulus unknown

Leftmost label spanning rows J–L: **Other Reflexes (sometimes including flexion and extension)**

* Reproduced by permission of the authors and publisher.

X. MENTAL CHANGES FOLLOWING THE REMOVAL OF THE RIGHT CEREBRAL HEMISPHERE FOR BRAIN TUMOR [*][9]

Stuart N. Rowe, M.D.,[†] Pittsburgh, Pa.

During the past few years with the improvement of technical methods in neurosurgery, and with the development of increasing hardihood on the part of neurosurgeons, and perhaps their patients, a few cases

[*] Read at the ninety-third annual meeting of The American Psychiatric Association, Pittsburgh, Pa., May 10–14, 1937.

[9] Reprinted from *Amer. J. Psychiat.*, 1937, 94, 605–612. (Reproduced by permission of the author and the publisher.)

[†] From The Neurosurgical Service, Landon Surgical Clinic, The Western Pennsylvania Hospital, Pittsburgh, Pennsylvania.

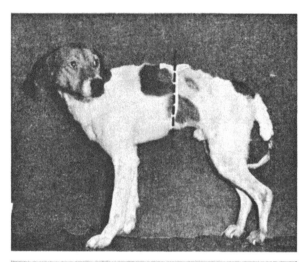

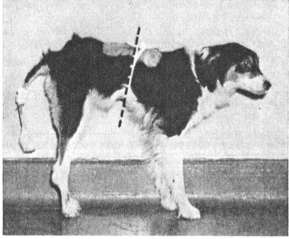

FIG. 50 Momentary standing of the chronic spinal dogs with complete transection of the cord between the first and third lumbar roots. The broken lines show the location of the lesion, and mark off roughly the "paralyzed" hind portion of the animals. In addition to standing, the dogs showed other integrated acts listed in the table. The photographs shown here were taken from one to three weeks following operation. (Kellogg, W. N., Deese, James, & Pronko, N. H. On the behavior of the lumbo-spinal dog.)

of very extensive cerebral ablation for brain tumor have been reported. Since the postoperative study of these patients may add to our knowledge of mental and neurological mechanisms, and since such cases are still not common, it seems quite proper to record them. In the present report, interest is centered particularly upon the effects on the mental status of the patient of the removal of a fairly large amount of cerebral tissue.

CASE REPORT

E. B., white female, aged 38. Hospital No. 5749.

SUMMARY. Headaches and the roentgenologic finding of calcification in the right frontal region led to the partial removal of a right frontal astrocytoma in January, 1935. Symptoms of increased intracranial pressure, epilepsy and mild mental changes appeared about six months later; and one year after the first operation a second more radical removal of the tumor was carried out. Ten months later (December, 1936), because of headaches and mental changes, a third operation was performed and most of the right cerebral hemisphere was removed. When examined six months after operation, the patient showed moderated emotional instability, slight impairment of recent memory, slight diminution in the normal inhibitions, but little, if any, deterioration in her intellectual ability as measured by mental tests.

PRESENT ILLNESS. The patient was first seen in January, 1935. At that time she gave a history of progressive, severe headaches for about one and one-half years. Examination showed only a very slight weakness of the left corner of the mouth, and a mild euphoria. X-rays demonstrated extensive calcification in the right frontal region.

FIRST OPERATION. January 31, 1935, a right transfrontal craniotomy and partial removal of a right frontal astrocytoma was carried out by Dr. Charles H. Frazier. A decompression was provided.

COURSE AFTER FIRST OPERATION. For four months the patient was symptom free. Headaches, petit mal and grand mal epileptic seizures, and more pronounced euphoria then slowly developed. Examination in February, 1936 (one year after the operation), showed some swelling of the right subtemporal decompression, slight haziness of the borders of the optic discs, marked impairment of the sense of smell on the right, hyperactive tendon reflexes in the left arm, and slight weakness of the left corner of the mouth and left arm. Mentally the patient was mildly abnormal in that she was markedly loquacious, excessively cheerful, and even jocose at times. Her intellectual ability on the Stanford-Binet scale was that of a superior adult with an intelligence quotient of 115.

SECOND OPERATION. February 7, 1936, a craniotomy was carried out (by the author) and about two-thirds of the tumor removed before the patient's reaction became so severe that the operation had to be terminated. The mass of tissue removed measured 6 x 6 x 3 cm.

COURSE AFTER SECOND OPERATION. Complete relief of symptoms was experienced for about six months. The immediate improvement in the patient's psychic state was marked. She became more calm, less talkative and jocose. On a repetition of the psychometric examination, she improved slightly upon her previous score.

About seven months after the operation, however, bouts of severe headache, and more pronounced mental changes began to appear. At times she was greatly depressed about her condition and would discuss various methods of suicide in a half-serious and half-jocose manner. On several occasions she reviewed her various symptoms and problems and future outlook at some length and with the utmost frankness on rather unusual occasions—such as in the course of a telephone conversation with a casual acquaintance, and at a bridge party. She was greatly worried over the prospect of further surgical treatment, but was equally distressed when she contemplated continuing life in her present condition. The over-talkativeness and lack of inhibition grew steadily worse. Nevertheless, the patient's sensorium and general intellectual resources remained fairly normal, although she complained of difficulty in remembering names and dates and even occasionally recent events.

After a discussion with the patient and her family of the risks and possible sequelæ of a third and more radical attack upon the tumor, operation was once more decided upon.

THIRD OPERATION. December 7, 1936. To provide a wide exposure, a small additional bone flap was reflected posterior to the original one. The tumor was found to lie principally in the frontal and temporal lobes and an effort was made to remove these areas without injuring the motor cortex, but tumor was encountered extending subcortically back into the parietal lobe. Accordingly, this procedure was abandoned, and the entire right hemisphere with the exception of the basal ganglia and a small medial portion of the temporal lobe was removed. In the frontal portion of the tissue remaining, there was some suggestion of tumor infiltration. This was removed as widely as seemed possible without encroaching dangerously upon the basal ganglia. [Figure 51.]

COURSE AFTER THIRD OPERATION. The cavity, filled with bloody spinal fluid, was aspirated daily. During the second and third postoperative weeks a staphylococcus infection occurred in this fluid, but the patient recovered with no change in therapy other than repeated aspiration and a transfusion. Her convalescence was also slowed by a low-grade osteomyelitis which developed in the small bone flap and necessitated its removal eight weeks after the operation.

The patient was completely hemiplegic on the left side for about seven weeks. At that time she began to make efforts to walk, with support on both sides, and discovered that she was obtaining a return of motor power in the left leg. This improved slowly and with the aid of a brace to support the left knee and ankle, she could walk with only slight aid ten weeks after operation. Touch sensation was lost on the left as well as two-point discrimination, stereognosis, sense of position, sense of motion and vibration, but pain sensation was preserved to some extent in scattered areas and was fairly well localized. The patient showed some limitation of conjugate eye movements to the left and upward for about eight weeks, and had of course a left homonymous hemianopsia (which spared the macula). The hearing was normal on both sides to ordinary testing (watch, whispered voice).

For a number of weeks after operation, the patient's mental state was considerably influenced by a number of changing factors—the operative shock, the blood in her cerebrospinal fluid, changing intracranial pressure, the post-operative infection, the prolonged hospitalization—and was correspondingly variable and difficult to evaluate. For the sake of completeness, however, this period may be briefly reviewed.

The patient showed marked lack of normal inhibitions for some weeks. She was highly euphoric at times, joking excessively, and sometimes very wittily, and always talking with very little restraint. Her mood varied widely and rapidly from time to time and she was occasionally extremely despondent. Her thought content was largely limited to her own situation for a time. The events since operation were poorly recalled, if at all, although older events and even such items as addresses and phone numbers were accurately remembered.

In the course of three or four weeks the patient's reactions became much more normal. While still displaying some lack of restraint in her speech, her inhibitions improved so much that her behavior and conversation were more natural than they had been prior to the operation. Her stream of talk was much less active and her restlessness decreased. The patient's emotional control, though improved, continued to be inadequate (presumably on the basis of operative trauma to the basal ganglia, or their injury in the course of the infection). She occasionally lost control of her voice or broke into sobs, though these outbreaks almost always accompanied a depressing thought content and were not altogether illogical or involuntary. Her outlook broadened so that she took a normal interest in her personal appearance, her home and family, her friends, and the activities of the world at large as portrayed in the daily papers.

PRESENT NEUROLOGICAL STATUS. Six months after operation. The cranial nerves are entirely normal with the exception of the left homonymous hemianopsia. The patient is only able to raise the left arm about six inches from her lap, but as the result of considerable

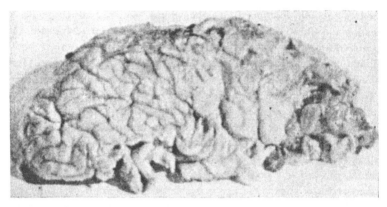

FIG. 51 Specimen removed at operation. The tumor presented on the surface anteriorly and infiltrated the parietal lobe subcortically. (Rowe, Stuart, N., Mental changes following the removal of the right celebral hemisphere for brain tumor.)

physiotherapy, the extremity is only moderately spastic and shows no contractures. The power in the left leg is about 75 per cent of normal on individual movements, but with the aid of a brace, the patient walks about the house by herself quite comfortably. The sensory changes are essentially the same as at the previous examinations—pain sense being preserved in irregular areas and being fairly well localized.

PRESENT MENTAL STATUS. 1. General appearance and behavior. The patient is quite particular about her personal appearance, is neat in her dress and toilet. She remains at ease and cooperates well throughout the examination. There are no special mannerisms [Figure 52].

2. Stream of talk and activity. The patient's physical activity is still considerably limited by her hemiparesis. She is out of bed about 12 hours daily, walks about the house freely, spends some time on a small

terrace out of doors, and goes for a daily walk or ride in the car. She can walk three to four blocks with slight aid from one person without excessive fatigue. In general she fatigues more easily than formerly, but manages to carry out the above program with little difficulty.

Mentally the patient is quite active. She is in charge of the management of the household (6 members), plans the meals, directs the cleaning, the buying, etc. She spends several hours daily working with her

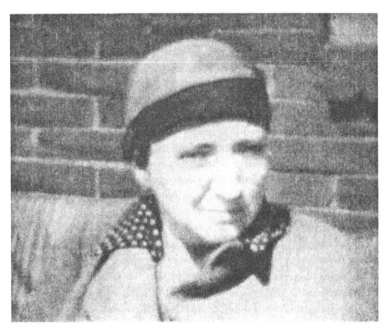

FIG. 52 The patient six months after operation. (Rowe, Stuart, N., Mental changes following the removal of the right celebral hemisphere for brain tumor.)

daughters on their school work and is normally worried over the failure of the younger (whose achievements in school are only average) to keep up with her sister (who does superior work). She takes a keen interest in the current events of her neighborhood, the happenings recorded in the newspapers, and reads several popular magazines fairly completely. Her retention of what she reads is sufficient to permit her to enjoy a continued story in a monthly magazine, but she has taken relatively little interest in books as yet. Rather frequent callers at the house occupy much of the patient's time, and with them she converses at some length, with some tendency to loquacity and to dominate the conversation. She maintains an active interest in her neurological and mental progress, as well as in the physiotherapy which she receives three times weekly.*

3. Mood. Emotionally the patient is still somewhat unstable. At times she becomes depressed very easily about her condition, and perhaps once in 24 hours she may weep without any real cause. When her attention is occupied with other matters than herself, she maintains a very even, cheerful mood.

4. Thought content. So far as can be determined, the patient has no abnormalities of her thought content. No compulsions, delusions or hallucinations have occurred at any time since operation.

5. Sensorium and intellectual resources. The patient is well oriented in all spheres. Her ability to concentrate in carrying out a test seems about average, but in the course of ordinary conversation she tends to shift fairly rapidly from subject to subject.

Some difficulty in recalling events of several days or weeks previous is at times experienced by the patient, but on testing recent memory and immediate recall there is no deficiency.

As measured by the Stanford-Binet tests, she still is in the superior adult group, with an intelligence quotient essentially the same as that found on the examination one year before.

6. Insight. The patient is aware of her emotional instability, and of the occasional memory difficulties, and is constantly trying to overcome them.

Finally, it seems worth emphasizing that the patient's mental status is still changing—at present improving. What progress or regressions may occur in the future is, of course, unpredictable.†

COMMENT

In this patient, the only mental changes six months after removal of most of the right hemisphere were (1) mild loss of normal inhibitions

---

* The patient received physiotherapy for six months under the direction of Dr. J. M. King. This prolonged and careful treatment certainly contributed much to the recovery of motor power by the patient.

† Eight months after operation the patient has made some further gains. The strength in her left leg has improved sufficiently to enable her to discard the brace and still get about the house easily and take a short walk daily. The patient's mental attitude is considerably improved. She is quite optimistic and cheerful and has a far better emotional control, so that the outbursts of weeping which formerly troubled her, now occur very rarely. She has begun to read books with more enjoyment and seems to have less difficulty with her memory.

with a tendency to over-activity of speech, (2) some impairment of recent memory, and (3) moderate emotional instability.

Unless one assumes a very extreme dominance of the left cerebral hemisphere in man these changes seem astonishingly mild after such severe cerebral insult. A brief review of previous experimental and clinical studies however, makes them seem more plausible. It is true that Lashley [1],* in his elaborate studies with rats found that loss of learning ability following injury to the brain occurred in direct proportion to the mass of cerebral tissue destroyed, without regard to the location of the lesion. But the careful work of Fulton, Jacobsen and their associates, [2, 3, 4] with chimpanzees and monkeys showed that in the primates unilateral frontal lobe lesions have little if any effect upon the higher mental processes, while bilateral frontal lobec-tomy caused a profound change—particularly upon mental activities demanding integration over a period of time. Furthermore, in these animals cortical ablations of equal or greater size (even when bilateral) which did not involve both frontal lobes failed to produce a similar mental picture. No evidence of dominance of either hemisphere was found.

The rather meager data as yet available from human cases tend to coincide with those obtained by these latter studies. A few cases of extensive unilateral cerebral ablation have been reported. Dandy [5] has recorded five cases of hemispherectomy for brain tumor. Three of these patients died within relatively short periods so that no estimate of their postoperative mental states could be obtained. One patient lived three and one-half years before dying of a recurrence of his tumor. Of him Dandy wrote, "There did not seem to be any obvious mental impairment. He was always happy and grateful for his exten-sion of life." The fifth patient was described two months after opera-tion as rational at all times, well-oriented, having a good sense of humor, and seeming normal mentally. The patient reported by O'Brien [6, 8] and by Gardner [7], who lived five years after hemispherectomy, was said to have shown no mental abnormalities whatsoever, although no exact studies of her intellectual level before or after operation were carried out.

In addition several studies of bilateral frontal lobe lesions are avail-able. Ackerly [9] studied carefully the psychic changes in a case operated upon by Spurling—a woman whose left frontal lobe was severely com-

---

* The numbers in brackets refer to the numbered items in the bibliog-raphy on pp. 441–442.

pressed by a large mid-line meningioma, and whose right frontal lobe was removed to permit the extirpation of the lesion. In this case, two years after operation there was no significant diminution in intelligence, no disturbance in the emotions or in general behavior, except a certain lack of distractibility, or tendency to an increased concentration upon the task at hand. It is not known of course, how much function may have returned in the injured frontal lobe following the removal of the tumor. One reason for suspecting the return of function on the left is the report of much more incapacitating mental deterioration in the case studied by Brickner. [10] This patient, both of whose frontal lobes were removed by Dandy, showed as his fundamental defect a quantitative diminution in the ability to synthesize—which in turn led to considerable loss of intellectual power and great alteration of the personality.

Finally, the operations carried out by Moniz [11, 12] and by Freeman and Watts [13, 14], for the relief of certain abnormal mental states involve the bilateral destruction of varying amounts of frontal lobe white matter. The procedure is reported to have greatly improved the psychotic states (particularly agitated depressions), without any marked change in the intellectual level, and with only occasional transitory effects on other mental functions. It is of considerable interest that these relatively small bilateral frontal lesions should produce such marked psychic alterations.

In summary, it would seem that the evidence available at present suggests that the higher cerebral functions in man are less dependent upon the integrity of the cortex as a whole than upon the preservation of the frontal lobes—a conclusion which is supported by the effects of hemispherectomy in the case here reported.

SUMMARY

1. A case of removal of the right cerebral hemisphere for brain tumor is reported.

2. From a neurological standpoint, the return of considerable motor function and some sensory function on the opposite side of the body is of interest.

3. Mental changes including impairment of recent memory, emotionality instability and diminution in the normal inhibitions, are present six months after the operation, but the patient's intellectual resources, personality and ability to meet the demands of her daily life have not been greatly altered.

4. The relatively mild mental changes resulting from hemispherectomy in this case are in keeping with previous experimental and clinical studies which indicate that in primates and man the higher cerebral functions are more severely altered by bilateral frontal lobe injury than by corresponding or even more extensive lesions of any other areas.

BIBLIOGRAPHY

1. LASHLEY, K. S. *Brain mechanisms and intelligence.* Chicago: Univ. of Chicago Press, 1929.
2. FULTON, J. F. & JACOBSEN, D. F. The functions of the frontal lobes, a comparative study in monkeys, chimpanzees and man. 15th Annual Congress, *Advances in Modern Biology*, 4, 113, 1935. Moscow: State Biological and Medical Press.
3. JACOBSEN, C. F., WOLFE, J. B. & JACKSON, T. A. An experimental analysis of the functions of the frontal association areas in primates. *J. nerv. ment. Dis.*, 82, 1–14, July, 1935.
4. JACOBSEN, C. F. Functions of frontal association areas in primates. *Arch. Neur. Psychiat.*, 33, 558–569, March, 1935.
5. DANDY, W. E. Removal of right cerebral hemisphere for certain tumors with hemiplegia. *J. Amer. Med. Ass.*, 90, 823–825, Mar. 17, 1928.
6. O'BRIEN, J. D. Removal of the right cerebral hemisphere. *Ohio St. Med. J.*, 28, 645, September, 1932.
7. GARDNER, W. James. Removal of the right cerebral hemisphere for infiltrating glioma. *J. Amer. Med. Ass.*, 101, 823–826, Sept. 9, 1933.
8. O'BRIEN, J. D. Further report on case of removal of right cerebral hemisphere. *J. Amer. Med. Ass.*, 107, 657, Aug. 29, 1936.
9. ACKERLY, SPAFFORD. Instinctive, emotional, and mental changes following prefrontal lobe extirpation. *Amer. J. Psychiat.*, 92, 717–729, November, 1935.
10. BRICKNER, R. M. Interpretation of frontal lobe function based upon study of case of partial bilateral frontal lobectomy. *Proc. Assoc. Res. Nerv. & Ment. Dis.*, 13, 259–351, 1932.
11. MONIZ, EGAS. Essai d'un traitement chirurgical de certaines psychoses. *Bull. Acad. de Med. Paris*, 115, 385–392, Mar. 3, 1936.
12. MONIZ, EGAS, & LIMA, ALMEIDA. Symptomes du lobe prefrontal. *Rev. neurol.*, 65, 583–595, Mar. 5, 1936.
13. FREEMAN, W. & WATTS, J. W. Prefrontal lobotomy in agitated depres-

sion; report of case. *Med. Ann. Dist. Columbia*, 5, 326–328, November, 1936.

14. FREEMAN, W. & WATTS, J. W. Prefrontal lobotomy in the treatment of mental disorders. *South. Med. Jour.*, 30, 23–31, January, 1937 [pp. 605–612].

XI. AFTEREFFECTS OF BRAIN INJURIES IN WAR
N. H. Pronko

Dr. Goldstein [10] has studied about 2,000 soldiers with skull and brain injuries caused by gunshot wounds in war. From a comparative study of wounds caused by high-velocity bullets and those from close distances or by other missiles, he makes the following generalizations:

The defects caused by gunshots fired from great distances and with great force produce relatively smaller functional disturbances than those produced by close shots. In the first place, the projectile, gathering momentum with distance, travels through the brain and leaves the skull on the opposite side of the head with such speed that no severe permanent damage is produced, sometimes even when the projectile traverses regions of functional significance. I have seen men who, after a short period of unconsciousness, have stood up and walked a considerable distance with no symptoms other than headache, after a high-velocity bullet had passed through both frontal lobes. Moreover, disturbances did not develop at a later period. Similarly, a shot entering the forehead, and emerging via the occiput, may leave the victim relatively unharmed. It must be remembered, however, that this applies only to injuries caused by high-velocity bullets. With all other missiles, the effect is much more serious. The superficial rebound shots that seem to the external view to do so little damage can have very severe sequelae; usually the internal table breaks and hemorrhage occurs [p. 24].

In damage to the motor area which has connections with the arms, legs, and other movable portions of the organism, we are informed that complete hemiplegia (paralysis involving the side

---

10 GOLDSTEIN, K. *Aftereffects of brain injuries in war.* New York: Grune & Stratton, 1942. Pp. 244. (Quoted by permission of the author and the publisher.)

of the organism on the side opposite the brain injury) is "rare and usually appears as a transitory occurrence" [p. 36]. Bladder disturbances are common shortly after injury but seem to be of short duration, disappearing usually after a few weeks. Some forms of paralysis involve corresponding parts of the hand and foot, for example the thumb and the big toe. "Such distributions are not comprehensive from a purely anatomic point of view."

As for perceptions, all are affected but only temporarily. "A total loss of sensation, however, is very rare and always transitory" [p. 43]. Nor are they equally affected, pain and touch being less disturbed than deep sensitivity, sense of position, or discrimination.

Visual reactions may be impaired in lesions which are not necessarily connected directly to the eyes, such as the frontal lobes or from diffuse blows on the head, in which cases they clear up. Unusual fatigue may also interfere with vision.

If the injury of the occipital lobe is extensive, there is frequently total blindness shortly after injury. However, even in very extensive damage of both lobes, the blindness is never permanent. It seems that only one case has been observed in which blindness persisted [p. 45].

OTHER BEHAVIORAL CHANGES. Unsteadiness and falling to one side upon closing the eyes occur only under these circumstances or when the patient with an injured cerebellum is confronted with a situation requiring very exact equilibrium, but disorganization of walking is seldom observed because patients with this type of brain damage usually die. "If they survive, the disturbances can be compensated very well" [p. 62].

Patients cannot be said to be lacking in "memory, attention and interest." While there are doubtless situations where this occurs, there are other situations where patients remember things and appear attentive and interested [p. 61]. Even familiar tasks are sometimes properly performed, at other times not. While the common tendency has been to relate these to disturbances of general functions of the organism or to hypothetical brain areas, Goldstein believes that the patient's behavior is to be understood as the adjustment of an injured organism to a situation which makes demands upon him which he cannot meet because of his reduced effectiveness as an injured organism. Goldstein calls this behavior a "catastrophic reaction." Normal as well as brain-injured, fatigued, or diseased individuals avoid situations in which they are inadequate.

The sick man has a strong urge to meet all demands as well as possible; his existence is bound up with such an endeavor to a greater degree than the healthy man's. Therefore, it is still more important for him not to be exposed to catastrophic situations. There is a danger that the after-effects of these situations may deprive him, for a varying length of time, even of such power of performance as he would otherwise have.

The sick man can exist only when he finds a new milieu adapted to his changed structure. The very endeavor to find such a milieu in which he can avoid catastrophic situations produces a definite behavior pattern. Much that might appear to be a symptom of the existing pathology is really only the expression of the sick man's flight from catastrophic situations.

There are different ways in which the patient evades the threat of catastrophe [p. 73].

One way is to exclude the world and its dangers, an extensive degree of which is fainting or an epileptic fit. Another solution is resort to orderliness, such as keeping one's things in a certain fixed place, avoiding company and thus unexpected situations, and so on. In summary, Goldstein's views, based on actual behavior of brain-injured soldiers, is a far cry from the still-prevalent "brain spot" theory which holds that absence of certain reactions is to be searched for in a chunk of the injured man's brain.

XII. OBSERVATIONS ON A CASE OF FRONTAL LOBECTOMY BEFORE AND AFTER OPERATION [11]

A 52-year-old man, diagnosed as having a tumor in the left frontal lobe, was examined 4 days before as well as 4 days after operation and was re-examined 14 months later. Striking changes in the direction of behavioral improvement were noted. These are reported directly from the observations of the psychologists concerned in the case.

---

[11] ELONEN, ANNA S. & KORNER, ANNELIESE F. Observations on a case of frontal lobectomy. *J. abnorm. soc. Psychol.*, 1948, 43, 532–543. (Reproduced by permission of the authors and the American Psychological Association.)

On the Revised Stanford-Binet the patient earned an IQ of 62 pre-operatively; four days after the operation he attained an IQ of 74; fourteen months later his IQ had risen to 111. The basal age on the first test was Year VI, while on the third test it reached Year XIV, and accordingly, the range was markedly narrowed. The verbal and spatial areas proved to be the most vulnerable to damage, and, therefore, the most diagnostically significant. The areas in which the greatest improvement appeared were those of retention, reasoning, and ability to generalize. The initial performance was characterized by highly unusual associations, and frequently by total disintegration of thought, as well as by marked perseveration and traces of aphasia. In the second performance, the bizarre language manifestations had disappeared entirely, but the perseveration remained especially marked in certain areas, and suggestions of aphasia were also persistent. In the final records, the patient was able to express himself entirely adequately, except in the Rorschach where some remnants of aphasic tendencies continued.

On the Kuhlmann the rise in IQ was almost as spectacular as on the Stanford-Binet, increasing from 53 to 80. Undoubtedly, these ratings measure more sensitively his functioning capacity in new situations than do the Binet ratings. His highest and most consistent achievement on both intelligence tests was his verbal facility, and this, coupled with his dependence on past learning as permitted by the nature of certain Binet items, accounted in part for the discrepancy between the test scores. Also, the Kuhlmann requires the organization of unfamiliar, impersonal material, presented in rapidly shifting patterns, so that his impaired flexibility was taxed beyond its productive limits.

All of the Rorschach records revealed marked interference with general functioning as typically found in patients with severe organic pathology.

The last record reflected a vast improvement over the records given before and immediately after the lobectomy, which corresponded with the improvement noted on the intelligence tests. In the third record, although there was residue of organic pathology, a striking increase in productivity, ability to project, and versatility was noted.

The patient's emotional adaptation to his impairment was one of acute anxiety, which he could not control shortly before and after the operation, and which he later managed through the mechanism of suppression [pp. 542–543].

The case reported here shows an individual's mode of reaction to a stress situation. The particular difficulty of this person is localizable in his tissue conditions. They may be viewed as *interference* rather than *causal* conditions which *prevent* him from performing adequate behavior rather than *producing* the reactions involved.

This individual had been going along presumably adequately until the expanding tumor became a definite setting factor in his behavioral responses. Reactions to stimuli did not then go off in the customary manner. Without necessarily realizing the particular condition involved, the patient began to worry, and this complex of factors prevented satisfactory performance on intelligence tests as well as in other areas. Once the "foreign body" was removed, the patient was again permitted to behave more effectively. Although in the case reported here the interfering condition was a biological one, we need make no distinction *in principle* between factors localized in the organism and economic, social, and geographical conditions. All operate as participating factors in behavioral events.

XIII. HOW DOES SHOCK THERAPY WORK IN SCHIZOPHRENIA (ALSO CALLED DEMENTIA PRAECOX)?

N. H. Pronko

It is generally agreed that a thumbnail description of a schizophrenic should include two chief characteristics: withdrawal and a compensatory "fantasy" behavior. The individual so labeled meets with some insurmountable difficulty in his life circumstances to which he cannot adjust. The result is a compensatory "adjustment" of a chronic daydreaming sort that leads to a progressive "insulation" of the patient from the rest of the world. Some of these patients go into a complete stupor from which they may or may not come out.

It has been observed that schizophrenics have occasionally shown "spontaneous recovery." Without any deliberate therapy, patients by their own means recovered the psychological status which they had had prior to their hospitalization.

Recently Rubé [12] systematically examined the records since 1928 of all patients diagnosed as dementia praecox or schizophrenia, the diagnosis having been verified by several psychiatrists. Since the patients were confined in wards where one physician was in charge of from 300 to 500 patients, it was practically certain that medical attention of any sort was hardly more than a myth. Nevertheless, 12 to 15 per cent of these schizophrenics showed "spontaneous recovery." We shall return to a consideration of them later.

In regard to treatment of schizophrenia, when the malarial treatment of paresis resulted in its cure, practitioners resorted to biological treatment of schizophrenia. Orientation of workers varied. Some went about devising techniques in a purely empirical fashion; others assumed some unknown bacillus, and still others felt that shock had a selective action on some hypothetical portion of the organism.

The wide variety of treatments that were used showed one remarkable fact that had been commonly overlooked, namely, that no matter what treatment was used, as long as it was carried out persistently and seriously, the percentage of patients showing improvement was between 30 and 40 per cent. Furthermore, again regardless of method employed, there was a progressive decrease in "cures" which eventually became stabilized at around 12 to 15 per cent, close to the percentage of "spontaneous recoveries."

Breaking up the records into three different periods, Rubé made an analysis of results with patients submitting to sulfotherapy at Saint Anne Hospital in Paris with which he was associated. The approximate results of his study are shown graphically. Puzzled by the decreasing effectiveness of sulfotherapy over the years, Rubé checked the medication itself, satisfied that it had remained constant over the years. This was true for the technique of administration as well as the general and local reactions of the patients.

Apparently, some variables other than biological ones were involved in both the differential results over the years and in those for men and women patients. Gradually, the hypothesis was de-

12 Based on an article by Rubé, P. Healing processes in schizophrenia. *J. nerv. ment. Dis.*, 1948, 108, 304–346. (Reproduced by permission of the publishers.)

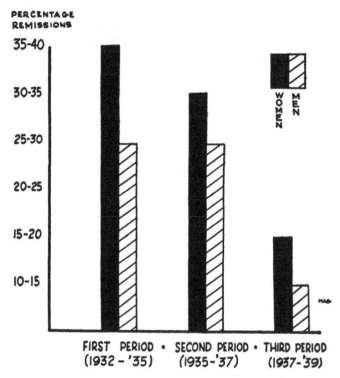

PERCENTAGE
REMISSIONS

35-40

30-35

25-30

20-25

15-20

10-15

FIRST PERIOD · SECOND PERIOD · THIRD PERIOD
(1932 - '35)   (1935-'37)   (1937-'39)

FIG. 53 Showing the percentage of successive groups of male and female schizophrenic patients recovering as a result of "shock therapy." Percentage recoveries are grouped according to the three periods shown. (Based on Rubé, P., Healing processes in schizophrenia.)

veloped that during the first period when the treatment was new these patients were assiduously attended. They received frequent inspection in order to follow the course of their treatment. At the first sign of improvement, they were quickly transferred, and psychological treatment was initiated. Every effort was made to establish contact with the patient and to promote more adaptive social reactions. But, in the later periods, fewer and fewer patients reached a stage where transfer was considered worth while, the reason being that an important psychological factor was missing that had been present earlier. The reader may well wonder how such a factor could operate while patients were practically inaccessible to human contact.

However, evidence forces us to acknowledge that the only factor submitted to any modification during this first phase consisted not so much in the manner of treatment as in the way which the staff hovered over them. This is how things might be interpreted: during the second, and especially during the third period, the physicians' interest veered toward new therapeutic methods. In order to devote more time to these methods, the physicians had regulated sulfotherapy according to a program to be followed by personnel who were certainly conscientious but devoid of the faith and enthusiasm which had inspired the original initiators of this program. Moreover, the number of laboratory tests for these patients had abruptly decreased. This category of patients assigned to sulfotherapy had moved away from the center of interest.

In the absence of any other factors, we concluded that the element capable of modifying prognosis in this treatment need not be sought elsewhere. According to us, this element of faith and enthusiasm carried with it into the patient's atmosphere a psychotherapeutic influence, which, although it remained unconscious on the part of those who brought it, nevertheless was of primary importance for its beneficiaries. We believe that this was the element which had brought the percentage of remissions during the first period up to 40% in the women's division and to 29% in the men's division [p. 314].

But how explain the discrepancy in the results of men and women patients? The most likely explanation involved an obvious variable in the area of nursing care. Women patients were attended by female nurses and men by male nurses. Apparently, through their superior nursing skills, female nurses were more successful in establishing a favorable rapport with their patients, thus facilitating their recovery toward an adequate social adjustment. In essence, what was done amounted to a series of mild jolts or "shocks" that turned the patient's attention successfully toward life and away from exclusive preoccupation with the subject matter of his "fantasies."

Further light is thrown on the details of shock therapy by noting certain features of insulin shock treatment. With this type of therapy, patients have frequently reported deep anxiety or fright following injection of this potent drug. It is very likely that this deliberately provoked anxiety in itself has important consequences by starting off a chain of reactions. Note that, for the first time, the patient is successfully invaded by a stimulus situation that is entirely outside his fantasy system. It is so compelling that the patient is forced to deal with it. Being afraid, he is now socially dependent. Eventually, the need for reassurance and comfort opens the door that leads back to a life within society. He is "cured."

Essentially then, the same kind of "shock" therapy principle may now be applied in understanding the cases of "spontaneous recovery" referred to earlier.

The only phenomenon which appeared during the course of evolution of these cases [of spontaneous recovery] is a change in environment. This new fact in itself produced a series of important psychologic phenomena: first of a negative sort, such as the disappearance of conditions which entertain either a state of conflict, or a state of affective overwork, or situations which perpetuate inferiority feelings, frustration or inhibition with all of their consequences. Secondly, of a positive kind, such as the appearance of a series of new reactions provoked by the establishment of relations with the members of another social group [p. 339].

We have shown to what extent the psychologic factor constitutes the very foundation of healing processes in schizophrenia. The manner in which the patient is first approached, the way in which the therapist "takes possession" of him and orients his mental functions on the way to recovery toward a level corresponding to normal functioning, is an essential part of the entire treatment of schizophrenia, and is just as important as the posology of insulin and shock. Psychotherapeutic action is no mere accessory to the treatment. It holds first place, and perhaps, from a certain point of view, it may be considered to constitute the only really effective factor [p. 338].

Records of villages and towns in medieval England show payment to a constable for administering a beating to pathological people, believed to be possessed by an evil spirit. Such treatment occasionally resulted in "cure." Here was the first "shock therapy." Later techniques included ducking the patient in a pond, rotating and trephining (boring a hole in the skull). More recent methods use Metrazol, electric shock, "brain insult" surgery, acetylcholine, carbon dioxide, antityphoid vaccine, yeast, sterilized milk, gasoline, oil of turpentine, and fever. In our opinion, it matters little what one uses from a psychological viewpoint. The essential feature is to "get a rise" out of the patient—to recall him to behavior within society, as was done with Dr. Rubé's patients. This seems to be the essence of "shock therapy."

XIV. THE RELATIONSHIP OF BRAIN INJURY TO PSYCHOSIS
N. H. Pronko

While to the layman, every psychotic must act and can act peculiarly only when there is something wrong with his brain, actually, over two thirds of psychotic patients have no demonstrable brain pathology. It does not occur to the layman that the presence of worries, frustrations, guilt feelings, and the like, over the patient's economic, domestic, and moral problems is an adequate explanation for his maladjustment. Yet an increasing number of attempts in such a pioneer orientation toward problems of psychopathology are being made.

Among others, Gallinek[13] takes issue with the viewpoint coming down to us from the last century to the effect that the psychoses in the aged are "produced" by hardening of the arteries and other changes in their brains. That this old viewpoint must be discarded is proved by the actual demonstration that the brains of patients who had died in advanced senile dementia often showed very few of the *expected* anatomic characteristics. The converse has also happened. Brains of elderly persons who were psychologically normal up to the time of their death showed "marked senile and arteriosclerotic changes . . . of the type which allegedly is the underlying pathology for senile and arteriosclerotic psychotic states" [p. 294]. In other words, serious psychopathology may occur without serious brain pathology, and serious brain pathology may be present in a normal aged person.

Rather than the fruitless approach outlined above, Gallinek suggests that actual investigation of patients diagnosed as arteriosclerotic will show a number of such psychological factors in their previous history as a lack of social adaptation, bad breaks, financial insecurity, and domestic and hygienic conditions.

---

[13] GALLINEK, ALFRED. The nature of affective and paranoid disorders during the senium in the light of electric convulsive therapy. *J. nerv. ment. Dis.*, 1948, 108, 293–303. (Reproduced by permission of the author and the publisher.)

Furthermore, if permanent brain damage is the underlying basis for the psychoses of the aged, then the kind of treatment called electric convulsive therapy (ECT) or shock therapy should have no effect. Among 230 consecutively treated patients, Gallinek administered electric shock therapy to 36 patients 60 years of age and over, the oldest patient being 84 years old. Almost all of these patients would have been diagnosed as psychosis with cerebral arteriosclerosis or senile psychosis. The behavioral picture was one of depression and paranoia (false, bizzare beliefs). A few were agitated, and one was definitely manic. Most patients received considerably less than ten treatments with the consequence that most of them showed good and lasting results.

The author concludes that the favorable outcome of these cases indicates that these behavioral reactions are *reversible*, many permanently so, and almost all of them at least temporarily.

Their reversible character militates strongly against the concept of close causal relationship between the undoubtedly irreversible [anatomic] pathologic changes of senile degenerative and arteriosclerotic nature and the psychoses, and, on the other hand, favors the concept that these conditions are not strictly definable disease entities, but reaction types or syndromes of depressive, paranoid-depressive and manic-depressive symptomatology. A constellation may be the pathologic anatomic factor, but more than this one element seems to be necessary for the appearance of the psychosis, and the continued presence of the pathologic anatomic factor does not stand in the way of the cure of the psychosis [p. 301].

NAME INDEX

SUBJECT INDEX